AF323667

THE NEW BIG 5

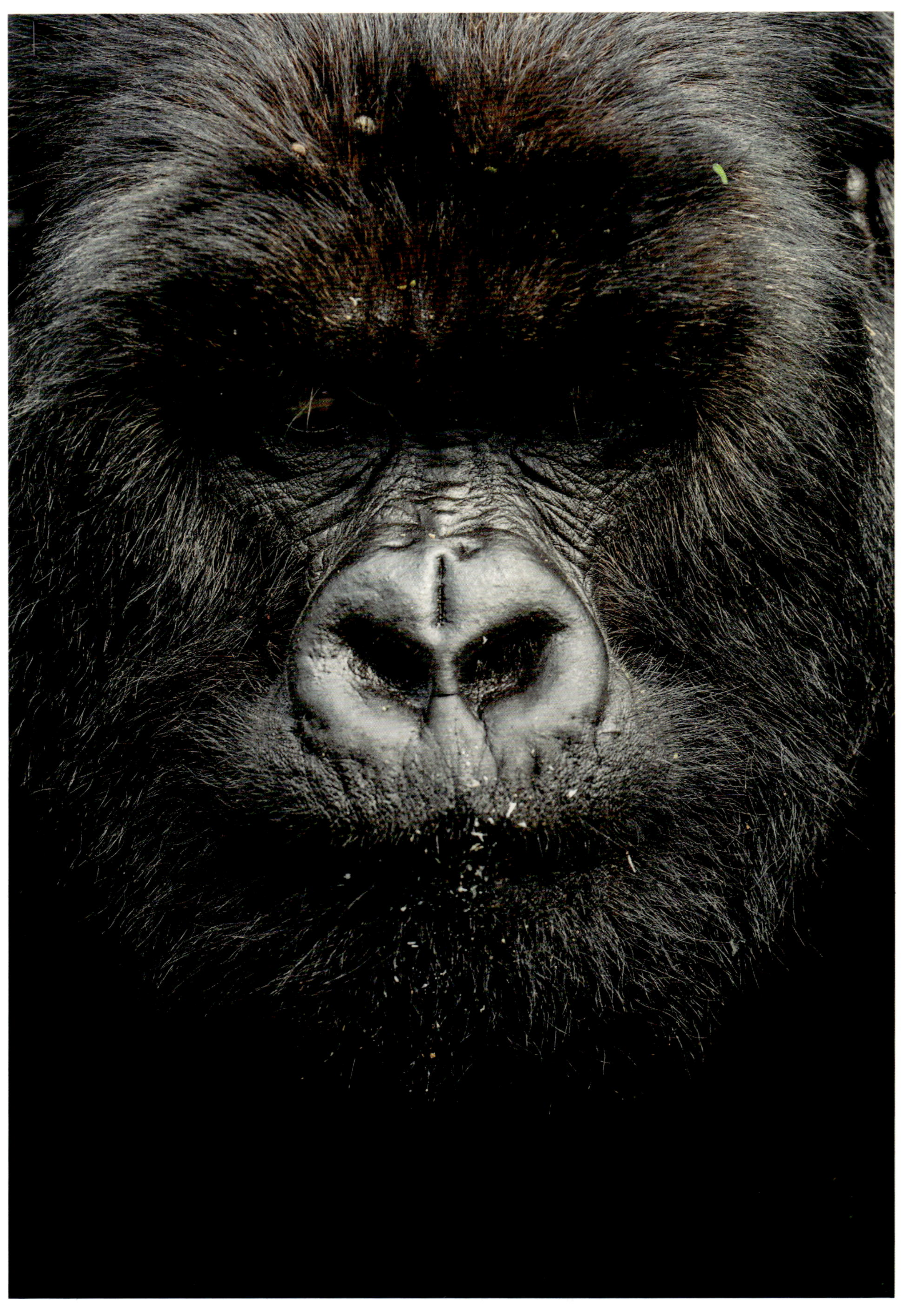

Graeme Green
Mountain Gorilla
Volcanoes National Park, Rwanda

THE NEW BIG 5

A GLOBAL PHOTOGRAPHY PROJECT FOR ENDANGERED WILDLIFE

GRAEME GREEN

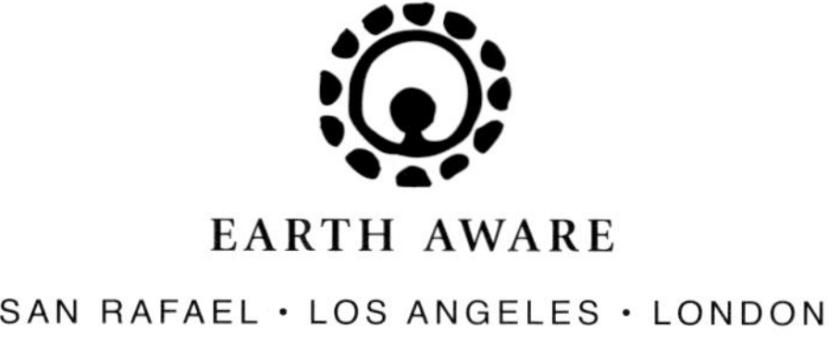

EARTH AWARE

SAN RAFAEL · LOS ANGELES · LONDON

For Andrea and Leo

CONTENTS

A Changing World

Dr. Paula Kahumbu
CEO, WildlifeDirect

THE BIG FIVE WAS THE NAME BIG-GAME HUNTERS IN AFRICA gave to the five animals that were most difficult to shoot and kill: elephant, lion, leopard, black rhino, and Cape buffalo. The New Big 5 are the five animals, selected by an online vote, that people around the world most like to photograph and to see in photographs: elephant, lion, tiger, polar bear, and gorilla.

The New Big 5 project is an inspiring initiative, created by British photographer Graeme Green, that has brought together hundreds of leading wildlife photographers and conservationists from around the world, all united in their passion for wildlife and their commitment to highlighting the many threats facing the natural world. This book celebrates the animals, the photographers and their work, and the many conservationists working to secure a future for the world's wildlife.

The featured photographers are a community of storytellers whose images communicate the wonders of the natural world. But they, and we, are also part of a longer story, of how economic and technological development have altered our relationship with the natural world. It is also a story of changing attitudes and a growing awareness of our responsibility as humans to care for wildlife. We are all protagonists in this story, and how it plays out will depend on us.

Comparing the two lists, there are many similarities. All the animals on both lists are big, dangerous, and inspire awe in us. The original Big Five were all from Africa and were still common in Kenya when I was growing up there as a child. Of the New Big 5, two and a half are from Africa (since "elephant" on the new list includes both the African and Asian elephant), while the others are from Asia and the polar regions. All are becoming scarcer or are even threatened with extinction. All of them were and, in many cases, still are targeted by trophy hunters.

Hunting is older than human history itself. Hunting by early humans was for subsistence and was made possible by technologies—slings, spears, and bows and arrows—that compensated for the deficiencies of the feeble human body. Hunting skills embodied (almost exclusively) masculine prowess and courage, as in the case of the Maasai, for whom,

until recently, killing a lion was part of a young man's coming-of-age ritual. Recreational hunting developed as a status symbol, signaling membership into an elite group that no longer needed to hunt for subsistence. Soon, these elites decided that hunting afforded more pleasure if other people didn't get in the way. When White trophy hunters expelled Africans from their lands to create the first game reserves, they were following in the footsteps of their ancestors, who in the Middle Ages had cleared villagers from the royal forests in England.

We can be sure that, from the earliest days, hunting provided the inspiration for stories. For tens of thousands of years such stories existed only in oral traditions, as the spoken word. But vivid cave paintings allow us to imagine how exciting these stories must have been for the listeners, crouched around fires in the caves. Much later, similar tales were told by trophy hunters, seated in drawing rooms and clubhouses, with the trophies on the wall providing visual props for the stories of their adventures.

Technological advances, such as the large-caliber elephant guns used by trophy hunters, opened up new possibilities for killing big and dangerous animals. But it was a completely new technology, photography, that was to prove transformational. Many of the earliest wildlife photographs were of trophy hunters posing with the animals they had killed. The idea of photographic safaris, where travelers shot with a camera instead of a gun, caught on slowly. My dear friend, the late Richard Leakey, was one of the first to offer photo safaris in Kenya, as a teenage entrepreneur in the early 1960s. Wildlife photography requires similar skills to hunting, including patience, perseverance, and tolerance of difficult conditions in remote habitats, and, unfortunately, until recently remained very much a White male preserve. In the meantime, we became much more compassionate animals and the age of trophy hunting waned as modern people found it gruesome, cruel, and inconsiderate to fellow sentient beings.

However, the most transformative impact of photography has been on storytelling. This new technology has opened up the production of images to everyone, without the need for a cave painting or an oil painting, and given rise to new forms of storytelling, such as the photo essay. This book and the photography and articles on the New Big 5 website (www.newbig5.com) are a testimony to the power of photography. Photography celebrates the lives of animals rather than the moment of their death. Thanks to modern communications technology, these photos and the connected stories and issues can reach millions of people around the world almost instantly.

With this new power comes new responsibilities. Most listeners of the stories told around a fire or over drinks at sundown had personal knowledge of the animal protagonists. Modern viewers of wildlife photographs may never encounter the animals they depict and many have little contact with wild animals of any sort in their daily lives. As the only source of knowledge about wildlife for many people, photographers and the makers of wildlife documentaries have a responsibility to tell it like it is.

It's no accident that, although it is a global list, three of the New Big 5 are found in Africa. Here, we are incredibly lucky to be living on a continent where megafauna still thrive in habitats that are relatively accessible to photographers. In many other parts of the world, such as North America and Western Europe, much of the native megafauna was exterminated long ago. Elsewhere, such as in parts of Asia and South America, magnificent but hard-to-see animals persist in remote habitats.

In Africa, our protected areas provide vital refuges for hundreds of threatened species. Wildlife tourism, much of it based around photography, makes a vital contribution to local economies in wildlife-rich areas. But animals outside protected areas and, increasingly, even within them are under threat. The incredible photos and documentaries of wildlife in these pristine habitats that we all love to see only tell half the story. The challenge for modern storytellers is to use photography and filmmaking to also create compelling stories about hard-to-see animals and threats to wildlife.

These threats, described in detail in this book, affect the New Big 5 in different ways. Climate change is melting the ice cover on which polar bears depend. Habitat loss is confining the few remaining tigers and gorillas to ever smaller forest enclaves. The slaughter of elephants and tigers lines the pockets of criminal gangs who control the illegal global wildlife trade. Population growth creates and exacerbates human-wildlife conflict, for example, when humans respond to crop raiding by elephants and gorillas, or predation of cattle by lions. It is a tragic irony that when so many people crave contact with wildlife, those who live in the proximity of wild animals often perceive such wild animals as a threat.

The challenge for wildlife photographers is to devise ways of telling stories that inspire hope and highlight the continued search for solutions, like those that are showcased in this book. It's important to tell stories that speak of the courage of wildlife rangers, who risk their lives every day to protect threatened wildlife, or of the ingenuity of people such as the young Kenyan Richard Turere, who devised a system called Lion Lights to keep cattle safe from lion attacks at night.

Looking ahead, a further challenge is the diversification of wildlife photography. Women wildlife photographers are now, thankfully, a force to be reckoned with, but aspiring photographers from Africa and countries elsewhere in the developing world still encounter many barriers. In this respect, the New Big 5 project is taking a lead in promoting diversity and representation within the profession.

Beyond this, the latest technological developments mean that we can all become wildlife photographers. Many readers of this book might never have the chance to see any of the New Big 5 for themselves. But anyone can use their smartphone to take great pictures of wildlife they might encounter.

The New Big 5 project and the powerful ideas behind it have captivated wildlife lovers around the world, as this book will now do. The photographers featured in these pages have shared their beautiful work generously to spread the love of wildlife. I am humbled and moved by their photographs and inspired to pick up my own camera once again.

Introduction

Graeme Green

I FIRST HAD THE IDEA FOR A NEW BIG 5 A DECADE AGO, on assignment in Botswana's Makgadikgadi Pans. I'd heard people talk about the original Big 5 before and heard people use the word *shooting* for taking photos before. But this time something in my mind clicked, combining the two to turn the original Big 5 idea on its head. I thought a Big 5 based on photography, rather than hunting, was something that should exist.

It started out as what I thought was a cool idea. But talking to other photographers and conservationists about the concept, I felt it could be more than just a way to celebrate the remarkable animals we share the planet with. It could also be a way to shine a light on the crisis facing the world's wildlife.

The Earth is in the midst of a sixth mass extinction event, the first in history caused primarily by humans. The age of the Anthropocene that we're living in is marked out as one where human activity—agriculture, deforestation, urban development, pollution—is significantly and negatively impacting the climate and ecosystems across the planet. In 2021, a United Nations Environment Programme (UNEP) report described how we're "waging war on nature," and how our failure to get to grips with climate change, biodiversity loss, and pollution are posing a grave threat to all life on Earth, both wildlife and people. To continue on such a catastrophic course was marked out as "senseless and suicidal."

As a photographer and journalist, I've seen firsthand many of the problems causing declines in wildlife populations, from Tanzania to Peru to Nepal. I wanted to use the New Big 5 project to raise awareness on issues like habitat loss, the illegal wildlife trade, and climate change.

In 2019, I started producing a series of podcasts, articles, interviews, photo galleries, education packs, and more for the New Big 5 website (www.newbig5.com), looking at issues such as human-wildlife conflict, plastics, food sources, and the trafficking in animal body parts, as well as solutions, from cutting-edge technology to female ranger teams. Using the original New Big 5 concept, which captured people's attention, we could look at situations facing all kinds of animals, from lions, pangolins, and rhinos to hornbills, sloths, and stick insects.

One by one, I contacted photographers, conservationists, and wildlife charities around the world who loved the New Big 5 idea and came on board to be part of the project and support the mission.

After months of intense work, the project launched in April 2020, inviting people around the world to vote on the website for their five favorite animals to photograph and see in photos. Voting ran for a year, a hit of positivity during the long, dark, difficult days of the COVID-19 pandemic. When the results were announced a year later, in May 2021, the New Big 5 project became global news, covered by TV channels, newspapers, magazines, and websites, including the BBC, CNN, Sky, *The Guardian*, *Forbes*, *National Geographic*, the *South China Morning Post*, and many more, not just announcing the animals in the New Big 5, but also talking about the threats the five species and many others face.

The New Big 5 of wildlife photography, as decided by the public vote, are the elephant, polar bear, lion, gorilla, and tiger. It's a powerful list. What's striking is that even these five incredibly popular animals are facing threats to their existence, from lost habitat to the international trade in body parts (ivory, skins, bones…). The animals in the New Big 5 are just the tip of the iceberg, symbols that can stand for all the world's wildlife. They're a stark reminder of the many other thousands of species living in forests, deserts, grasslands, on snow-covered mountains, and in the deepest oceans, at risk of disappearing from the face of the Earth if we humans don't quickly take action. If we're unable to save these five animals, it's difficult to feel optimistic that we can save so many other less globally treasured species from extinction. The New Big 5 should remind us all of what we stand to lose.

The project was never intended to target trophy hunting itself, just to create a new, positive alternative, one that celebrates the natural world—a Big 5 that's about life and creativity, rather than death and suffering.

But as the project ran, it was interesting to realize how many people had heard and used the original Big 5 term without knowing what it meant. Many had assumed it stood for Africa's biggest animals, forgetting animals such as giraffes and hippos, both of which are larger than

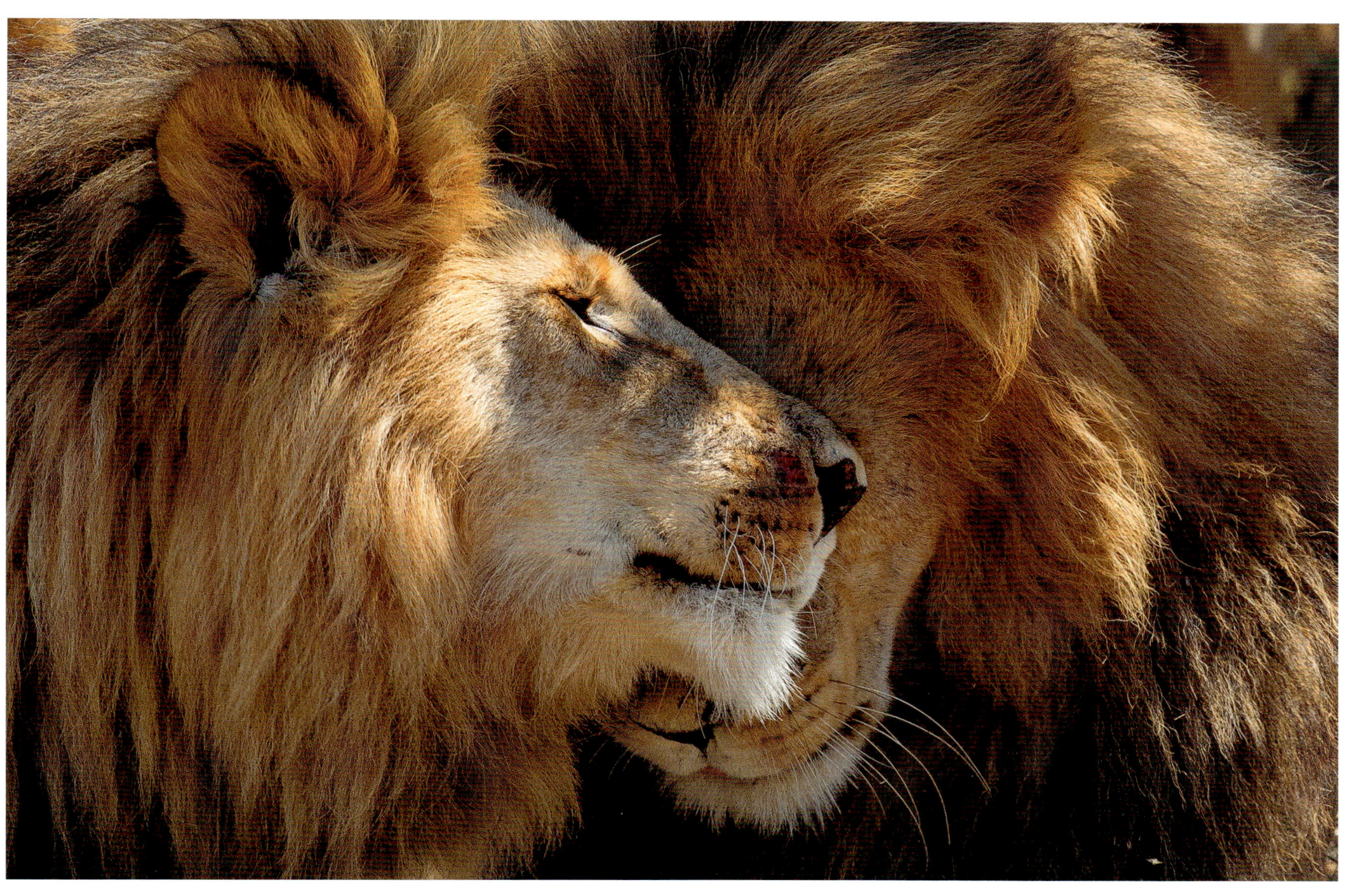

Graeme Green
African Lions
Mara Naboisho Conservancy, Kenya

leopards or lions. Others thought it meant the most dangerous or lethal, forgetting animals like hippos (which kill more than double the number of people each year than are killed by lions), crocodiles, snakes, scorpions, or mosquitos. Still others believed the list was based on the most popular or charismatic animals, which is an odd thought; there are clearly many animals (cheetahs, gorillas, giraffes, zebras, chimps…) that have a more powerful hold on people than the humble Cape buffalo.

I heard from many supporters of the project who detested the original Big 5 idea, including camp owners and safari managers who'd banned staff from using it. A "butcher's term" is how one camp owner described it to me. Conservationists I talked to felt it was an insult to their work trying to stop endangered animals, like rhinos, elephants, and lions, from going extinct for a term to still be in use that's directly connected to the hunting that decimated numbers of Africa's wild animals.

The Big 5 isn't the only term connected to Africa's violent past. *Safari* is a Swahili word, meaning "journey," from the Arabic *safar*. Used by Arab traders in Africa, the word *safari* was adopted in the 1800s by White hunters, mainly from Britain and other parts of Europe, to describe their hunting expeditions, or hunting safaris, where they'd shoot animals, such as lions and elephants, for trophies. That creates a strange state of affairs today, with many wildlife lovers paying to take safaris (a word rooted in the hunting that wiped out millions of wild animals across Africa) to see the Big 5 (the list of animals most prized by trophy hunters).

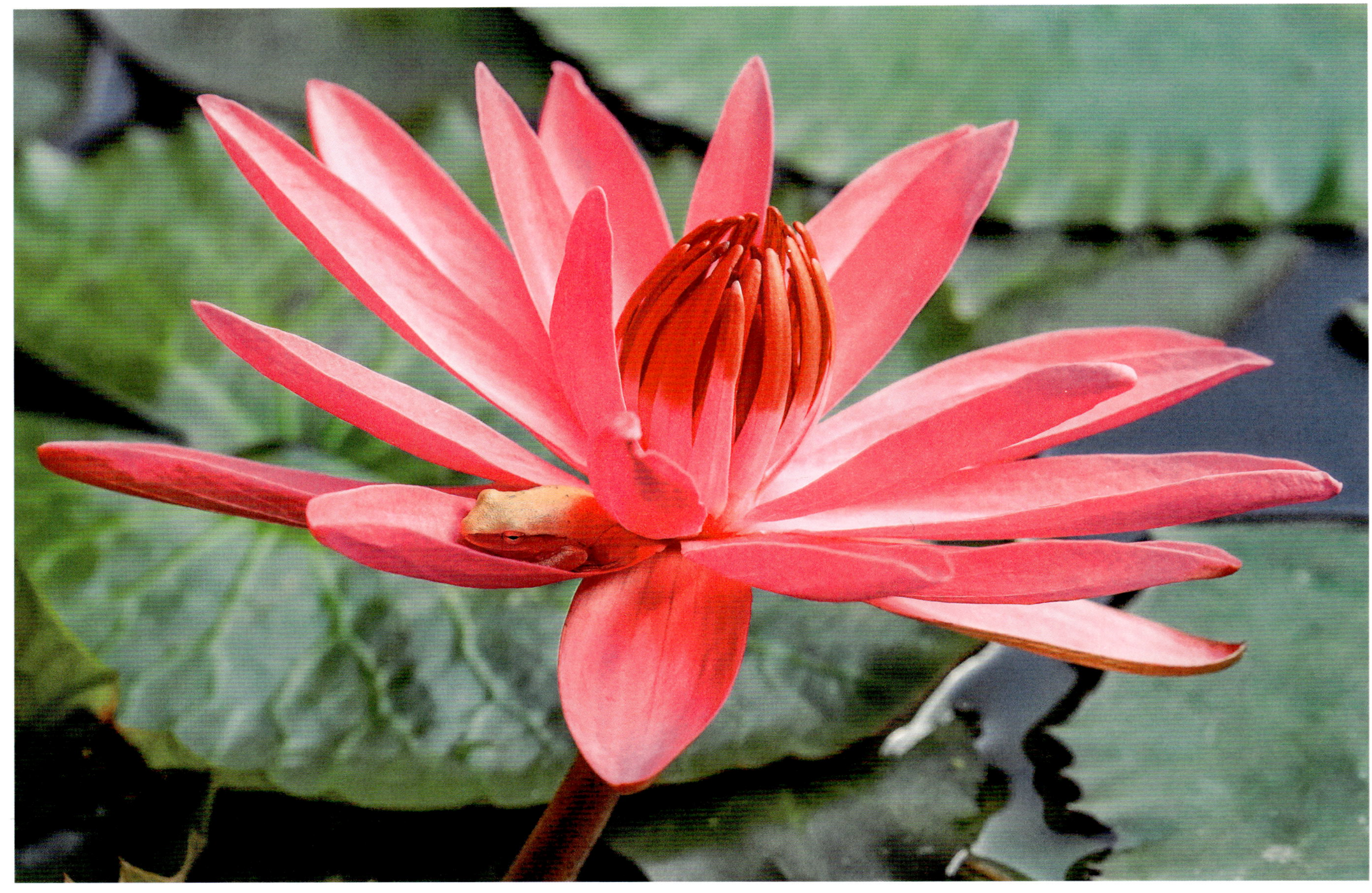

Graeme Green
Golden Tree Frog
Langkawi, Malaysia

It's interesting to look at language and how it's used. In books about Africa, there are stories of great "explorers" and "adventurers." It turns out that many of these men were not driven to explore new lands and cultures, but instead were motivated by the massive profits to be made in the ivory trade, Africa's "white gold" rush, and to satisfy what appear to be psychopathic levels of bloodlust. White hunters with powerful rifles sometimes killed more than a dozen elephants or rhinos in a day or boasted of killing more than 500 elephants in a year. Having killed all the elephants in one location, they would search out new populations, ignoring warnings that elephants were being wiped out. The reckless levels of colonial-era hunting shaped the African continent and are a major factor in why there are so few of some species left alive in Africa today. There are many more suitable words for these people than "explorer" or "adventurer."

I've never used the words "game" or "big game" for animals, sensing this was a language that belonged to people different from me. "Game" or "sport" suggest two equal sides, both with an equal chance of winning, rather than a one-sided attack on an unsuspecting animal. For hunters to reduce the often painful and drawn out death of an animal to "sport" or a "game" says a great deal about how they view other life.

Likewise, the word "trophy" suggests a heroic, noble battle, a victor displaying the "spoils of war," rather than the miserable, painful reality of an animal being killed. It's absurd to imply that animals, like elephants or leopards, are an enemy that needs to be conquered.

Personally, I'd like to live in a world without trophy hunting. I've never been able to understand why anyone would want to harm or kill an animal for "fun," whether it's fox hunting, dog fights, or dancing bears. These are living creatures, capable of intelligence and emotion, able to feel physical and mental pain. To make an animal suffer for pleasure, for a hobby or entertainment, is indefensible. The debate over trophy hunting is fierce. To me, trophy hunting is outdated, pointless, and cruel, and should be resigned to the past. If the New Big 5 can be a small part of a shift in thinking and a move toward a world without trophy hunting, I'm happy for it to be.

But there are far greater threats and causes of suffering to wildlife today than trophy hunting, and it's those that are the focus of the New Big 5 project. As I did with the New Big 5 website, this book combines incredible photography with facts, insights, expertise, and ideas from conservationists and other experts. The following chapters look at existential threats, such as habitat loss, fragmentation and degradation, the global wildlife trade, and global warming, offering hopeful ideas and practical ways to move forward.

The photos in this book took me a year to collect and curate, selecting from more than 16,000 images submitted by many of the best international photographers working today, alongside new and emerging photographers. The photographers and the species they've photographed come from all over the world: the United States, Kenya, Japan, Mexico, Sweden, Botswana, the United Kingdom, China, and elsewhere. All the photos were taken in the wild, and each photographer signed an agreement confirming that the animals were not baited and that their pictures were not taken at zoos, "sanctuaries," places where animals were forced to perform for the camera, or any other situation likely to cause them stress or harm.

The chapters dedicated to each species in the New Big 5 are powerful tributes to these remarkable animals. As a photographer, I'm as interested in frogs, lizards, and birds as I am the charismatic giants, and it was always my plan to use the New Big 5 project to shine a light as far and wide as possible on all kinds of diverse species. The final chapter of the book focuses on species that are endangered. For this section, I mainly worked from the International Union for Conservation of Nature's (IUCN) respected Red List. Many species on the Red List face severe threats, including those listed as Vulnerable (VU), Endangered (EN), or Critically Endangered (CR), the three highest categories before extinction.

It wouldn't be possible to study all 8.7 million species on Earth or, with 100 percent accuracy, to categorize all the species that have been newly discovered, lost, declared extinct, rediscovered, or are still unknown to science, meaning any list is bound to be flawed. To give a fuller picture, I also drew from other lists, including from governments and non-governmental organizations, looking at endangered or threatened species.

My intention is to show the sheer range of wildlife in diverse geographical locations and habitats facing serious threats to their existence, from iconic animals—such as rhinos, orangutans, and whales—to less famous "unsung heroes," each one equally valuable and deserving of their right to live. These images represent a drop in the ocean. Pictures of the creatures facing extinction on our planet could fill entire libraries. But this collection of photos gives a strong sense of what is at stake.

Looking through the photos in this book is an emotional experience. It's clear that humans are causing devastation right across the natural world.

Urgent action is needed. This message is at the heart of the New Big 5 project, and I hope it's what people take away from this book. Every creature deserves to exist. From bees to blue whales, from tigers to termites, all wildlife is essential to the balance of nature, to healthy ecosystems, and to the future of life on our planet.

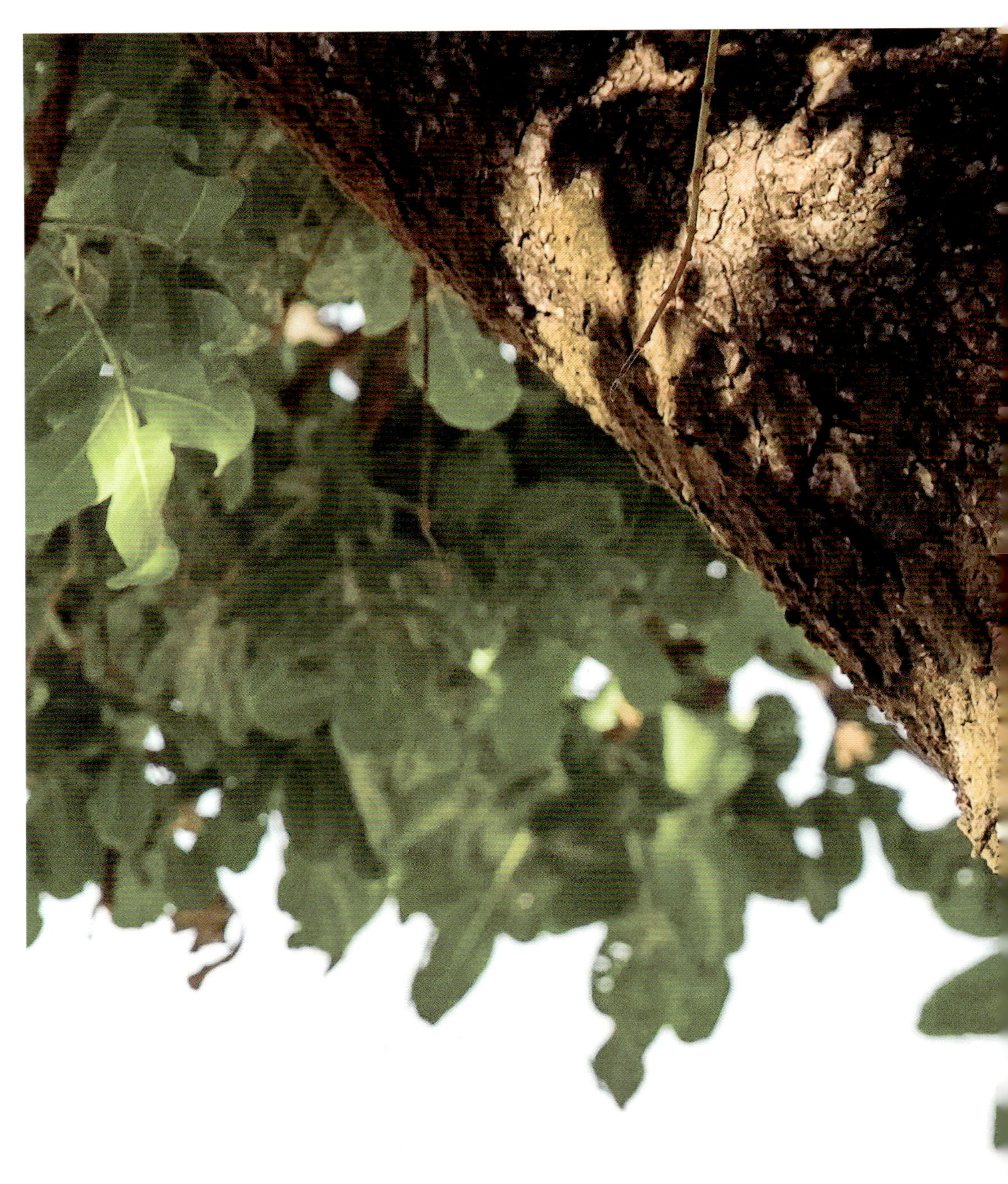

Graeme Green
Leopard
Ruaha National Park, Tanzania

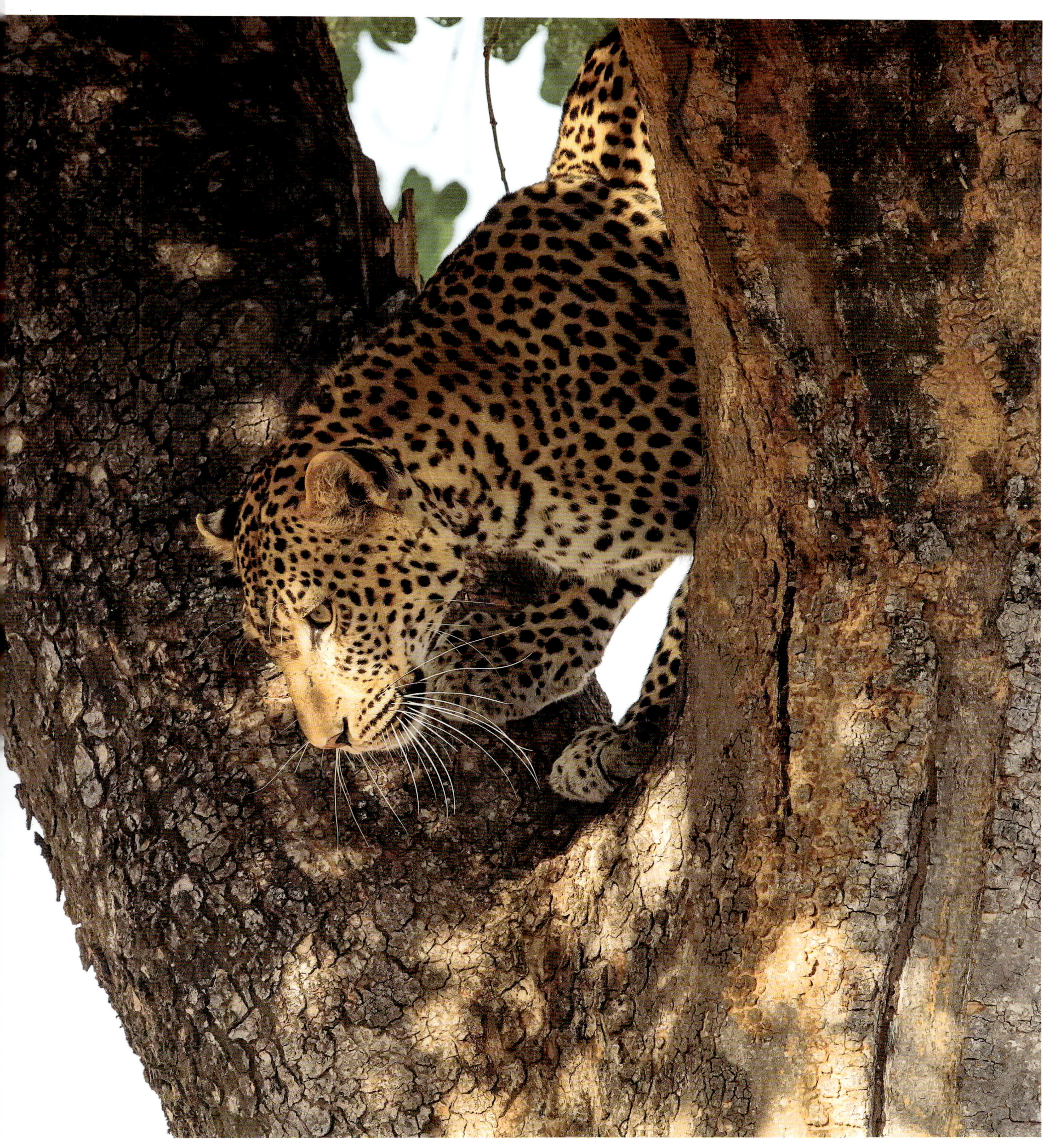

The Blink of an Eye

Graeme Green

ONE EVENING, IN THE REMOTE WILDERNESS of Ruaha National Park in Tanzania, I watched a lone bull elephant as it fed at a giant baobab tree. The sun was setting, turning long grass and the baobab golden, as the elephant used the tip of its trunk to reach the high branches that smaller animals couldn't get to and bring fresh flower buds down to his mouth.

The thought that went through my mind, as it does every time I watch an elephant in the wild, is how extraordinary life on Earth is. From the towering giraffe to the bright orange and blue rock agama to the deep-sea anglerfish that produces its own light, we live alongside creatures that are a match for anything science fiction writers have imagined to populate alien worlds.

Elephants are the world's largest living land mammal, an animal that can weigh more than six tons and consume 550 pounds of food per day. But, with their padded feet, they're able to move silently through forests, like ghosts. Intelligent, emotional animals with strong family bonds, they can map and remember pathways across vast areas, and pass the knowledge on from generation to generation.

With around 40,000 muscles (more than there are in the human body), their trunks are powerful enough to tear branches from trees, but dexterous enough to pick a seed up from the ground. I've seen elephants use their trunks for affectionate greetings and to give younger animals encouraging shoves, to blast themselves with a cooling shower, and to suck up a good drink (a trunk can hold up to two gallons of water). Their tusks, which have brought so much destruction on them, can be used to strip bark, to dig into the ground, or to defend themselves.

"Elephants are the product of about 60 million years of evolution," says evolutionary biologist Professor Richard Dawkins. "It's incredible. Their trunk is an astonishingly clever, sensitive instrument. Early elephants would've been smaller, with no trunk or a small trunk, like a tapir. The trunk would've lengthened gradually over time. The tusks are also remarkable. Tusks started out as incisor teeth and grew out gradually."

The elephants we see today are the result of minute changes that occurred over the equivalent of 750,000 human lifetimes. "Every living creature is the result of evolution," Dawkins explains. "Evolution is about gradual, gradual change. It's spectacular, in that it has produced an astonishing array of diversity and, at the same time, a shattering level of complexity. In each generation, tiny improvements were favored in reproduction, so the genetic basis of those improvements got passed on down the generations. The elephant is no exception. There used to be many elephants at one time all over the world. Over millions of years, what we see is change in multiple branches. With elephants, there are just two branches left: in Africa and Asia. The whole process of evolution is a slow, gradual, ramping up of change."

It's tragic to compare the patient, peaceful process of evolutionary creation with the rapid, violent destruction humans are causing in the natural world. The number of African elephants once reached upward of 30 million. Today, only around 400,000 remain, their numbers decimated mainly by the ivory trade. In the 1800s, it's estimated that 100,000 elephants were killed in East Africa each year, the trade in tusks running alongside, and often intertwined with, the horrific slave trade, as colonial powers wreaked devastation across the continent.

Despite international conservation efforts and ivory bans, the killing has continued. An estimated 100,000 elephants were killed in Africa during the poaching crisis between 2010 and 2012. The International Union for Conservation of Nature (IUCN) recently listed African savanna elephants as Endangered and African forest elephants as Critically Endangered. Asian elephants are also under threat, having declined by at least 50 percent in the last three generations, leaving around 45,000 in the wild. In evolutionary terms, it's as if an artist spent a lifetime producing a masterpiece with thoughtful, tiny brushstrokes only for an angry child to punch their fist through the canvas. "It takes no time at all to drive a species extinct," says Dawkins. "It takes orders of magnitude longer to build it up. That's the tragedy. Every time a species goes extinct, especially something like an elephant, you're wiping out tens of millions of years of evolutionary research and development in the blink of an eye."

Elephants are "ecosystem engineers," spreading seeds and modifying landscapes, turning woodland and scrub into grass savanna, which brings in herbivores. Predators can then hunt and feed, and scavengers can clean up.

All these animals are part of what Angolan poet and politician Agostinho Neto called "the perpetual alliance of everything that lives." Humans were part of that alliance, too. But we broke out, evolving too far ahead of the pack, to stand alone, outside the natural order, to the

Graeme Green
African Elephant
Ruaha National Park, Tanzania

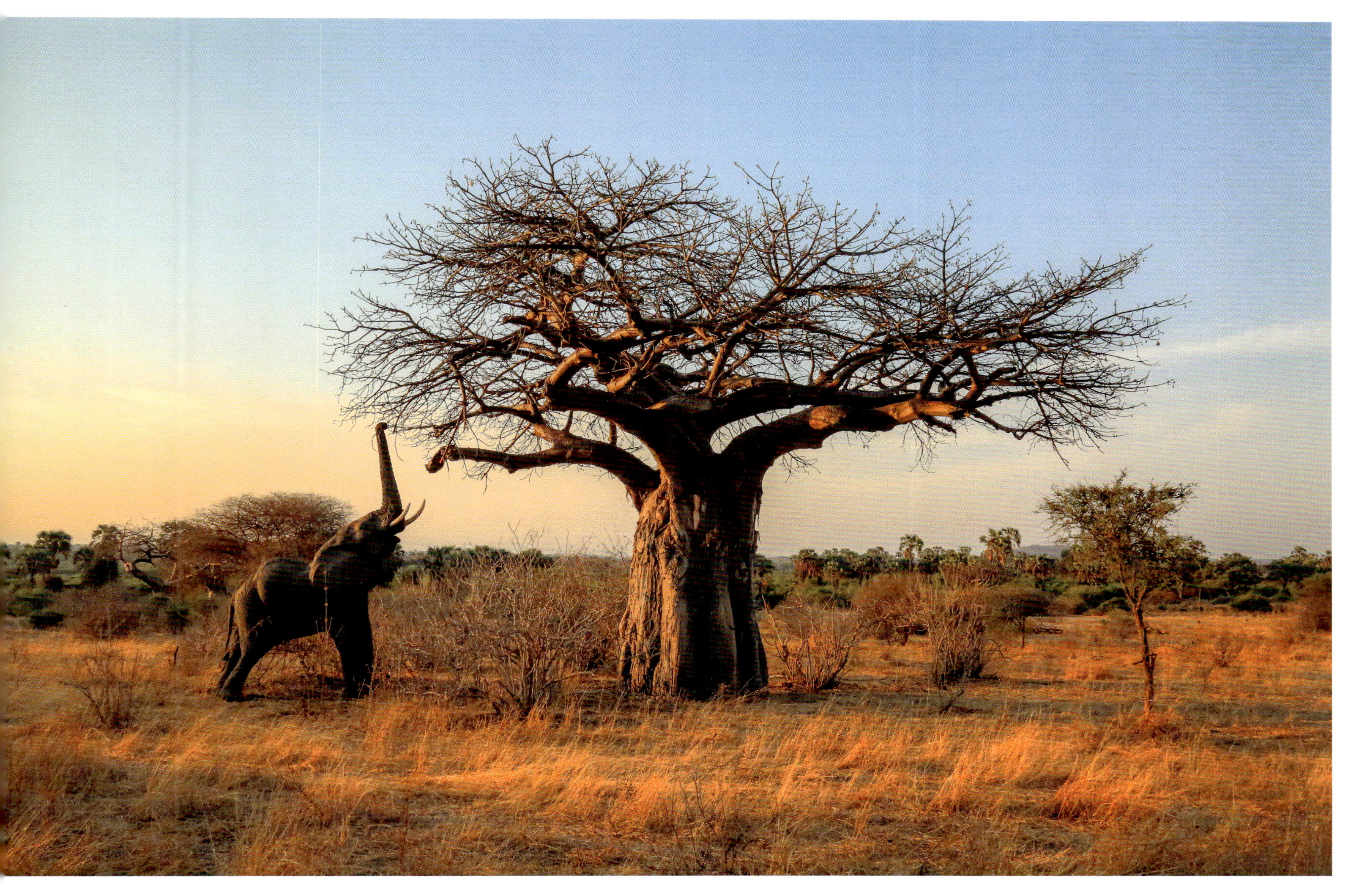

15

detriment of every other living creature. No other species dominates the planet as humans do. No other species can cause the death and suffering of so many others, from felling forests and damming rivers to industrial farming and hunting with rifles right through to altering the planet's temperature by extracting and burning fossil fuels.

Our control over the planet and our use of its resources—for food, fuel, and for leisure and luxury items—has disrupted the balance of nature across the planet and now threatens humanity and all life on Earth. "The big change—agriculture—only happened 10,000 years ago," says Dawkins. "Before that, we were hunter-gatherers, pretty much like other animals, surviving in our own ecosystems. Then, we invented agriculture, and there was a big explosion of human numbers and the efficiency with which we could kill and domesticate animals. Now, we dominate the world with technology and machines, amazingly so."

A DECADE AGO, I TRAVELED TO INDIA to report on the rapid disappearance of the country's vultures. Local dumps, where the birds would normally be feeding on cattle carcasses, were empty. The primary cause of vulture deaths was diclofenac, a toxic anti-inflammatory drug used by vets and farmers to treat cattle, which the vultures ingested from the carcasses. The drug caused catastrophic declines across Asia, with 50 percent losses year-on-year from 1992 to 2003.

Often seen as ugly and dirty, or associated with death, I have a soft spot for these birds. Nature's "clean-up crew," the scavengers dispose of domestic and wild animal carcasses, stopping the spread of diseases, such as rabies and tuberculosis, to other animals, including feral dogs, and to humans. Vultures have existed for more than 20 million years. But in the space of a decade, countries lost up to 99 percent of these birds. In Asia and Africa, more than half the resident vulture species are now listed as Critically Endangered.

A few years earlier, I spent time with marine biologists off the southern coast of Belize. We set lines to catch sharks, to take samples, and tag them, in order to monitor the population, shark movements, and average size. Between work, we'd swim, sometimes sharing the water with nine-feet-long nurse sharks.

Sharks were, and still are, being killed in huge numbers. Shark's fins have no nutritional value or flavor, but the desire for this status item among China's growing middle class and in other parts of Asia is helping to send sharks to oblivion. The researchers in Belize were working to show the impact of eliminating sharks from their ecosystems, known as a "trophic cascade," where a top predator is removed and there are knock-on effects throughout the food chain. Here, it was ultimately leading to too many grazing fish and lifeless coral systems. The scientists'

goal was to produce evidence to persuade governments to create Marine Protected Areas to maintain healthy marine systems, not least so people could still fish to eat and make a living.

Sharks have swum in Earth's oceans for around 420 million years. But the global abundance of oceanic shark species has declined by 71 percent over the past 50 years, another blink of an eye. Overfishing, as bycatch and for their meat and fins, is the main driver.

Vultures and sharks were early lessons for me in the balance of nature and the importance of all living creatures to their ecosystems. Apart from a few politicians, every creature on Earth has a purpose or a role to play in the big picture. Remove one and it's difficult to predict what will happen, but the outcome is rarely good. Vultures and sharks were also both lessons in how quickly human activity can obliterate large numbers of a species.

Shortly before his death in 2021, I spoke to Professor Thomas Lovejoy, the "godfather of biodiversity" and founder of the Amazon Biodiversity Center. "The world's biodiversity is in perilous condition," he warned. "All the recent reports show that major elements of life on Earth are driven toward endangerment and extinction. In my lifetime, the rate of extinctions globally has clearly accelerated. The biggest driver of extinctions is human activity. The human population has tripled, agriculture has spread around the world, and forests have disappeared. It's mostly a thoughtless destruction of nature to fulfill immediate human desires— sometimes it's "needs," but mostly it's just "desires." The good news is that a lot hasn't gone over the cliff yet, but we're pretty close to the edge."

The impact has been felt everywhere. Rhinos have roamed the Earth for 50 million years. At the beginning of the 1900s, there were half a million. Today, there are around 28,000, with three species listed as Critically Endangered, mainly due to poaching for their horns, which are used in traditional "medicine," despite having no medicinal value. Pangolins, the world's most trafficked mammal, have existed on the Earth for 80 million years but some species could disappear in the next few decades, the animals used for meat in Africa and Asia, their keratin scales also sold for traditional "medicine" in Asia.

Tiny, out-of-sight creatures often receive fewer headlines. But losing miniscule creatures would have many impacts, including the removal of a base layer of food for other species. For example, scientists are concerned about the impact of climate change on tiny phytoplankton that krill feed on—losing krill would be felt right up the food chain, from Antarctic fur seals, penguins, and albatrosses to humpback whales. More than a third of freshwater fish species are also threatened with extinction currently, a food source to billions of people and a crucial part of bio-diverse ecosystems.

Scientists also warn of a possible "insect apocalypse," which would alter life on Earth. More than 40 percent of all insects are declining, by rates of at least 2.5 percent each year, with threats including climate change, habitat loss, invasive species, and pollution. Insects perform vital roles, from cleanup operations to pollinating plants, as well as serving as a food source to other species. "If all mankind were to disappear, the world would regenerate back to the rich state of equilibrium that existed 10,000 years ago," as American biologist E. O. Wilson said. "If insects were to vanish, the environment would collapse into chaos."

The 2019 Global Assessment Report on Global Biodiversity from the Intergovernmental Science-Policy Platform on Biodiversity and Ecosystem Services (IPBES) found that more than one million animal and plant species are at risk of extinction. That's from an estimated 8.7 million species that currently exist on the planet. Species extinctions aren't new, but the speed and scale of extinctions and population declines is. "The crisis is very serious, deep, and pervasive," says Professor Sandra Díaz, Professor of Ecology at Argentina's Córdoba National University and co-chair of the IPBES Global Assessment report. "The fabric of life on Earth is unraveling fast. Some species that are extinction-prone are crucial for ecosystem-engineering, nutrient-transport, and for sustaining other species, so we should be expecting large changes in the fabric of many ecosystems."

Humans are taking a big gamble: that we can live without the species that are disappearing. "Pollinators are essential for many of the plants we eat, and plankton, for the fisheries we exploit," says Díaz. "But from a different philosophical perspective, one can say that every creature on Earth has the right to be alive and we humans have no right to cause its disappearance. We can't afford a loss of the living world of the magnitude that's predicted. Some of the damage is already beyond repair. Some species have already gone extinct globally. Some ecosystems have already gone beyond the point of return. But the fact that these species are at risk is not destiny. If we act urgently, the future is still in our hands."

There's also a pragmatic, self-preservationist reason to save the world's wildlife. "Every drop of water we drink, every cubic inch of air we breathe, everything we eat… 100 percent of all those things comes from nature," says Jon Paul Rodriguez, chair of the IUCN Species Survival Commission. "We're so closely connected to nature for our own survival, so it doesn't make any sense for us to wipe it out."

We have no idea which species losses might lead to wider catastrophe. "I don't think there's any unimportant species," Rodriguez argues. "I firmly believe in drawing the line at zero further extinctions from our behavior. Every species matters. We don't know how many connections exist. Lots of creatures are dependent on each other. We need to try to prevent sudden changes in a system that come from one little tipping point. But maybe some of those tipping points have already been reached. I grew up on the Caribbean coast of Venezuela. In ten minutes, I could fish enough fish to feed us all, but now it's much more difficult. Tipping points don't happen suddenly—in a human lifetime, we see them gradually and get used to them. There are examples of forests that don't have predators, or coral reef replaced by invasive species. Many of these things are happening now.

"At the same time, we also see that if you let nature recover, she will recover," he adds. "In Central America, we see areas where there were cities and pyramids, which are now covered by trees. With horrendous scenarios like Bikini Atoll, where the atomic bomb was tested a few decades ago, there are beautiful coral reefs. It illustrates that nature is resilient. In my lifetime, I've seen major declines in the world around me. But I'm convinced we have the motivation and the capacity to move the needle in the right direction."

THE GREATEST CHALLENGE TO WILDLIFE around the world currently is habitat loss. It's identified as the main threat to 85 percent of species described in the IUCN's Red List. Because of changes, including industrial agriculture, deforestation, urban development, and new human settlements, many animals no longer have a safe home or space to roam, hunt, move between grazing land or water sources, or to find mates. Lions, for example, now occupy just 8 percent of their historic range, their numbers cut by 50 percent in the last 25 years to 20,000 or fewer. Animal habitats are also being polluted, degraded, and fragmented by roads, canals, power lines, and pipelines.

Industrialized countries have destroyed so much of their nature to make way for farming, housing, factories, and energy production. The United Kingdom is one of the most depleted countries in the world, having lost almost half its biodiversity since the Industrial Revolution. Developing countries now face similar pressures, especially as populations continue to expand. In 1900, there were just 1.6 billion people on the planet. Today, there are around 8 billion, which is predicted to rise to nearly 10 billion people by 2050.

Population numbers alone aren't the issue. Human consumption of food, fuel, and other natural resources is the greater problem, especially levels of consumption in Western counties. We lose 64 million acres of forest each year, mostly tropical rain forest, largely for agriculture and meat production. Beef accounts for 41 percent of global deforestation, with forests also being lost for cocoa, palm oil, and timber. About half the world's original forests have disappeared and they're still being removed 10 times faster than any possible level of regrowth. About 80 percent of terrestrial animals depend on forests for their survival.

With less space to live in and human populations encroaching into previously wild areas, there's been an increase in human-wildlife conflict, from Colombia, where ranchers lose up to 5 percent of cattle to jaguars, to Canada, where polar bears, driven by sea ice losses, are spending more time around human settlements. In Africa, animals, such as elephants and buffalos, raid people's crops, while predators, such as lions and leopards, target livestock. There can be human casualties, but more often it's animals that are injured or killed, with retaliatory or preemptive poisonings of big cats, or villagers defending their homes and crops from elephants with spears and arrows.

"Imagine yourself as a farmer living in a rural village in Africa," says Sam Shaba, Program Manager for Tanzanian wildlife charity Honeyguide. "You and your family have cultivated three acres of corn, hoping it will feed your family for a year, and maybe you'll be able to sell some and send your child to school. One night, you wake up and there's a herd of elephants wiping out the last remaining crops. This is the life of thousands of people living next to wildlife where we work in northern Tanzania. People lose up to 70 percent of their crops to elephants and sometimes have up to 40 livestock killed by predators in one night. Imagine that amount of pressure."

As human populations grow, so does the potential for conflict. "Our national parks aren't fenced, and wildlife depends on community lands outside national parks for dispersal areas, seasonal grazing, passage, and sometimes breeding," Shaba explains. "It is possible for humans and wildlife to coexist, especially in the case of pastoralist communities, because their land uses are compatible with conservation. But the benefits must outweigh the losses for people living with wildlife. For the relationship between people and wildlife to be sustained, local communities need to be involved in decision-making."

Necessity is driving solutions, from Lion Lights (flashing lights that keep predators at bay) to beehive fences (bees can scare away elephants, with the upside that honey can be produced to eat or sell). Other tactics range from bomas that keep animals safe at night to compensation schemes for owners who lose livestock. "Governments, NGOs, and other conservationists should help provide solutions for human-wildlife conflicts," says Shaba. "These need to be tools that are proven to work and that the community can make or buy themselves. Some effective methods we've tried include strobe lights, blow horns, chilli crackers, Roman candles, and chilli fences. Intelligent elephants quickly figure these out, so there needs to be a constant variety of methods. We're still experimenting."

ANIMALS ARE ALSO BEING DELIBERATELY TARGETED in Africa and around the world for the global illegal wildlife trade, which is estimated to be worth around $23 billion, possibly more. Criminal gangs trafficking wildlife are connected with the drug trade and human trafficking. Across Africa, there's been a rising number of cases of animals being killed for their body parts for use in belief-based rituals, motivated by the idea that vulture heads or lion claws will bring power, strength, good luck, or magical spirits. Bushmeat, to eat or to sell, also drives the hunting of wild animals, which increased during the global COVID-19 pandemic, as many people struggled to survive.

Animals are also trafficked around the world as exotic pets, or turned into ashtrays, boots, belts, jewelry, and useless trinkets. "I've seen all kinds of weird stuff, like guitars made out of armadillos," says Peter Knights, CEO of WildAid. "There's no end to the imagination of what people can put animals into as products. For an incredibly beautiful animal to be rendered down to a rag, a bone, or a necklace is tragic, especially when you know how few of these animals there are left."

The wildlife trade is a global problem. But Asia's demand for illegal wildlife products is one of the main drivers wreaking devastation on the natural world. Body parts, such as highly valuable rhino horn, tiger bones, and pangolin scales, are used in traditional Chinese "medicine," a tragically absurd situation where endangered animals are being wiped out for products with no medicinal properties, just to serve irrational, anti-scientific beliefs. The source of the COVID-19 pandemic is also believed to have been a disease passed to humans from animals, such as pangolins or bats, at China's food markets.

As with drugs, while the demand exists and huge profits can still be made, the global wildlife trade will continue. "You have to change the society," says Knights. "If a person buys rhino horn to cure cancer, you can't appeal rationally to that person. But you can appeal to their grandchildren or neighbors and show it's antisocial, that they're destroying our planet. The person buying the product is driving the whole process. The hunter might be poor and just doing something to feed their family—they may not have a choice. But the person who buys ivory or other animal products has choices. When the buying stops, the killing can stop, too."

The killing of wildlife robs people of the income that wildlife tourism can bring in and steals futures. But it's about more than economics. "The illegal wildlife trade threatens public health, biodiversity, our culture and heritage, and the rule of law," says Takudzwa Mutezo, Head of the Legal Department at Tikki Hywood Foundation, which targets

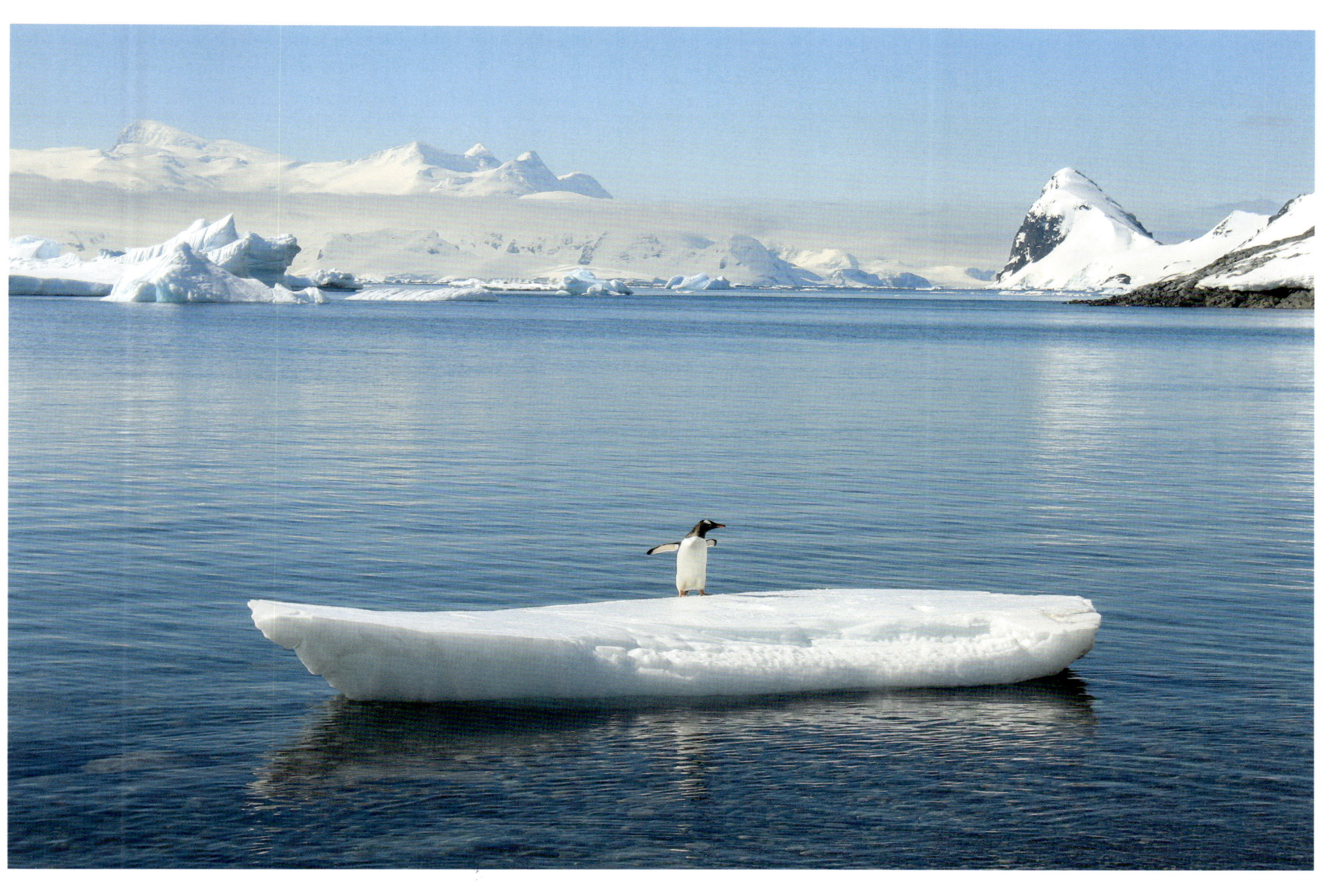

Graeme Green
Gentoo Penguin
Wiencke Island, Antarctica

wildlife crime in Zimbabwe, South Africa, and Cameroon. "In Zimbabwean culture, we have totems, a family symbol passed on from one generation to the next. My totem is a moyo-chirandu, the heart of an animal, so it's my responsibility to protect wildlife. It's sad that one's culture and spirit animal can be reduced to mere trinkets for the benefit of so few people."

Laws to protect wildlife already exist. They just need to be used. "For the law to be effective, it must be understood, implemented, and enforced," says Mutezo. "The establishment of specialized courts for environmental and wildlife crimes could make a real difference. This would allow a new wave of law enforcement, prosecutors, and judiciary who are specially equipped to deal with the complexities involved in environmental and wildlife crime."

The law needs to reflect the fact that many of those illegally killing animals, for bushmeat or other animal products, are poor. "Poverty is an undeniable driving force for the illegal wildlife trade, which is fueled by members of the wealthy elite from demand countries who seek to benefit from wildlife at the expense of the poor," Mutezo says. "Attention should be paid to the major benefactors of the illegal wildlife trade, to avoid criminalizing the less privileged."

Wildlife trafficking wouldn't be possible without high-level corruption throughout the supply chain route, from the source to where it's sold, including national parks, ports, shops, law enforcement, and other government agencies. "Corruption is the main enabler behind every cog in the illegal wildlife trade," argues Jamie Joseph, founder of Saving the Wild, who works to expose high-level corruption in South Africa, which she says allows the killing of rhinos to continue. "If we lose the war on corruption, we lose the war on everything."

While poachers are sometimes caught and imprisoned, it's rare for corrupt politicians or officials to be prosecuted, a sign of a lack of international will to investigate criminal activity, such as looking into bank accounts. "We need to pursue high-level targets and expose and eliminate

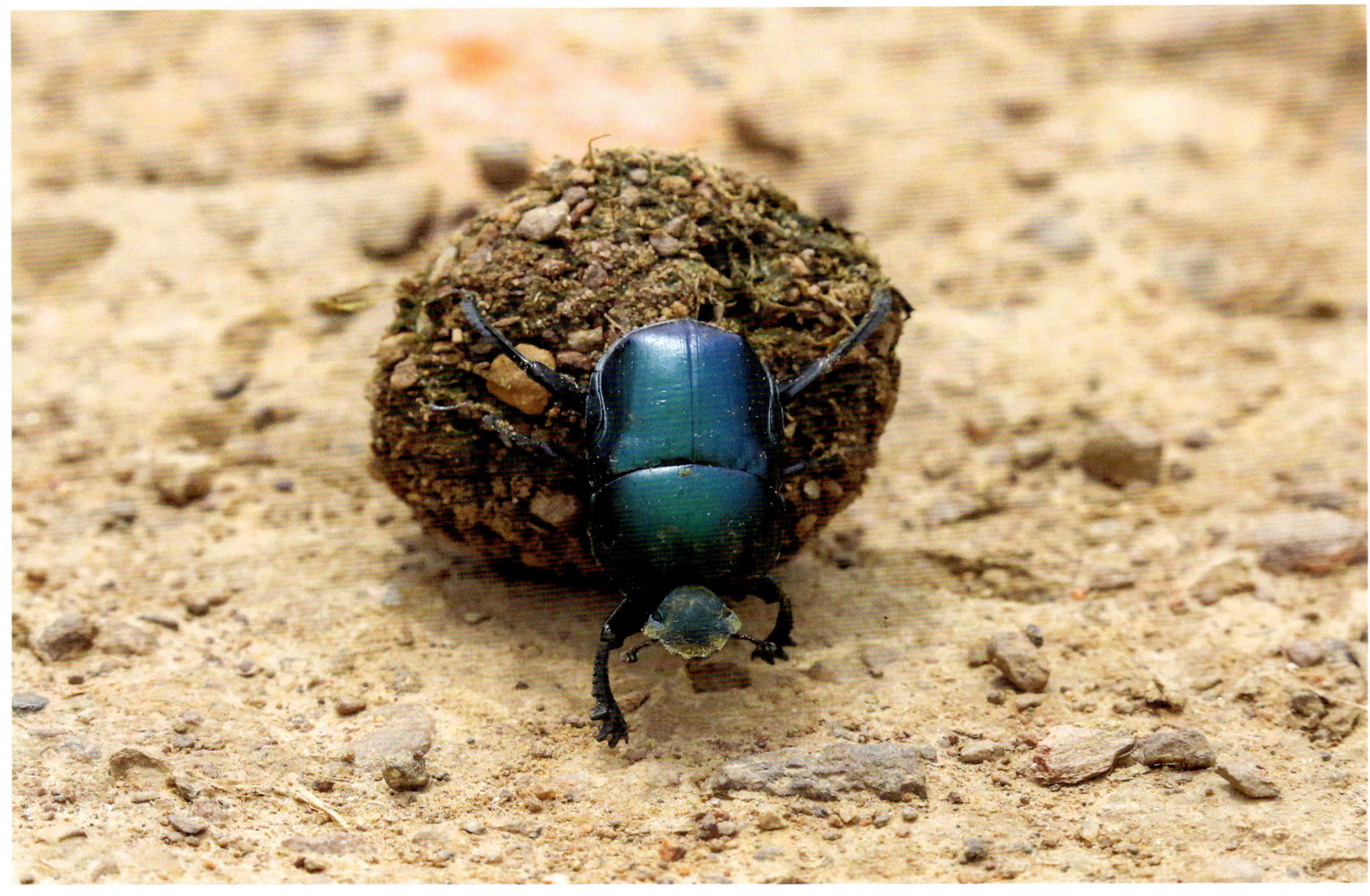

Graeme Green
Dung Beetle
Akagera National Park, Rwanda

the corruption that enables rhino poaching and other crimes," suggests Joseph. "Globally, the narrative needs to change from the 'poaching problem' to the 'corruption problem.'"

The fight to protect wildlife is one that costs lives. "I always start my day with a prayer," says ranger Gracien Muyisa Sivanza, who works in Virunga National Park in the Democratic Republic of the Congo (DRC). "We live each day knowing it could be our last."

In January 2021, six rangers were killed by local militia in Virunga, one of the last remaining habitats for mountain gorillas. Another attack, in April 2020, saw 12 Virunga rangers and five civilians murdered. "It's a very painful experience to lose so many people—brothers, fathers, and husbands—all at once," Sivanza tells me. "When I see their families at funerals, tears always flow. But then I pull myself together and life goes on."

For more than 20 years, eastern DRC has suffered instability and conflict, creating armed groups that work to exploit natural resources in Virunga. The fight to protect Virunga isn't just about gorillas or elephants—it's for the future of the country. "The park's responsible for development projects that promote peace and create jobs," Sivanza says. "Millions of people depend on tourism. My fellow rangers who passed away are the heroes of conservation. To honor their memories, we continue the fight we started together. They didn't die in vain."

THERE ARE MANY OTHER REASONS WHY wildlife numbers are dropping, from poisonous pesticides to plastics clogging the oceans to invasive species being introduced. But over everything, there now hangs the specter of global climate change. The world isn't on track to meet the Paris Agreement's goal of limiting global warming to below 3.5°F above preindustrial levels.

"In the same way humans are going to find their habitats and homes destroyed by floods and fires, and human food sources will be compromised by drought, the same things will happen to animals," says Dr. Paul Johnston, head of Greenpeace International's Science Unit. "Their habitats might cease to exist. Animals might be killed by extreme events. They could be made locally or globally extinct. There's also the possibility of dislocation in time and space, so things no longer line up—for example, plants and pollinators may not emerge at the same time or even be in the same place at the right time."

I've grown up hearing experts pleading for urgent action on the climate emergency. We've had decades of global leaders denying reality or dragging their heels. Just as there have been calls to protect elephants since the 1800s, or decades of efforts to save rhinos or protect the Amazon, it seems humans are capable of staying on any course, no matter how destructive, as long as it's profitable.

The language on climate has changed over time, from avoiding disaster altogether to a more resigned acceptance that we'll have to adapt to the worsening effects. We're already living with the consequences, including an increase in wildfires, storms, drought, and flooding. Recently, there have been unprecedented heat waves at both the North and South poles, with the 745-square-mile Conger ice shelf collapsing in Antarctica. We haven't been short of warning signs.

"There's evidence that coral reef systems will be very seriously threatened," Johnston says. "We're already seeing changes in forest environments, where higher temperatures and drought lead to a greater numbers of fire days. We've seen heat waves in Siberia and other cold regions, where permafrost is thawing. We know species are being affected. The polar bear is running out of natural habitat, due to the reduction in sea ice, for example."

The Australian government recently listed koalas as officially endangered. Disease, habitat destruction, and road accidents all contributed, but the major factor was the intense bushfires, brought on by climate change. The 2019–2020 "black summer" killed around three billion animals in Australia, including bats, birds, kangaroos, and more than 60,000 koalas.

Climate change's impact on wildlife will have knock-on effects on the planet's ability to provide food, clean air and water, and other services humans rely on. "If you look at bee pollinators, they're under a lot of threats—not just climate change, but the impact of man-made chemicals," says Johnston. "The loss of pollinators would leave a hole in the system and the food we're able to produce. You don't know what onward effects there are going to be to any species going extinct."

To limit the effects of global warming, governments and businesses around the world would need to make massive, systemic changes of the kind they've repeatedly failed to achieve for half a century. "We need to radically get greenhouse gas emissions under control and start reducing atmospheric levels of carbon dioxide and other greenhouse gases," says Johnston. "The first link in the chain is to completely remove our reliance on fossil fuel energy sources, to substitute fossil fuel energy sources for renewable energy sources. It may be that we're too late to reverse some of the impacts, though."

It's a dispiriting picture. Record levels of deforestation, rising oceans, and extinctions make it look like the war is being lost. But battles are being fought and won all the time to save species and habitats. Seemingly unstoppable tides of destruction have been turned back. Each one of these battles matters. Each one will help determine the kind of world we'll be living in and the animals still living alongside us after the next blink of an eye.

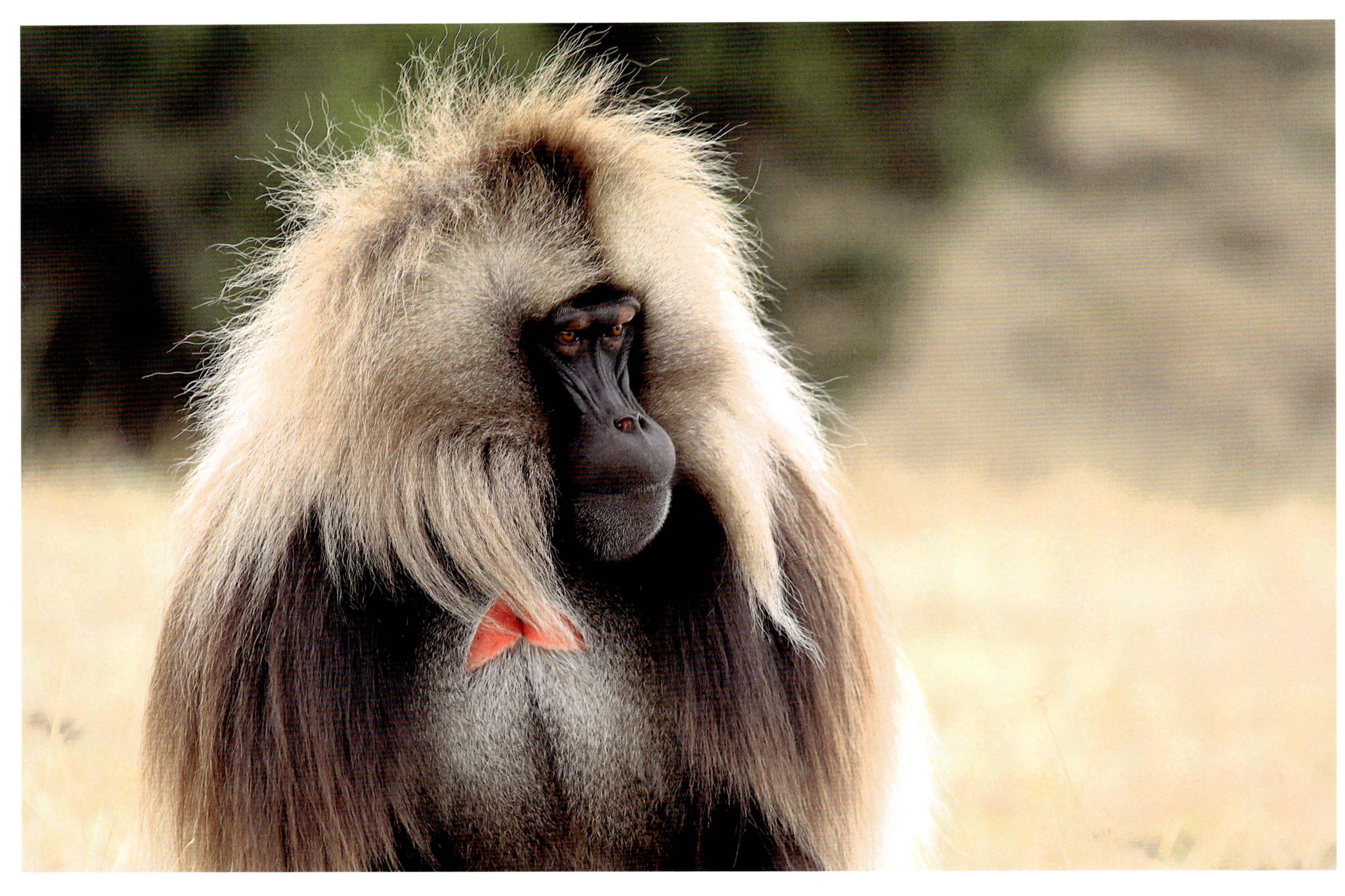

Graeme Green
Gelada Monkey
Simien Mountains National Park, Ethiopia

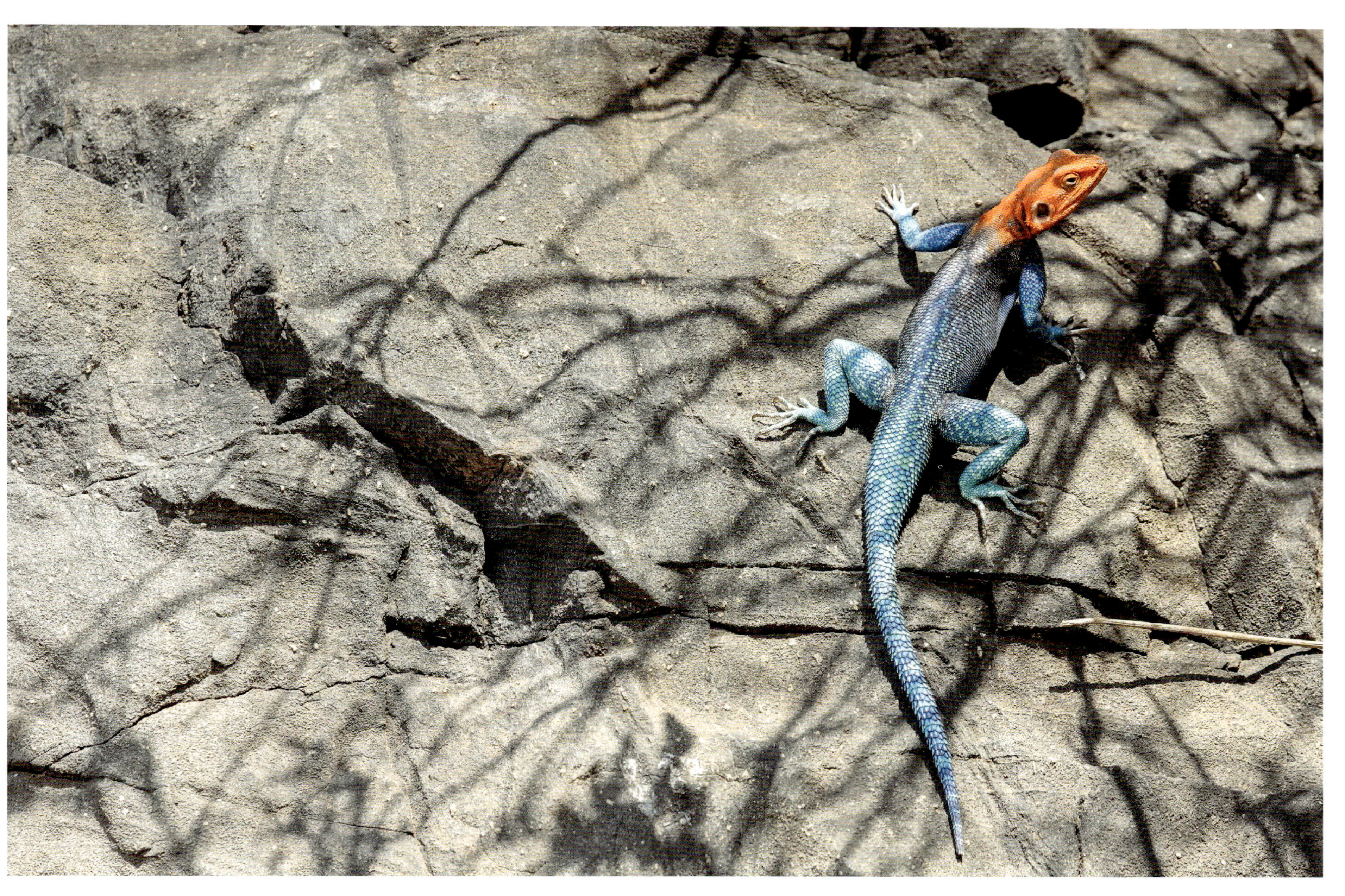

Graeme Green
Red-headed Rock Agama
Ruaha National Park, Tanzania

A Wilder, Fairer World

Graeme Green

IN 2011, I TRAVELED ON A NARROW WOODEN MOTORBOAT deep into the Peruvian Amazon to report on the Ashaninka's fight to protect their homeland. Brazilian energy company Eletrobras planned to construct a 541-feet-high hydroelectric dam across the Ene River, which forms part of the headwaters of the Amazon, part of a larger scheme to build 60 hydroelectric dams in the Brazilian, Peruvian, and Bolivian Amazon, and export the electricity to Brazil. The Ashaninka, who owned the legal titles to the land, feared the dam would be forced on them, flooding 456 square miles of land, displacing more than 10,000 people, and destroying their homes, food (fish, forest animals, and plants), and livelihoods.

The following year, I took a bus down to the Aysén region of Chile to cover Patagonia Sin Represas' (Patagonia Without Dams) campaign to stop the construction of five hydroelectric dams on the Rio Baker and Rio Pascua, Chile's two biggest rivers by volume, which would send electricity 1,550 miles north to mining operations in the Atacama desert. Local people argued the dams would irrevocably damage the environment, pollute their drinking water, force people from their homes, and open Chilean Patagonia up to other commercial interests, such as mining and logging, as well as threatening endangered wildlife, including the huemul deer. "Who owns the rain?" Don Julio, an 81-year-old sheep farmer, memorably asked me. "When a company owns the water system of Chile, do they own the glaciers? Do they own the rain? What do they own?"

In both cases, the energy produced was intended to be sold elsewhere. In both cases, local people would see little benefit but have to live with the negative consequences. Coming away from both situations, I didn't feel hopeful. I feared local people would be steamrolled over by governments and energy industries because of the vast profits to be made. But in both cases, I was proved wrong. The dams were stopped.

With an avalanche of bad news stories, it can be difficult to remember that a lone voice or a small group of campaigners often make a stand and win. "Anger can drive people to take action," says Farwiza Farhan, environmental activist and founder of Forest, Nature and Environment Aceh (HAkA), who fought palm oil company Kallista Alam in Indonesia's Supreme Court in 2015. Kallista Alam was forced to pay $26 million for illegally setting fires and clearing land for palm oil plantations in the Leuser Ecosystem, 6.4 million acres of biodiverse rain forest habitat, the only place in the world where the Sumatran orangutan, rhino, tiger, and elephant still live in the wild.

Leuser remains at risk from deforestation and commercial exploitation. But the unprecedented fines handed down to the company (which, Farhan suggests, happened because so much international attention was focusing on the case) showed the Indonesian government would punish illegal environmental destruction. "We can't look toward the future and have the spirit to move forward if we always assume the worst will happen," says Farhan. "Seeing the realities on the ground can be disheartening, but we have so much we can win back. None of us can do it alone. Our legal victory can bring hope and strength that, if we work together, this battle is winnable."

Conservation successes are responsible for the fact that many animals still exist. It was feared mountain gorillas would be extinct by the turn of the last century. But, thanks to interventions in Rwanda, Uganda, and the DRC, their numbers have steadily risen to more than 1,000.

Commercial whaling wiped out two million whales in the nineteenth and twentieth centuries, but, since whaling was banned in 1986, humpback whale populations have recovered in the South Atlantic ocean from just 440 in the 1950s to 25,000 today.

West African giraffes plummeted to near-extinction, just forty-nine left, before Niger's government and communities rallied. They're now standing tall at around 600.

Siberian tigers, Jamaican rock iguanas, Checkered skipper butterflies, Nassau groupers, sea otters, and Hula painted frogs are among the many other species saved from extinction by people taking action.

From the Churah Valley kukri snake to the Star octopus, new species have been described by scientists, with others thought to be lost to history rediscovered. New national parks and Marine Protected Areas have been created or expanded. Dams have been destroyed, restoring free-flowing rivers, so freshwater fish populations can thrive again. Planes have been loaded with rhinos and lions, moved from country to country to create new strongholds. Breeding centers have helped increase numbers of struggling creatures, such as pandas, marmots, and condors.

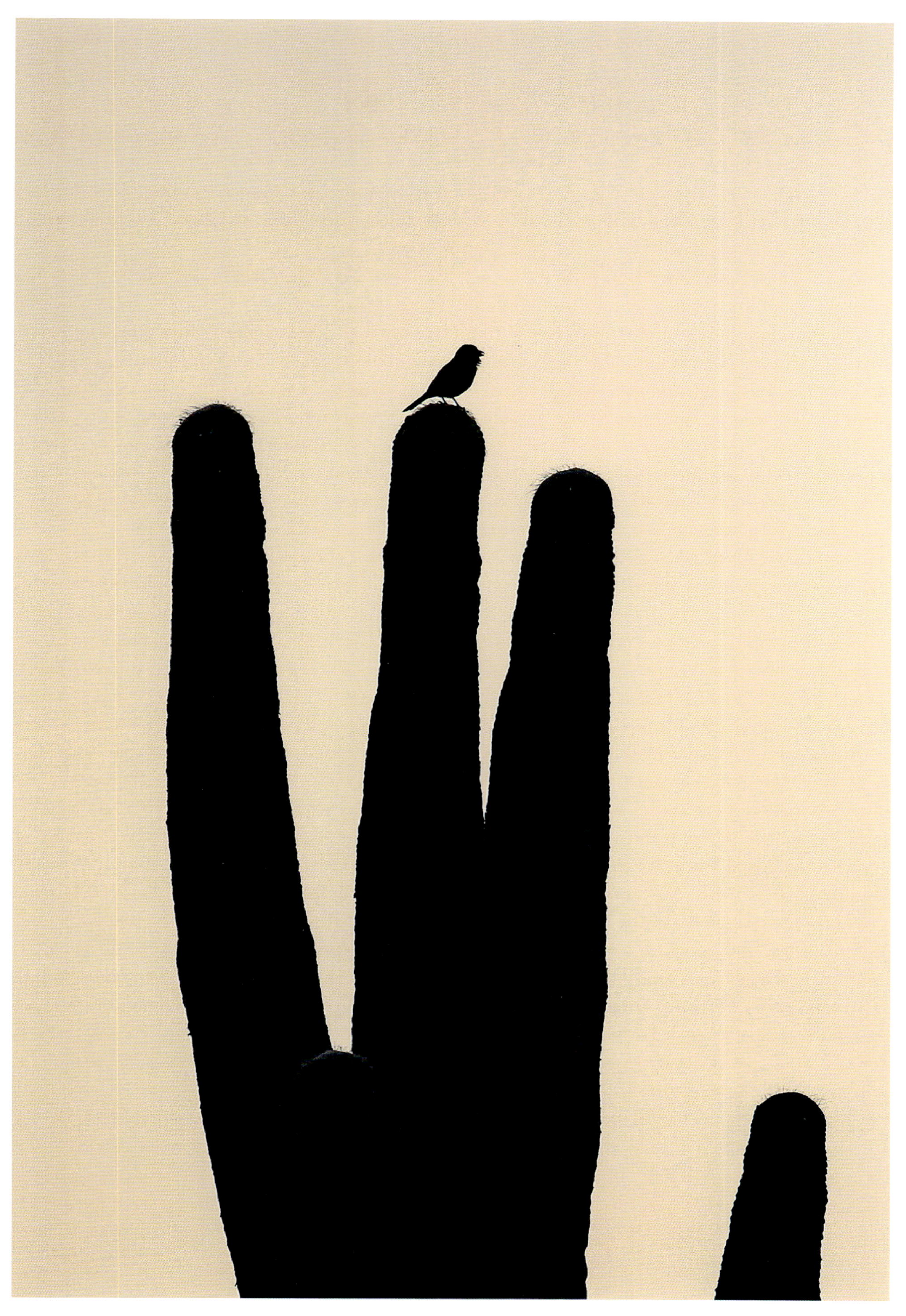

Graeme Green
House Finch
Helia Bravo Hollis Botanical
Garden, Mexico

 "There is no silver bullet to save the natural world," says Frans Schepers, Managing Director of Rewilding Europe. "But rewilding gives nature the opportunity to heal itself and bounce back to create wilder, more biodiverse habitats. According to the United Nations, we need to rewild an area the size of China globally."

Rewilding Europe has returned European bison to Romania's Southern Carpathian mountains and worked on projects with beavers, eagles, pelicans, and deer in Portugal, Italy, Sweden, and elsewhere. But rewilding is about more than reintroducing animals or planting trees. It means restoring intact healthy ecosystems with the full former range of wildlife and plant life. "Rewilding can bring a huge amount of benefits for people," explains Frans. "Our ecosystems need to recover. We need keystone species, including top predators and large herbivores, which drive ecological processes. For people, naturally functioning ecosystems are better at providing us with clean air and water, preventing flooding, storing carbon, and better for physical and mental health. And people are starting to see that nature is one of the best ways to mitigate climate change."

"By 2030, we want to see rewilding practiced extensively across Europe. We'd like to see large numbers of herbivores roaming our landscapes, with carnivores and scavengers living off them. We'd like to see insect populations recover, a food source for birds, amphibians, and reptiles. We'd like to see many dams and dikes removed, bringing back fish to rivers and wetlands. We'd like to see our remaining old growth forest being protected, and existing forest becoming much wilder. We'd like to see large areas protected so wildlife can breed and recover."

So much nature has been destroyed across Europe, the US, and elsewhere. Developing countries across Africa, Asia, and Latin America are now being asked to avoid the mistakes industrialized countries have made and to instead develop via "green economies." Rewilding is one way to address that imbalance. "It's a moral responsibility," says Frans. "If we ask people on other continents to protect what they have, we should protect what we have. In Europe, we're still losing nature. We're still losing old growth forest with illegal and legal logging. How can we say the Amazon should be protected if we don't protect what we have? Everyone in the world realizes we need to restore nature because our systems are broken."

I've seen the impact of rewilding around the world, including Patagonia Park in Chile, a restored ecosystem with Andean condors, rheas, guanaco, and rare huemul deer, and plants, like the bright-red *neneo macho* shrub and bushy *coirón* grass, recovering after decades of overgrazing by sheep and cattle. Over the last 30 years, Kristine Tompkins and her late husband, Doug, who made their fortune with clothing companies (The North Face, Esprit, and Patagonia), have been buying up and restoring land, then returning it to the governments of Chile and Argentina. They've so far helped create fifteen national parks in Chile and Argentina, protecting 14.8 million acres of wilderness.

Rewilding Argentina (an offshoot of Tompkins Conservation) recently returned jaguars to Argentina's Gran Iberá Park in Argentina's Iberá wetlands, the animals last seen there in the 1930s, before habitat loss and hunting drove them to extinction. "Seeing the jaguars walk out into freedom was one of the most emotional days of my life," says Kristine Tompkins, president and cofounder of Tompkins Conservation. "Jaguars are a keystone species, so they're incredibly important to a fully functioning ecosystem. It also sets a standard for what's possible in rewilding. It tells us that, given the right circumstances, you can bring back almost anything."

Tompkins Conservation have also worked with white-collared peccaries, red-shouldered macaws, giant river otters, and other species. Restoring ecosystems protects the environment, preserves clean air and water, combats climate change, and creates jobs. But it's also an emotional mission. "The absence of beauty and wildness in our lives means we're missing a large portion of why our hearts beat," Tompkins says. "You can make all the scientific rationales for bringing something back, but it's about an emotional love of imagining a place functioning as it should, like wolves in Yellowstone or Iberian lynx in Spain."

Tompkins believes rewilding is key to the future of humanity. "Over the last 200 years, humans have wreaked havoc on natural systems and on one another. We're in the middle of one of the largest extinction crises known to man. Billions of people are suffering from the rapidly increasing effects of climate change. It's imperative that we don't accept this simply as 'the price of progress,' and instead move toward human dignity and the ethic that all life has intrinsic value. I feel tremendous sadness that we've learned nothing from records of the collapse of civilizations over and over again at great cost to everyone. Now, the collapse we face is at a planetary level. I want to live and die on the team that pushes against these trends."

"There is no world where human ingenuity and technology will 'fix' climate change. The protection and restoration of large-scale regions and the return of keystone species is essential for our ability to simply stay alive. If you talk to someone living in South Sudan or islands in the South Pacific, the effects of climate change are not events somewhere in their future. They are here."

THE NEED TO RESTORE NATURE is being met with grand ideas. Scientists from Arizona State University in the United States recently published a "geoengineering" proposal to restore sea ice levels in the Arctic. The $500 billion idea suggested building 10 million massive wind-powered pumps to pump seawater onto the surface of the ice in winter, where it would freeze and thicken the ice cap, helping protect Arctic ecosystems and bringing back a tool to combat climate change. It's an extreme measure for extreme times, just like the scientists who've harvested eggs from the last remaining female northern white rhinos in Kenya's Ol Pejeta Conservancy and flown them to a laboratory in Italy to create embryos using the sperm of dead rhinos—a Jurassic Park-esque effort to bring the species back from extinction.

Alongside efforts to turn back the clock, it makes sense to invest more money and time now to protect the animals and wild places we still have before they need to be brought back. We could, in the future, spend millions to recreate a pangolin in a lab, or we could stop all the world's pangolins from being killed now.

A wilder world, restored and protected, makes sense to me on an emotional, philosophical level. It's about the kind of world I want to live in: a world where I can still hear a lion roar, see birds of prey soaring in the skies, and swim with hordes of colorful fish at coral gardens, rather than a drab, lifeless planet. The world is a far better place for us to live with all this remarkable wildlife than without it.

Nature also provides food, future medicines, and the biodiverse systems we need to fight climate change, and turns the wheels of the global economy. "The cold, hard fact is that humanity is deeply intertwined with nature," says Dr. Bruno Oberle, Director General of the IUCN. "Up to 50 percent of global GDP is related to nature and biodiversity."

But nature is disappearing. Around 28 percent of more than 140,000 assessed species on the IUCN's Red List of Threatened Species are threatened with extinction. "The unsustainable extraction of natural resources leads to climate change and depletes the nature our survival depends on, driving biodiversity loss at rates unprecedented in human history," says Oberle. "Average temperatures have already risen 2°F in the past 100 years, leading to rising sea levels, more frequent and extreme droughts, floods, and wildfires. Inequality further exacerbates the issue."

The human and economic cost is already massive. The cost of doing nothing would be far greater than taking action now. "Go deep enough and you'll find nature stands at the center of our entire economy," argues Oberle. "Economic growth—the relentless pursuit of GDP—must be decoupled from resource use. Governments need to give nature the central place it deserves in decision-making. Sustainability and biodiversity must be firmly brought into the DNA of finance and business. With agriculture fundamentally dependent on nature, food production mustn't drive biodiversity loss. We must completely change how we produce and consume natural resources. We must also stop treating waste like a useless by-product to be hurled back into our ecosystems without consequences."

"Ultimately, we urgently need new means of production, new products, services, and infrastructures, and new ways of investing our financial resources. We must serve the needs of the planet, so it can continue serving our needs. All this has to be done bearing in mind the different requirements and abilities of different countries."

THE PROBLEMS THE WORLD FACES can't be solved in isolation. For me, there's no hope of tackling the global crisis in wildlife and nature without addressing poverty and inequality. In a world that produces enough food to feed the entire population and enough money sitting in bank accounts to eradicate poverty, addressing inequality should be a priority in its own right. But we also can't expect to look after wildlife and nature, or get to grips with biodiversity loss and climate change, as long as criminal levels of poverty and inequality are allowed to continue.

Over the last fifty years, the global economy has grown five times larger, mainly due to the tripling of natural resource extraction and the rapid increase in production and consumption, which created our global emergency. The food, fuel, and lifestyles of people in developed countries are the main drivers of deforestation, biodiversity loss, and climate change. But poorer people around the world are the worst hit by the consequences.

The world's ten richest men now hoard six times more wealth than the world's poorest 3.1 billion people, around 40 percent of the global population. The global COVID-19 pandemic has also increased poverty and inequality.

Africa is not a poor continent—it's an unequal one. The continent contains seven of the world's ten most unequal countries and is home to more than half of the world's extreme poor, with 413 million people living on less than $1.90 a day. The top 1 percent of Africans owns 33 percent of the continent's wealth.

In Nigeria, Africa's largest economy, which has vast oil reserves and other natural resources, one in ten children die before they reach their fifth birthday, and a quarter of Nigerians lack access to safe drinking water. More than 10 million children don't go to school, 60 percent of them girls. Yet, $24 billion, less than the combined wealth of the five richest Nigerians, could end poverty in the country.

The World Bank estimates 87 percent of the world's extreme poor will live in Sub-Saharan Africa by 2030. But poverty isn't just a homegrown issue. Inequality was built into the colonial system, where occupying powers took control of countries' resources and wealth, leaving the citizens poor. Inequality isn't an accident or something that's unavoidable. "The strength of the imperialist system as a whole rests on the necessary inequality of its parts," as Uruguayan journalist and author Eduardo Galeano wrote.

Colonialism in Africa created a legacy of inequality that has endured. Many African countries still see their natural resources—agriculture, fishing, minerals, oil, gas—and wealth siphoned out of the country, with little benefit to the population, except a few in positions of power who collaborate with foreign companies.

In the last few years, Canadian company ReconAfrica has begun oil and gas activity across a 21,330-square-mile area of northeast Namibia and northwest Botswana. African and international organizations, local Indigenous leaders, and campaigners, including Djimon Hounsou and Leonardo DiCaprio, are fighting to protect the pristine ecosystems of the Kavango region, a "natural paradise" with remarkable biodiversity, including savanna elephants, African wild dogs, black and white rhinos, Temminck's pangolins, and Martial eagles. Kavango East and Kavango West in northern Namibia are currently home to around 200,000 people, including the Indigenous San. The wider threatened area, encompassing the UNESCO World Heritage-listed Okavango Delta, provides livelihoods for more than one million people.

Environmental activists predict a catastrophe of the kind seen in the Niger Delta, including loss of wildlife, contamination of water supplies, air and soil pollution, reduced human rights, increased crime, and the loss of land and homes, and a wider environmental disaster for Africa. "The entire equation is colonial," says Nigerian environmental activist Nnimmo Bassey. "It's colonial extraction. It's happening across the continent. They found oil and gas almost everywhere across the continent, and all the pipelines go to seaports to feed other markets outside the continent. Africa remains useful for extraction. This has gone on for hundreds of years, and it's continuing. It plays out in a way that's attractive to politicians who use measures such as GDP to tell the world they're making progress, but really it's just a cover for global exploitation."

Stealing a nation's wealth, leaving a legacy of poverty behind, is a disaster for people and wildlife. Inequality is a major cause of political and economic instability and increases pressure on natural resources. Poverty also contributes directly to the loss of wildlife and environmental destruction. People who are struggling to survive are more likely to break into national parks and protected forests to hunt animals for food or to sell, for illegal fishing, or to collect firewood. No fence or ranger's gun will stop someone from trying to feed their family.

The killing of Rafiki, a silverback gorilla in Uganda's Bwindi Impenetrable National Park, made global headlines. But the gorilla's death was a reminder of the hardships people face, even in thriving tourist zones. "The man who killed Rafiki was a very hungry, desperate poacher," says Dr. Gladys Kalema-Zikusoka, Ugandan veterinarian and CEO of Conservation Through Public Health, who works in Bwindi. "He was among the most vulnerable in the community. He needed to eat and would have sold some of the meat. He wasn't poaching gorillas, but he came across Rafiki. It made me realize that we're not reaching everybody. We need to address hunger."

Poor people with crops or cattle to protect, who see no economic benefit from living alongside elephants or lions, are also more likely to attack wild animals. The poaching of animals for their horns, skins, or tusks is usually controlled by organized, well-funded criminal gangs, with the large profits meaning the trade would be likely to continue regardless. But poverty is a great recruiting agent to get local people involved with the illegal trade. In Namibia, studies of prison inmates locked up for poaching for the wildlife trade found that poverty and needing to feed their families were their main motivations. Reducing poverty would also make it harder for criminal gangs to find local people who don't care if animals are killed or not, especially if those locals were receiving direct benefits from those animals being kept alive and felt a sense of "ownership."

These aren't Africa-specific issues. Bolivia is one of the world's most unequal countries, with 20 percent of households living in extreme poverty. "Poverty is a determining factor in wildlife crime," says Tania Baltazar, cofounder and President of Bolivian NGO Comunidad Inti Wara Yassi (CIWY). "The lack of education and resources mean people find wildlife trafficking an easy way to make money. Those who know it's a crime don't see it as dangerous, as the penalties are lax and there's a low probability of being sanctioned. The common factor is poverty, living outside the margins of human rights, without electricity, potable water, and school education, with a lack of employability.…In recent years, there have been many cases of trafficking parts of jaguars, pumas, and ocelots, such as fangs, skins, and skulls, which have been sent to China, where they're used for 'medicine' or ornaments."

Solutions have come in the form of jobs in ecotourism or other sources of income, such as growing fruit. "Clear policies are needed against trafficking," says Baltazar. "You have to start with education and awareness, along with poverty reduction, employment, and alternative economic development."

THE GREATEST MISTAKE MADE IN CONSERVATION was to think animals could be protected by taking people out of the picture. In many parts of

Africa, the setting up of national parks has meant Indigenous people being dispossessed and excluded from ancestral lands. Protected areas were fenced off and guarded, with Indigenous Africans kept away from sources of water, food, firewood, and spaces to graze animals. Creating protected areas often wasn't an act of altruism or driven by a desire to look after animals, but a way for colonial occupiers to control valuable natural resources and the money to be made from trophy hunting, ivory, and, later, tourism. Under British rule, natural resources belonged to the Crown, not to Africans.

Whereas words like *adventurer* gave White hunting a positive spin, the word *poacher* was used to criminalize Indigenous African communities' traditional hunting, a racist way to discriminate and divide people on two sides of the fence: respectable and legal White European *hunters* with a right to hunt inside protected wildlife areas, contrasting with illegitimate, criminal, Black *poachers* on lands they'd lived on for centuries. Indigenous people were seen as a problem to be removed or to wage a war against. Traditional hunting, for meat, inside protected wildlife areas became a punishable offense. One of the first things colonial forces did was to build prisons. Illegal hunting by Africans was often blamed for declining wildlife numbers, rather than European hunters and the ivory trade. It takes a brutal kind of person to steal someone's land and then blame them for the crimes you commit on it.

"Colonialism introduced the concept of exclusion," says Paine Makko, executive director of the Ujamaa Community Resource Team (UCRT) and an advocate for Indigenous Peoples in Tanzania. "Indigenous people suffered evictions from their native lands to make way for exclusive conservation models. Take the example of the Maasai, who were moved from the Serengeti to Ngorongoro to create the Serengeti National park during colonial times. These communities were moved to either Loliondo or Ngorongoro, in what we now call the Ngorongoro Conservation Area. The people were promised not to be moved again. Yet today, the same people are being threatened to be moved out of these areas. There are many other cases where external forces make decisions with a top-down approach that fails to involve local communities."

Even after countries gained independence, controlling protected wildlife areas was a way for national governments and those in charge to keep their hands on the money generated from hunting and wildlife tourism, a huge source of revenue in countries such as Kenya and Tanzania.

From India to Ecuador, many of the world's national parks and protected areas have been created by removing tribal peoples.

Most serious wildlife organizations now work to make local people central to conservation initiatives. But even today, Indigenous communities across Africa, from the San to the Maasai, face arrest and eviction,

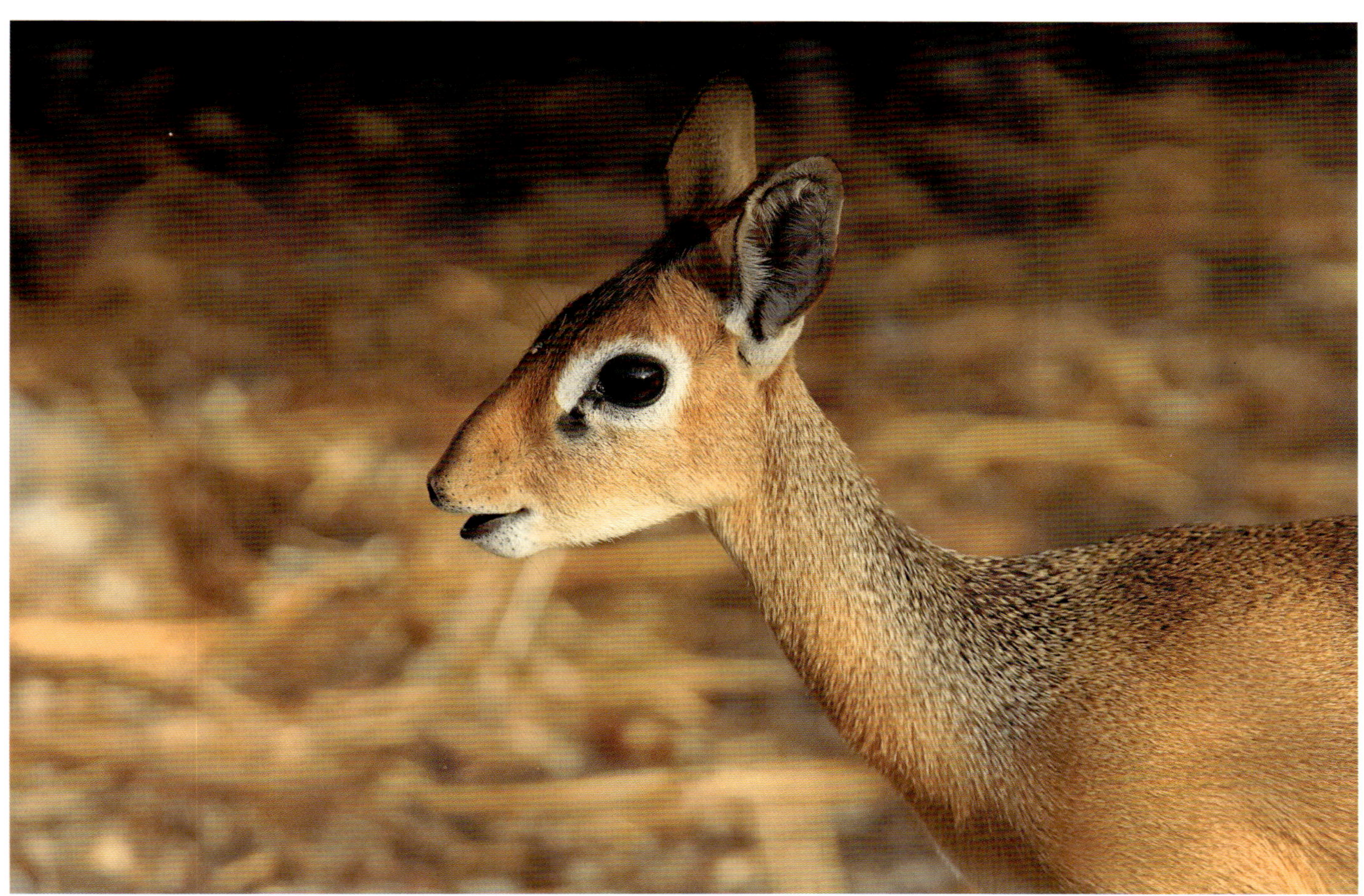

their homes and lands taken to make way for tourism, conservation, diamond mining, or trophy hunting.

This is not only an injustice, but also a shot in the foot for conservation by excluding local people and their knowledge of wildlife and nature. "Indigenous people have always thought of a communal way of living and coexistence as of great importance to them," says Makko. "Westerners may not entirely depend on nature for survival. But, as the livelihood and culture of Indigenous people depends on a healthy ecosystem, it's in their best interest to protect, manage, and sustainably use environmental resources."

Makko argues that having more Indigenous people involved in conservation would benefit wildlife and people. "Keeping areas open for local communities and Indigenous peoples' traditional way of living prevents unsustainable development, which threatens wildlife habitats, grazing areas, and corridors. Conservation is a very expensive process, and for African countries with limited resources, it's hard to finance. Indigenous and local communities offer a more sustainable solution. But they need recognition for their efforts and not to be seen as enemies of conservation."

Before the global pandemic, wildlife tourism contributed $29.3 billion per year to the African economy. There's big money to be made from wildlife, but too often the money flows out of an area or country, with too little going to local people. "There's a lot of inequality around resources and money generated from wildlife, and, in particular, the money that goes into the hands of the communities," says Makko. "As long as this inequality continues, poverty will continue in communities. Considering communities play a vital role in conservation, they should receive a fair share of resources generated through wildlife and conservation. Take the example of the Ngorongoro Conservation Area, which generates billions in money, yet the Indigenous people in the area live in extreme poverty."

Land ownership is also a crucial issue. "Land ownership is everything for Indigenous people," says Makko. "Land is their life. Owning land creates security and safety in the areas they reside in. It gives communities confidence for their survival."

Even well-intentioned conservation efforts have continued a strategy of protecting wildlife by using barbed wire fences and armed rangers to keep local African people outside of protected areas. Fences might be necessary to protect some highly valuable endangered animals. But in many places, creating guarded spaces that only wealthy tourists can enter has left a legacy of disenfranchisement and resentment.

"Communities have to be the drivers of conservation," says John Kamanga, cofounder and Director of SOLARO (South Rift Association of Land Owners) in Kenya. "Guns for conservation don't work. How many guns can we put out there to protect wildlife? In some cases, it's important to have a balance. But it's more encouraging to make communities the ones who want to protect wildlife. In Kenya, 70 percent of our wildlife resides in communal areas, which are not protected. In a lot of areas where communities live, wildlife has always been there. From a Maasai perspective, it's a lifestyle. They protect their forest because that's where they get their medicine and food from. We have come up with a new English word—conservation—but it's not a new concept to them."

Kamanga sees a future where humans and animals find ways to live alongside each other. But coexistence between people and wildlife is likely to become more difficult as human populations expand, new settlements are built, and land is taken over for agriculture or real estate, with wildlife habitats and ranges shrinking. "We have to look at things from an economic perspective," says Kamanga. "We have to see conservation and wildlife as a way to benefit people. Traditionally, tourism was where Whites would come and build a lodge, and they thought they would build a school or do something here or there. But actually, it's about doing business where Africans are part of it. For there to be poverty, while others make so much money, is wrong. The resources belong to the people. When outsiders come and take away everything, it's very wrong. Leaving the community that has this big asset in poverty is wrong. It's a social ill that has to be corrected."

ONE OF THE MOST ENCOURAGING SHIFTS I'VE SEEN in Africa is the expanding system of conservancies, which help protect and recover wildlife populations. In these privately managed areas, camp owners and tourism businesses pay to lease the land from the landowners, such as the Maasai, who are also often allowed to keep their livestock grazing within the conservancy. It's a precarious balance, but it means that Indigenous people, rather than being ripped off or kept on the outside, receive a decent benefit from wildlife tourism.

"Conservancies are improving people's and communities' lives by creating jobs, scholarships, schools, clinics, water infrastructure, and the regular income that comes from land-lease fees," says Daniel Sopia, CEO of the Maasai Mara Wildlife Conservancies Association. "We're also seeing rising wildlife numbers, such as lions, particularly in Kenya, where over 70 percent of wildlife lives on community land. In the Mara, community conservancies have the highest densities of cats, such as cheetahs and lions."

Local communities have been shut out in the past, but here they're involved in the decision-making process. "The situation is changing slowly in Kenya, where communities are now at the forefront, driving conservation, and the benefits are trickling down to the grassroots, unlike before," Sopia explains. "But I still see a big problem in other countries, such as in southern Africa, where people living with wildlife are experiencing terrible poverty and marginalization."

It's hard to defend situations where tourists in Africa might spend $1,000, $2,000, or more for a night in a safari camp, while local people are struggling to survive on a few dollars or less per day. "There has always been a mentality or perception from the West that local people don't deserve bigger pay, due to their capacity or their living standard, so they've been used as tools to cultivate wealth," says Sopia. "This mentality must stop if wildlife is to have a future on this continent. Equality and fairness must be the norm. Communities must be empowered and supported to work toward sustainability."

WILDLIFE DOCUMENTARIES AND FILMS are another huge money-spinner. But it's another area that Black Africans have historically been excluded from, the stories about their continent and wildlife often told by White Western TV hosts. Wildlife photography, too, has been dominated for decades by White, male photographers, something that's only now starting to change.

I've also spoken with Africans, Asians, and Latin Americans who have found themselves excluded from conservation in their own countries. But having African leaders and homegrown NGOs directing conservation "by the people, for the people" in Africa (and Asian leaders in Asia, and Latin American leaders in Latin America...) would mean better local understanding and communication, and more trust, which is likely to be more effective on issues such as poaching or family planning. "There's a greater sense of confidence and ownership when the people involved are from here and have a real stake," says Elizabeth Babalola, a Nigerian conservationist and Director of Talent Acquisition at the African Leadership University's School of Wildlife Conservation. "I'm more likely to believe they'll make decisions in my best interests. It's also about nuanced things, like language. If someone's in a negotiation with a person who speaks a different language, it's likely they'll miss out on the context. African leaders would be better positioned for these crucial conversations."

Babalola wants to see changes in the people making decisions for the future of Africa's people and wildlife. "It would be great to see at least 50 percent of leaders in conservation being women," she says. "Right now, it's about 30 percent. Many African-focused NGOs need greater diversity on their boards and in the senior leadership. It would be great to see the top five NGOs all run by African executives, with at least a 50 percent African board. I'd love to see more Africans in decision-making positions. It's more effective."

AROUND THE WORLD, people are demanding changes to power structures and those who get to make all-important decisions. In 2021, after years of legal campaigning, the Constitutional Court of Ecuador recognized the rights of Indigenous communities to have the final say on land rights, and oil, mining, and other industrial activities on their territory. "Indigenous peoples make up only 5 percent of the world's population but we're the custodians of 80 percent of the planet's biodiversity," says Ecuadorian politician and Indigenous rights activist Yaku Pérez, who ran for president in the country's 2021 election. "The right of self-determination for Indigenous peoples is recognized by the United Nations. One of the branches of self-determination is consent, the right of Indigenous peoples over their territories. We don't live off the Earth—we live *with* the Earth. The Earth is a living organism that gives us food, drink, shelter. She gives us life."

In Ecuador, as elsewhere, Indigenous peoples have been excluded from land, wealth, politics, and decision-making positions. Pérez has campaigned against mining in Ecuador's cloud forests and protected areas owned by Indigenous people. But Ecuador's government recently brought in decrees to make it easier for international companies to open areas up to mining, oil, and other extraction. "The mining decree is a declaration of war on the defenders of water and nature," Pérez says. "It's harmful to the rights of Indigenous and non-Indigenous peoples alike. Mining leaves environmental pollution, poisoned water, violence, dispossession. They destroy forests and ecosystems, which generates more greenhouse gases and global warming.

"We are already on a path of no return toward climate collapse, a crisis caused by the limitless greed of human beings. If we don't correct the path of the capitalist civilization, we're condemned to planetary ecological collapse. I hope that, by learning from the wisdom of our grandfathers and grandmothers, and from the evidence of the scientific community, we can make solidarity prevail over greed, and care for the planet, rather than plundering it. We need to be custodians of all species in the great miracle of creation."

The Amazon is one of the most biodiverse regions on the planet and serves as the "lungs of the Earth." Like many nature areas, it has been seen by many in terms of the profits it can provide, if exploited. "Over the last five centuries, since the arrival of the conquistadores, the Amazon rain forest has been seen by outsiders as a place to extract resources," says Indigenous activist Nemonte Nenquimo. "Our lands have been exploited for everything: gold, animal pelts, rubber, hardwoods and fine timbers, oil, cattle-ranching. This is impacting not just our communities, but all life on planet Earth."

The scale and pace of destruction has increased in recent decades, in Ecuador, Brazil, and elsewhere, as governments and outside companies take from the Amazon as much as they can. "This vision of resource extraction is bringing the Amazon to an ecological tipping point, a point we will not be able to return from," Nenquimo says. "Without protection of these territories and resources, the climate crisis will only get more severe."

Nenquimo is the first female president of the Waorani of Pastaza and cofounder of the Indigenous-led nonprofit organization Ceibo Alliance and Amazon Frontlines. In 2019, she and her Waorani Indigenous group took the Ecuadorean government to court over its plans to sell their ancestral territory in the Amazon to oil companies, without consultation or permission. A historic legal decision protected 500,000 acres of primary rain forest in Waorani territory. The ruling set a legal precedent for Indigenous rights.

The exclusion of Indigenous peoples from decision-making is harmful to the planet. Indigenous people, Nenquimo argues, tend to think and act according to a different set of principles than the take-all-we-can-get destruction and extraction that governs many global cultures: less consumerist, more sustainable, more likely to live in balance with nature. Deforestation rates on lands looked after by Indigenous communities tend to be 50 percent lower than elsewhere.

"We have a different perspective," Nenquimo says. "We have a profound, spiritual connection with Mother Earth. We would never act in a way to harm Mother Earth and our source of life. Our ways of life are based on reciprocity, not consumption, and the understanding that we are all related and connected. We rely on our ecosystems. It's our forests, deserts, mountains, and oceans that allow us to survive. We have seen how industrial civilizations have poisoned our rivers and territories, but why would you poison the air you breathe and the water you drink? We have seen forests destroyed, but why would you destroy your home, medicine, and food? But our knowledge and ways of life are even further at risk than many people think. By forcibly displacing us from our lands, we're facing a cultural tipping point. Our connections with the land are coming under immense pressure."

Having more Indigenous leaders in politics and other decision-making positions would strengthen humanity's collective gene pool of ideas and could create a global shift towards living more sustainably with nature, rather than the endless pursuit of economic growth. "The only way to confront the biodiversity and climate crisis is to restore our balance with nature," Nenquimo argues. "Our way of life protects the Amazon rain forest and our planet's climate. If Indigenous peoples around the world were given greater decision-making power, we could be even more effective in the protection of our territories and of the world's biodiversity and wildlife. We could also dedicate ourselves to healing and restoring our ecosystems, which have been so damaged by industrial civilization and reckless exploitation.

"Indigenous leadership is needed on a global scale. Only when our lands and waters are healthy can we protect the climate, prevent future pandemics, and ensure our planet continues to provide for human life. This can only be done if companies and governments worldwide respect our rights to sovereignty and self-determination. To continue to fight for the survival of the planet, we need to be respected and protected."

THE FUTURE CONTAINS A CENTRAL INJUSTICE: many of the people who are least responsible for causing the biodiversity crisis and climate change are expected to suffer the worst impacts, including Indigenous communities, the poor and marginalized, and women.

"Africa is bearing the irreversible brunt of the climate crisis, from the water crisis to food insecurity," says Nigerian climate justice activist Adenike Titilope Oladosu. "We are heading to a point of no return. In regions like Sub-Saharan Africa, climate change is fueling conflict between farmers and herders over the control of resources. In the Lake Chad region, where more than 10.7 million people's livelihoods have been decimated, it provides an environment that helps armed groups to gain ground."

In one of humankind's great acts of self-harm, women around the world have been repressed and excluded from decision-making in

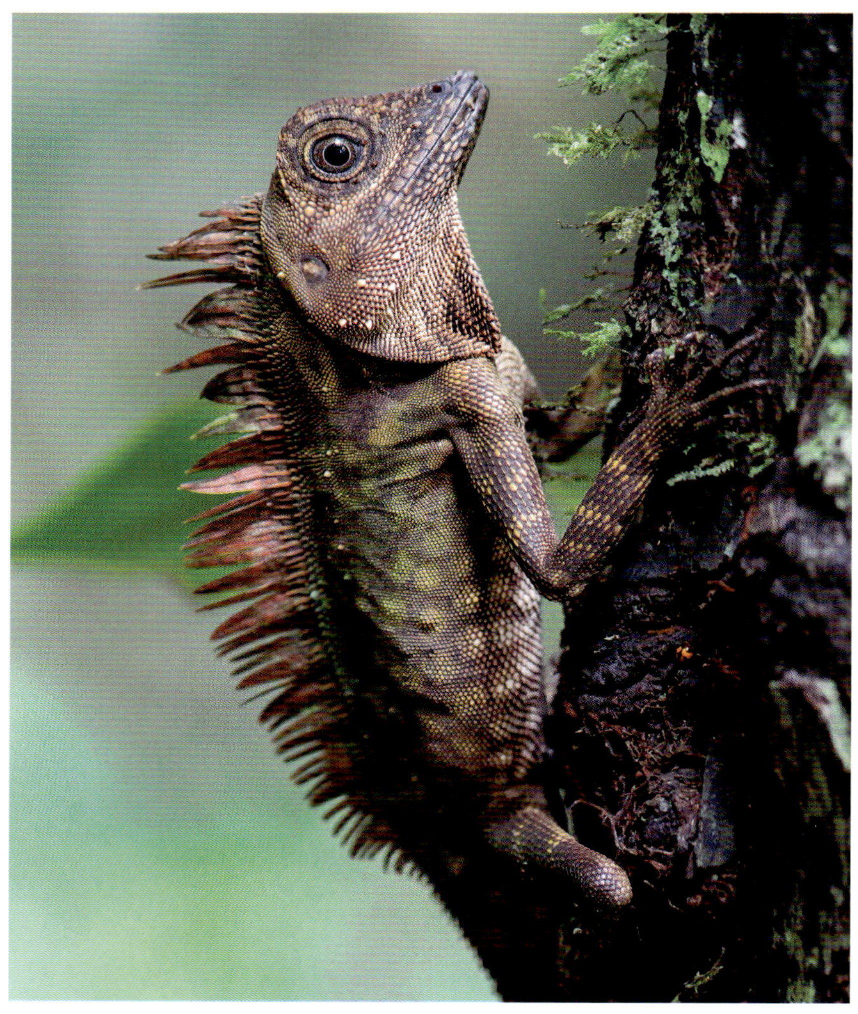

Graeme Green
Blue-eyed Anglehead Lizard
Gunung Mulu National Park, Malaysia

communities, companies, and governments. That will also need to change, not just because women's rights matter, but because women have been shown to make better, long-term decisions that benefit families and communities, and to be less prone to selfish or destructive thinking, less likely to be corrupted or bribed, and more likely to protect natural resources for future generations.

"Women and girls have been at the forefront of the fight for climate justice, yet they are the hardest hit by the climate crisis," says Titilope. "As an ecofeminist, I believe in a world where women and girls can exercise their rights without any form of injustice. I advocate for women's land rights because it will lead to women's empowerment, strengthen girls' education, increase women's bargaining power and gender equality, eradicate child marriage, hunger, and poverty, provide food security, and tackle climate change. In the Sahel region, 80 percent of the lands are degraded, and there are more than 20 million child brides. When women have fixed assets, such as land, they can transform those resources to the benefit of the society, while keeping them sustainable for reuse in future. Ultimately, it will lead to improvements in the lives of women and girls, and help tackle climate change."

IT'S THIS KIND OF JOINED-UP THINKING that holds the key to a wilder, fairer world. Climate change, biodiversity loss, and the pollution of air, soil, and water are all connected. But the struggle to stop the destruction of the natural world is also connected to poverty, inequality, Indigenous rights, women's rights, land rights, and human rights. We don't just need to transform agriculture, energy, and economic systems, but also to change worldviews, societies, and power structures.

Giving women more power and control over their lives not only improves female education and safety from sexual violence or forced marriage, but also reduces poverty, creates more sustainable ways of living, and means less destruction of wildlife, forests, and oceans, which, in turn, helps combat climate change. Likewise, if more Indigenous communities were fairly included in wildlife tourism, and conservation, not only would it help tackle poverty and improve lives, but less wildlife would be killed for bushmeat and the illegal wildlife trade, and forests, oceans, and other habitats would be more likely to be safeguarded, again meaning the whole planet benefits.

Clamping down on corrupt officials involved in the wildlife trade would not only reduce the animals being killed, but it might also lead to better politicians, more likely to work to improve the lives of their citizens than enrich themselves, which would reduce poverty and, in turn, decrease levels of poaching.

Transitioning to greener energy sources wouldn't just help mitigate the climate crisis, but it would also create jobs, reduce the numbers of refugees, and lessen our reliance on the oil and gas of human rights-abusing dictatorships, making countries more self-reliant, energy prices more stable, and conflict less likely. Each positive change can have a ripple effect.

The individual choices we all make matter. Eating less (or no) meat, for example, would mean less animals suffering in industrial farms and reduce global warming (meat production being one of the largest causes of greenhouse gas emissions), as well as making people healthier. But real change will require collective action.

Wildlife and nature need to be global priorities for governments. Developing countries will need support, while the countries who've profited so much from destroying the natural world should pay a fair price. Voices demanding change will need to become louder than those insisting on business-as-usual, persuading politicians to start making the right long-term decisions for the future, and pressuring global industries to stop destructive practices and to act in the best interest of all life on Earth, not just a profiting minority. There will need to be changes in farming, fishing, forestry, energy, and transport.

We need to restore and rewild, and to protect our remaining wild places, as well as to create greener cities. The next ten years are critical. But our collective track record so far isn't encouraging. Our leaders have repeatedly shown themselves not to be up to the challenge, either inadequate or corrupt. We've had decades of empty promises, with little action. Protecting the planet has been twisted into a Right vs Left issue, batted back and forth between parties, as the clock ticks down. The Internet swirls with anti-science and deliberate disinformation campaigns, slowing progress, and there are powerful individuals and organisations, who profit from the destruction of the natural world, with a vested interest in keeping us on our current path. I don't feel hopeful. But I've been proved wrong before by people working together to beat what seemed impossible odds.

In just the last few years, we've experienced global pandemics, massive wildlife declines, raging wildfires, heatwaves and other extreme weather, and glaciers melting and collapsing into the sea, far beyond what could be expected as "normal." The disasters that have been predicted are no longer far off in the future, but here in our present and getting worse.

If there was no solution available, just an impossible downward spiral to oblivion, we could be excused for throwing our hands up. But the Earth isn't experiencing a collapsing sun or a mysterious supernatural force. These are human-made problems. We've never had so much information and knowledge at our fingertips. We already know so many of the answers.

What happens next is a choice. But to have so many solutions in our grasp and fail to act to protect the world's wildlife and our planet is a crime that future generations won't be able to understand or forgive.

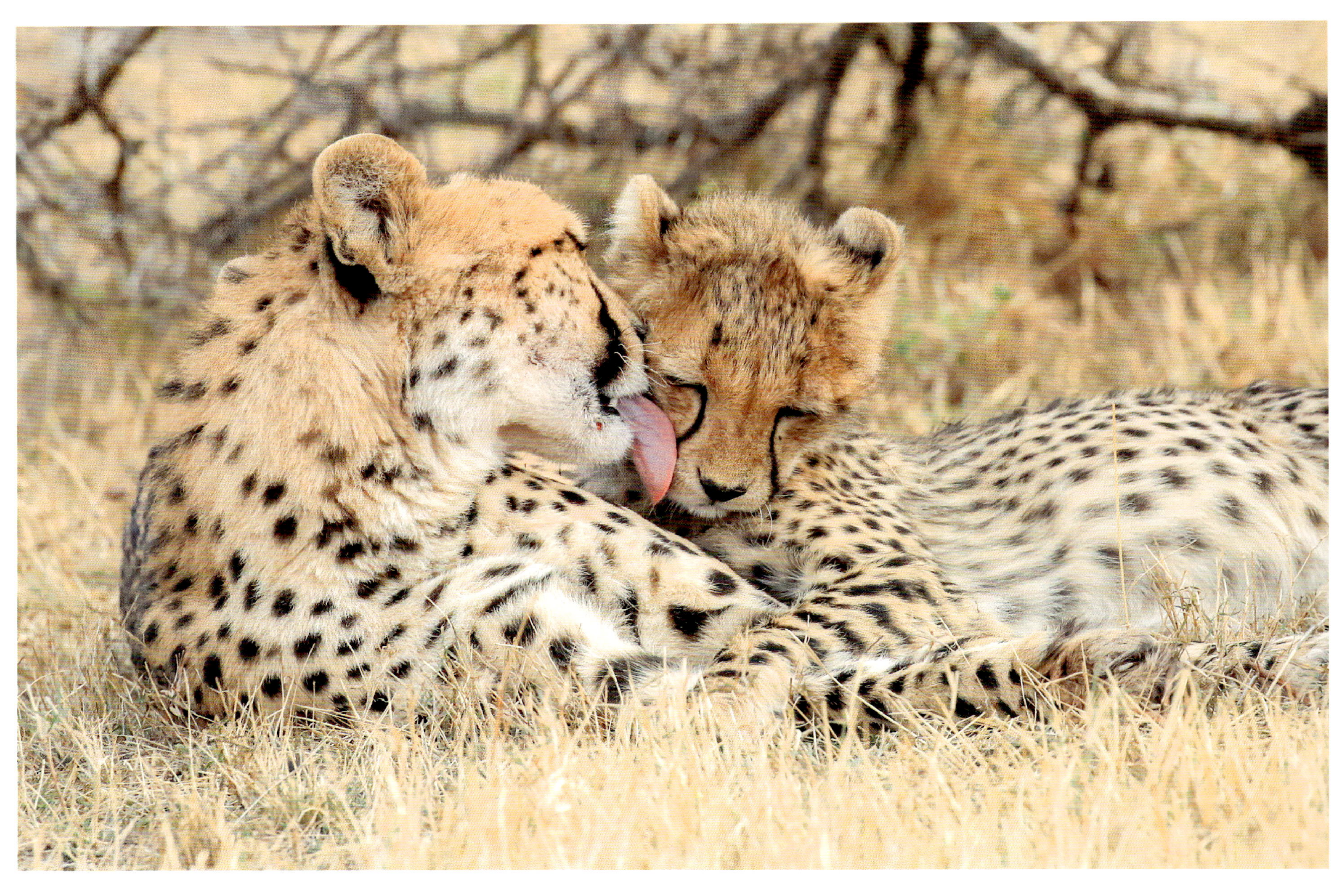

Graeme Green
Cheetahs
Mara Naboisho Conservancy, Kenya

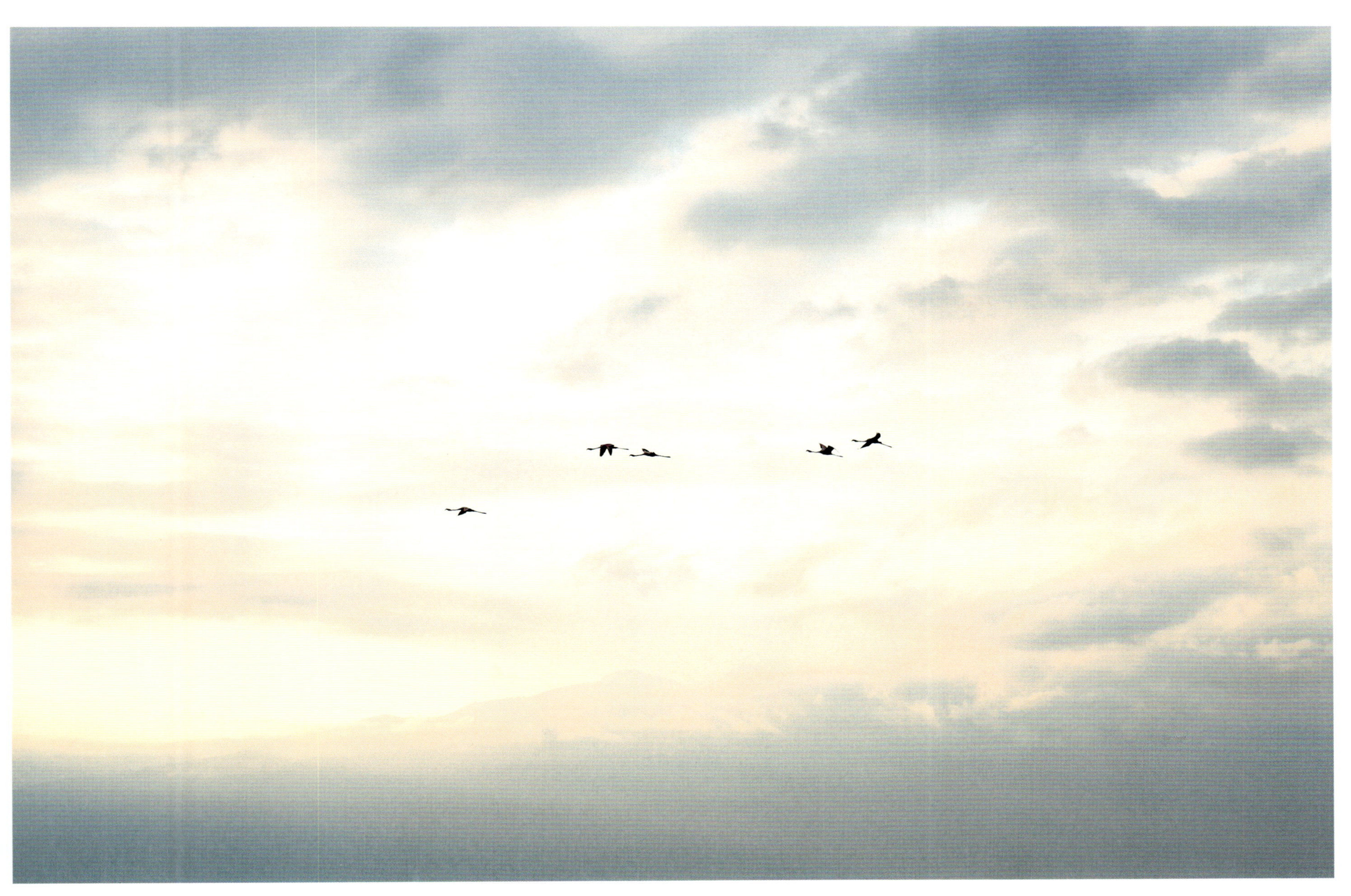

Graeme Green
Lesser Flamingos
Lake Natron, Tanzania

ELEPHANTS

Elephants

Dominique Gonçalves

Manager, Elephant Ecology Project at Gorongosa National Park

ELEPHANTS ARE SUCH MAGNIFICENT ANIMALS. The largest living land mammal on Earth, they live in family groups made up of multiple generations. The intergenerational association is important for the passing and sharing of knowledge to the younger generations. In an elephant society, older females are matriarchs and the guardians of wisdom, culture, and leadership. They invest time, patience, and effort in teaching the younger elephants how to survive, passing them all their cultural and social knowledge, as well as the knowledge they have about their environment. This continuous passing on of knowledge means it stays in families and is never forgotten.

The social bonds between elephants are highly complex. Like humans, elephants are capable of forming strong connections with their friends and family members. These relationships start at the core of the herd, between mother and calf, then radiate out. In Gorongosa National Park in Mozambique, where I work, it's common to hear a greeting ceremony when family groups meet each other after a long period apart. The males also create affinities with younger and older males, adventuring through the landscape together, the younger elephants learning from more experienced males.

Protecting the herd and keeping all members of the herd safe is the priority. I learned this firsthand when I came across a mother and her injured calf one day. The calf was limping, as its leg had been caught in a snare. The wound was very serious. As I waited for the veterinarian's help, the mother's agitation grew. She tore two small trees from the ground, then picked up a large stick with her trunk and began wildly thrashing it. Past the mother we could see the baby, hidden in the brush. We stayed for hours, hoping help would arrive in time, but the mother finally bolted into the brush with her wounded baby. Four days later, the mother was spotted, alone. Knowing the baby didn't survive, we were struck by how fiercely the mother had fought to protect her, much like a human mother might have behaved. The poor mother was trying to protect her baby. I still can't decide if she was trying to keep us away or if she was asking us to help. It taught me a lot about how elephants feel empathy and how much they grieve. You can read about it in books, but for me, only when I saw that situation did I really understand that each elephant is an individual, with complex relationships and emotions.

Spending time with elephants, I often think of these lines by the American writer Peter Matthiessen: "There is mystery behind that masked gray visage, an ancient life force, delicate and mighty, awesome and enchanted, commanding the silence ordinarily reserved for mountain peaks, great fires, and the sea."

Over the years, I've had many memorable experiences. On one occasion, I'd located a group of four bull elephants. One of them, whose name was Aloisio, moved toward us. At that moment I couldn't move. My heart was pounding. I was really scared for the first time, being alone in that situation. He came so close to me that when I looked at him I could see my face reflected in his eye. He seemed to bend his head down to get a better look at my face. That was quite a peaceful moment. Then he lifted his head and slowly led the others away to a nearby lagoon. It's moments like this that will stay in my memory for a lifetime.

Elephants are an important piece of the ecosystems where they exist. They disperse seeds, dig waterholes, create footpaths, fertilize the soils, and maintain the forests and savannas where they live.

I spend my time working with African elephants. But Asian elephants also teach us about humility—they show how a majestic animal can be worshipped as a god, but can also be seen as an enemy by others, or used by people who have mastered ways to break their behavior and spirits to use them as servants or workers.

In just the last few years, the International Union for Conservation of Nature (IUCN) listed the African savanna elephant (or African bush elephant) as Endangered, and the forest elephant as Critically Endangered, both for the first time, following population declines over several decades. The Asian elephant is also classified as Endangered by the IUCN. The total number of Sumatran elephants is estimated to be around 1,400, and it's believed that we have fewer than ten years to save the subspecies from extinction.

Threats to elephants are dynamic and complex, including ivory poaching, the loss of their habitats, and getting closer to people, the latter of which increases conflict interactions that can result in death or injury for people, or, more often, the elephant. Even though the general trend is one of population declines, in certain places elephant populations are increasing. But it all feels very fragile, and it will continue to be until the threats are eliminated, including the demand for ivory, land use, and reduced interactions between people and elephants.

Ivory is a major reason why elephants continue to be killed. It's sad to see how humankind has so often thought of nature only for profit or status, and sad to see that it's hard for humankind to stop when it must. Some of the results of this greediness can be seen in the faces of elephants, or the lack of their tusks. It shows not only in their faces, but also probably in their range, their behavior, and their communication.

As human populations expand, there is increasing contact between people and wildlife. Coexistence describes a situation where people and wildlife live in close proximity without attrition. Coexistence isn't easy, but it is worthwhile. People need nature to be healthy and thrive. But we have to navigate carefully where people and elephants live together.

Elephants need space and people need space. One of the first things I learned as a conservationist is that pragmatism works, while ideology does not. We need to listen and make practical decisions for each area, decisions based on the reality of the place. The communities' views, ideas, and desires must be respected, and their voices amplified so coexistence can continue. More support, including funds and other resources, technology, and knowledge-sharing, needs to be given to community-led strategies across the conflict landscapes.

Elephants are extremely intelligent. When we're looking at conflict with humans, we need to be ahead of the game. Elephants quickly adapt to our advances, so there's no one better than the people living next door to them to see the changes and to have the power to adapt quickly. The people living next to them are the ones who would bring the most long-term solutions, some drawing from traditional techniques that, with a sparkle of modernism and technology, change the system completely.

Losing elephants in Africa means nations would lose their pride and heritage, as well the integrity of their ecosystems. I'd like to see more African people have decent opportunities to care for their wildlife. I'd like to see local people's voices amplified and heard with the same level of importance and equity as international voices. Once we all listen and understand, rather than fighting about different ideologies and ways to use and profit from wildlife, then perhaps better decisions and actions can be made together for the benefit of both people and wildlife.

To protect biodiversity and ecosystems, we need more than just securing the integrity of the boundaries of a landscape. We need to see the value of comprehensive biodiversity knowledge and the creation of a detailed picture of life for the management and protection of biodiversity.

It would be useful to see solutions that encourage people to think about nature and people together, not only as a way to make money but also as a way of life, of coexistence. For that, we need to realize people and wildlife are part of the same system and they both need to learn to live together. As the world changes, we will need to become more nature-based and sustainable.

It's important to have local champions of biodiversity who look at all animals, regardless of their size or role in the ecosystem, because everything is interconnected. The creation and support of a new generation of local biodiversity specialists, researchers, and conservationists is of utmost importance because they're the ones who will help make sure biodiversity survives. It's an important step to work in partnership with communities to deliver solutions to our challenges, helping break the cycle of poverty and protect the biodiversity and ecosystems on which we all depend for a safe and healthy future.

I believe people are now recognizing that the natural world needs to be cared for. Nature needs its space and protection. It is not only an intrinsic right but also a necessary foundation for a healthy, sustainable, and prosperous world.

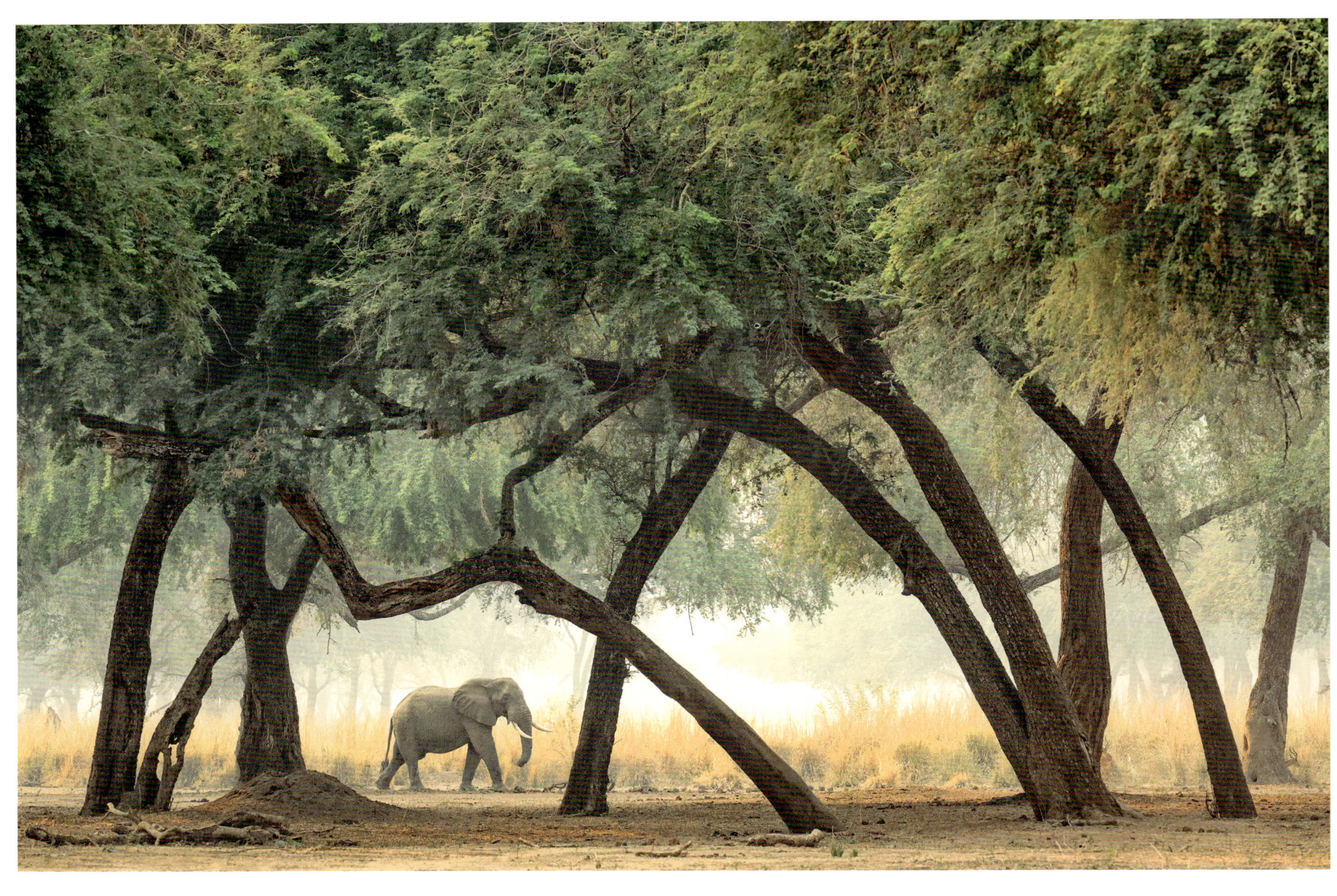

Marsel van Oosten
African Elephant
Lower Zambezi National Park, Zambia

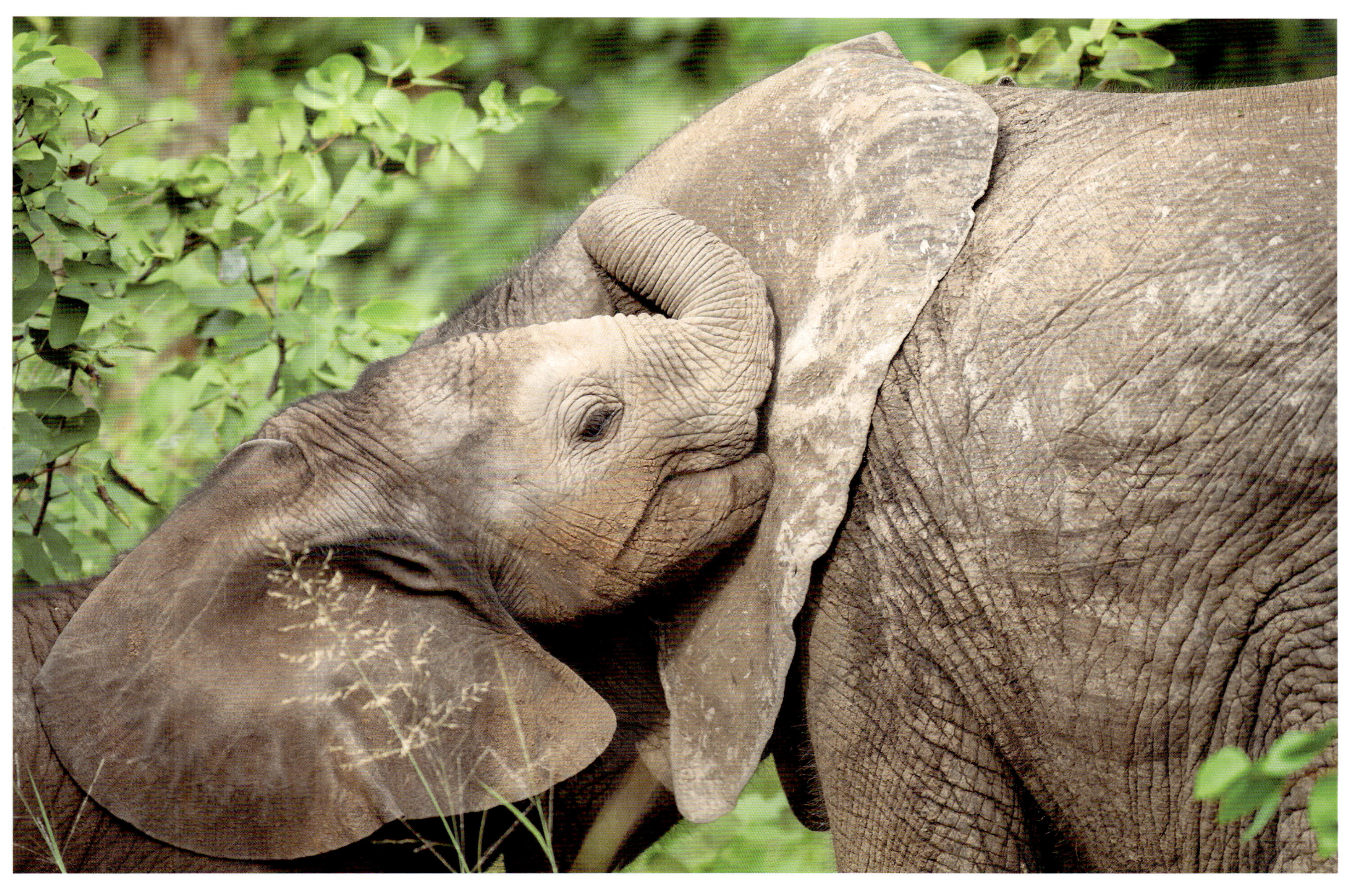

Berndt Weissenbacher
African Elephants
Kruger National Park, South Africa

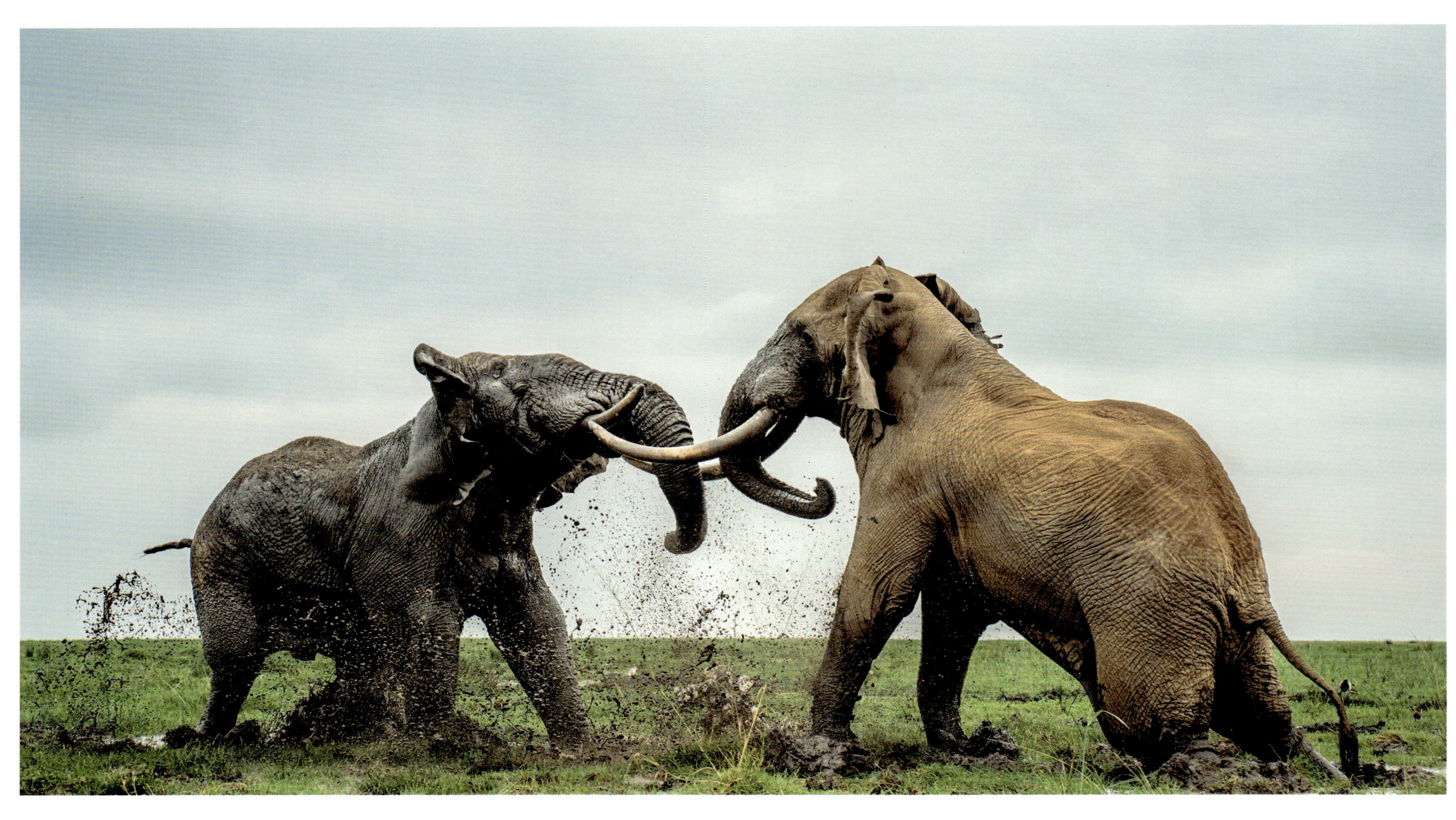

William Fortescue
African Elephants
Amboseli National Park, Kenya

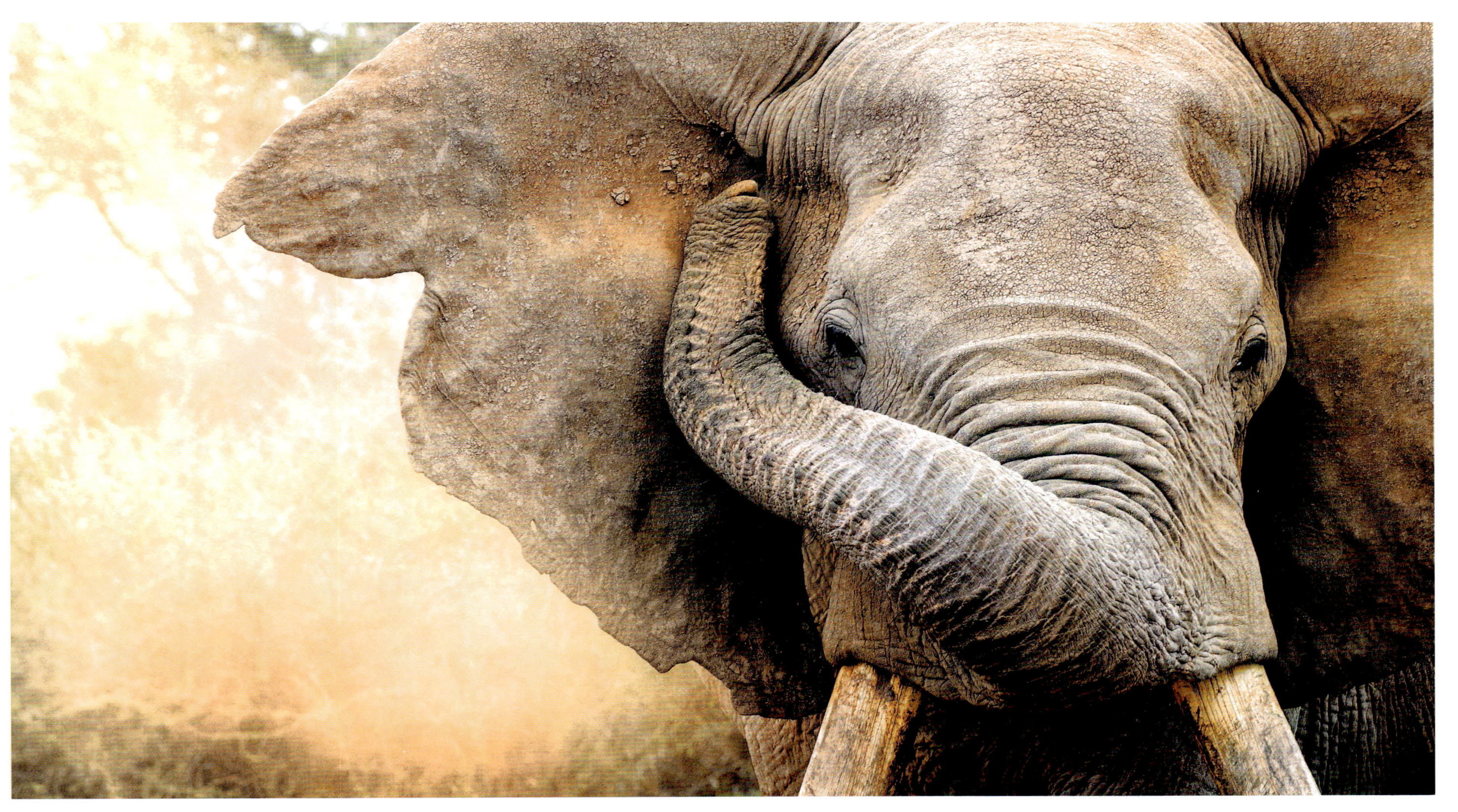

Vicki Jauron
African Elephant
Amboseli National Park, Kenya

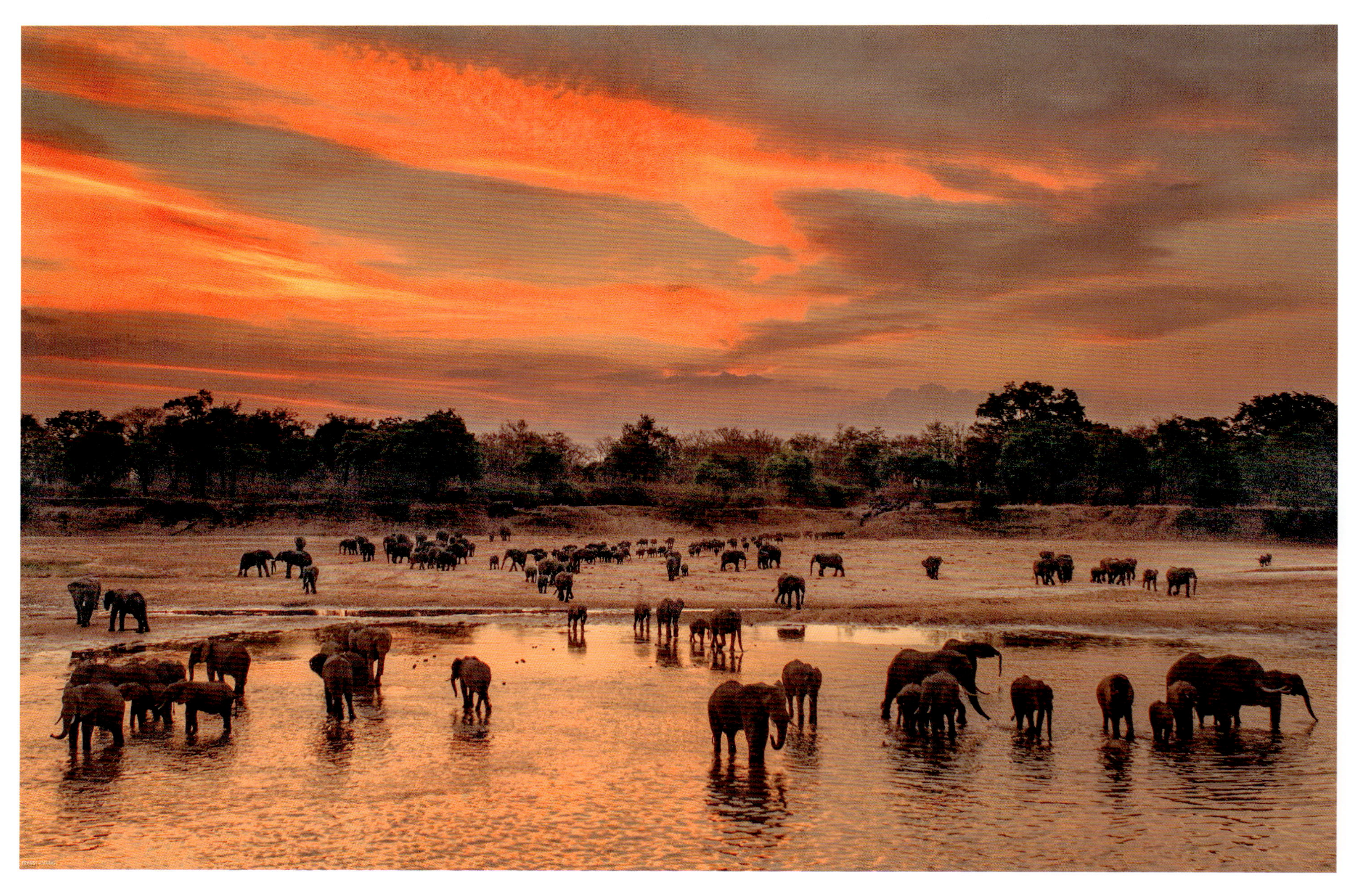

Frans Lanting
African Elephants
South Luangwa National Park, Zambia

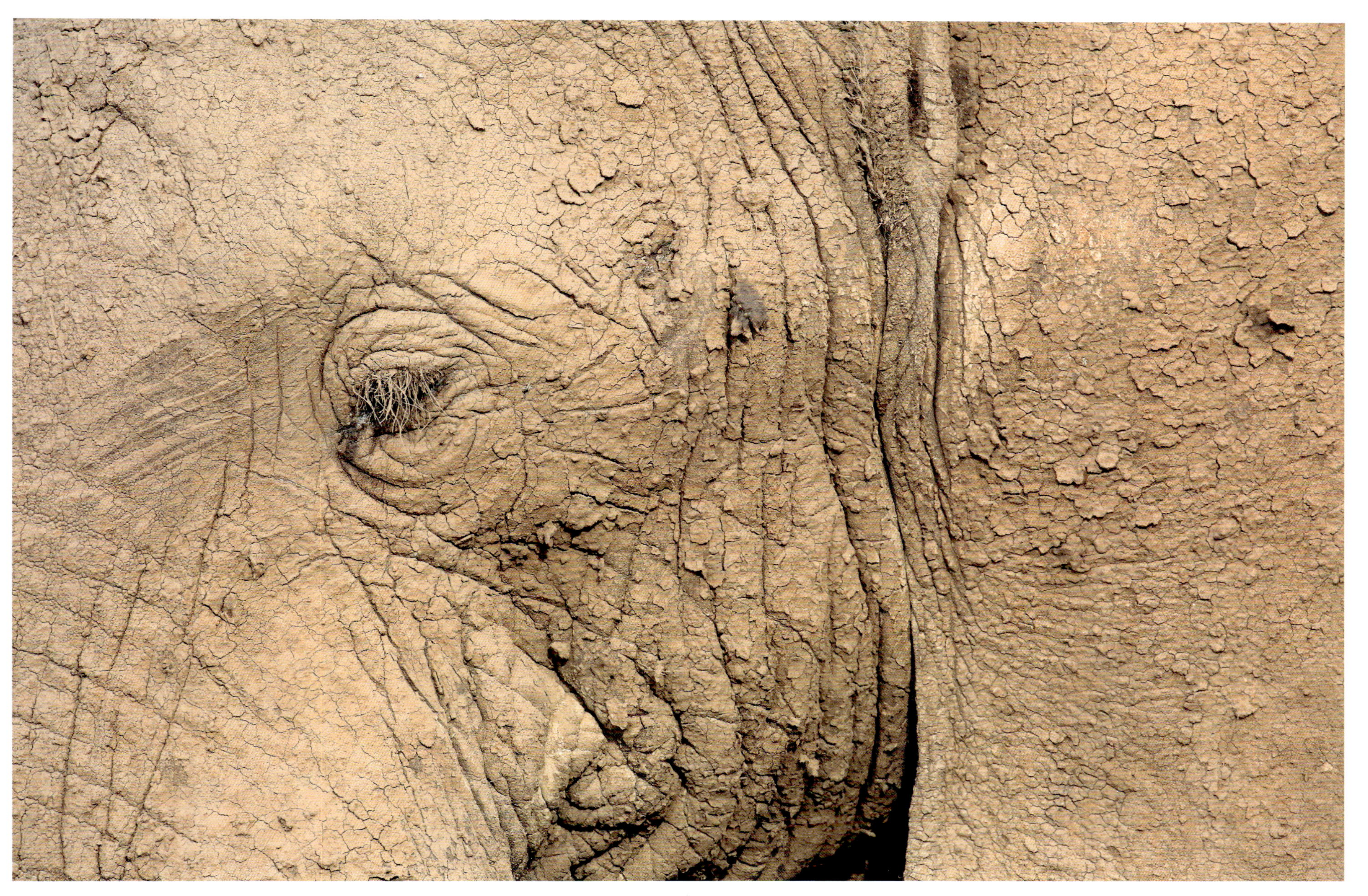

Graeme Green
African Elephant
Maasai Mara National Reserve, Kenya

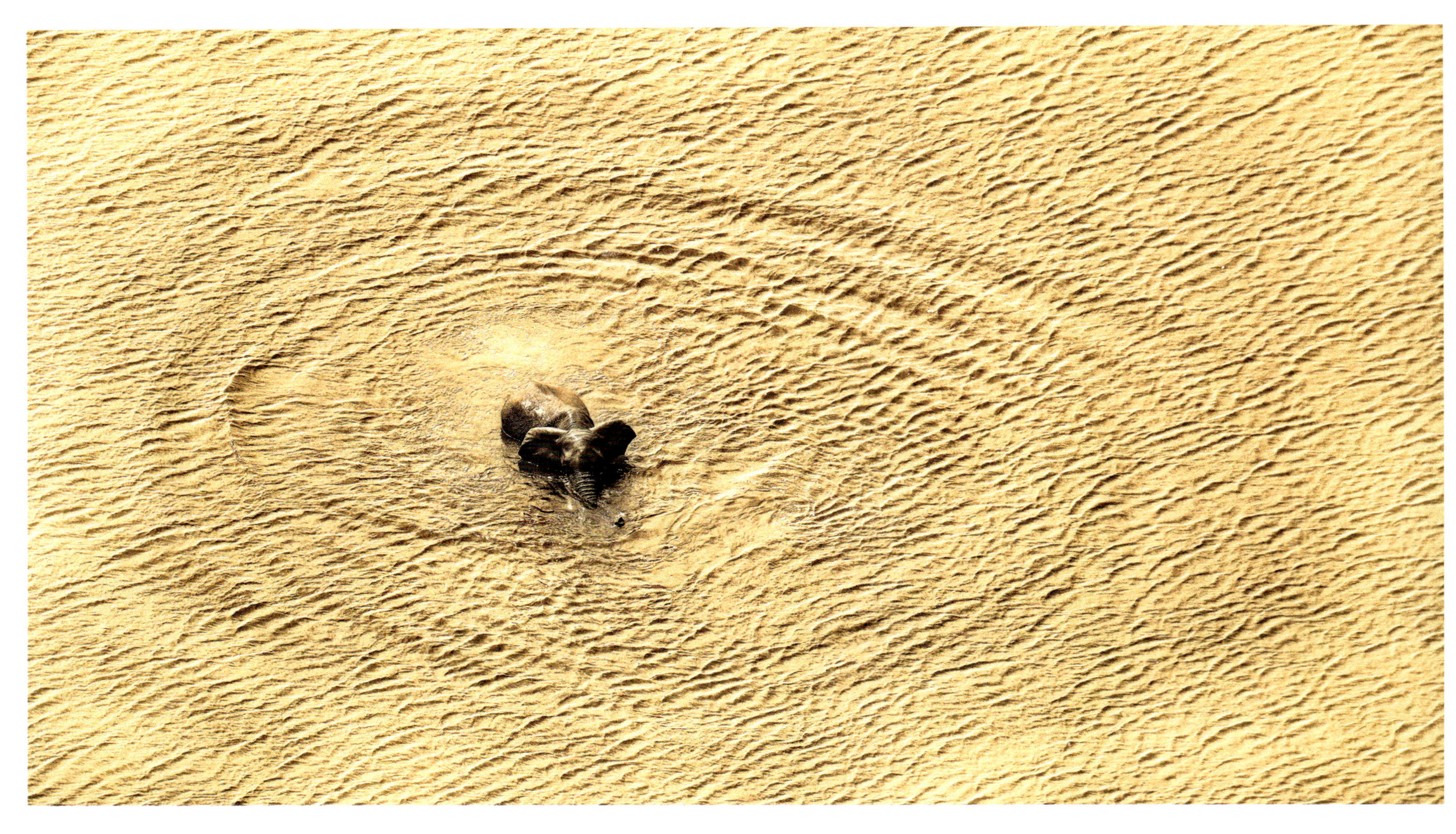

Beverly Joubert
African Elephant
Selinda Reserve, Botswana

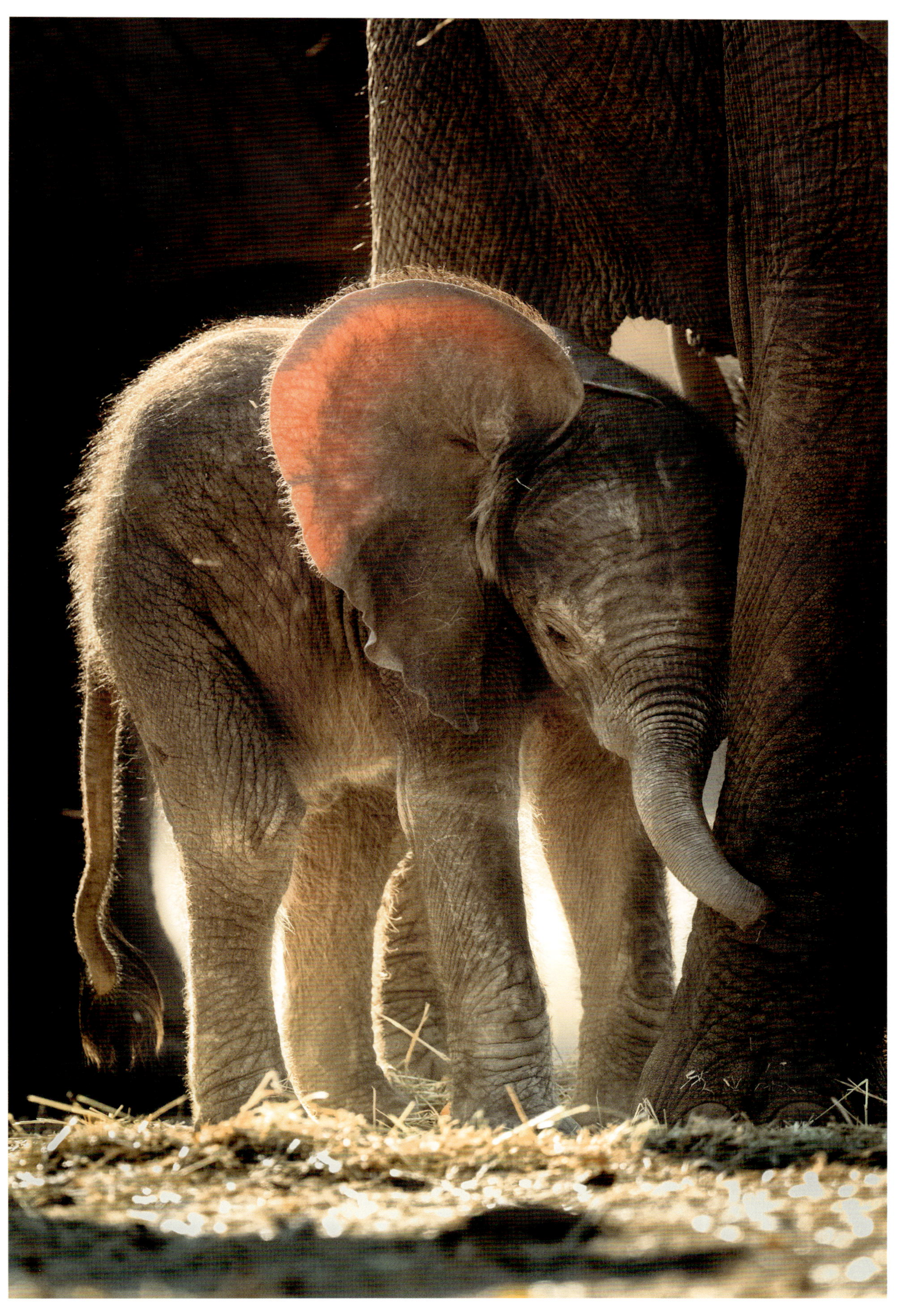

Carole Deschuymere
African Elephants
Mana Pools National Park, Zimbabwe

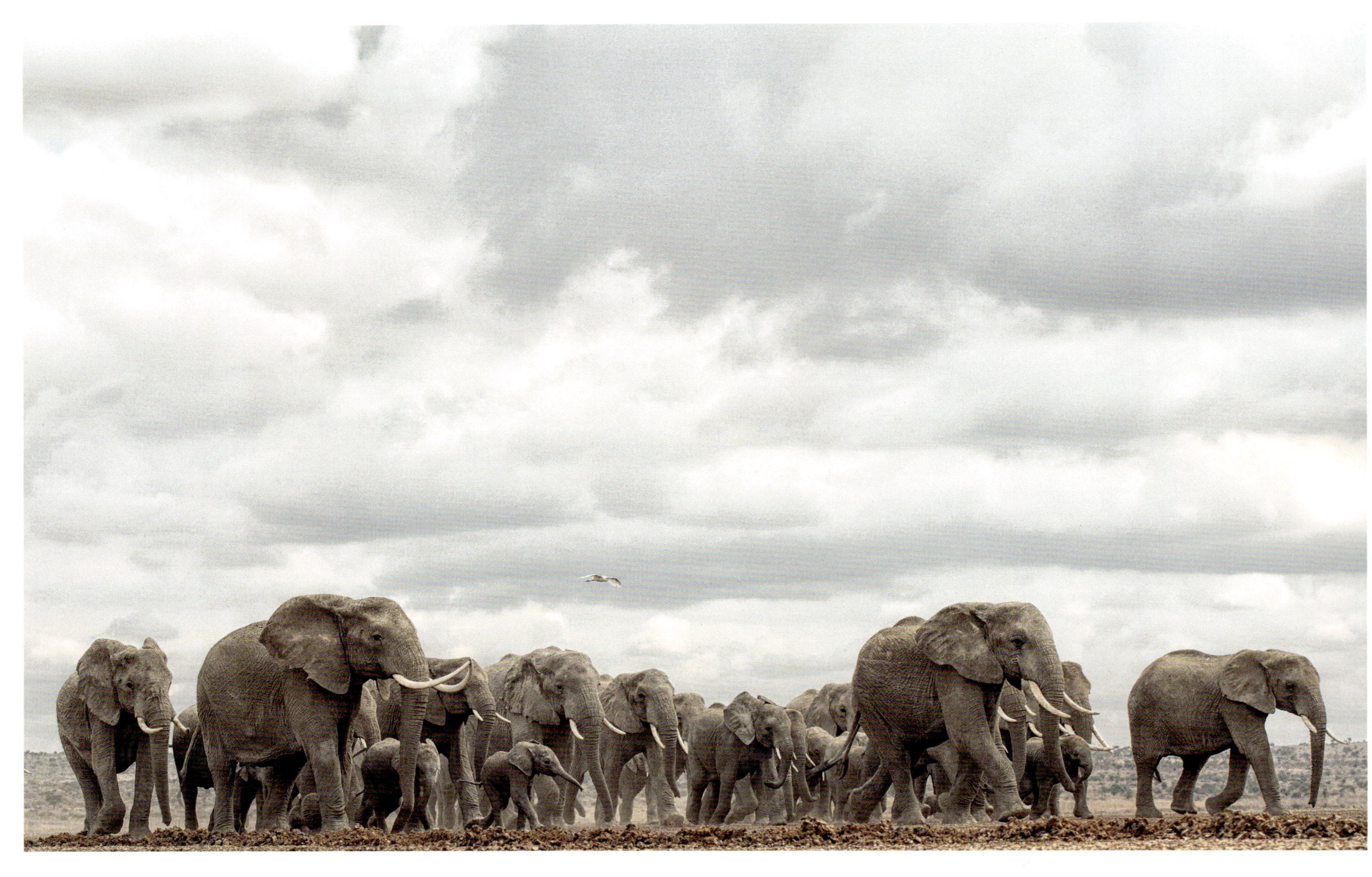

Chris Fallows
African Elephants
Amboseli National Park, Kenya

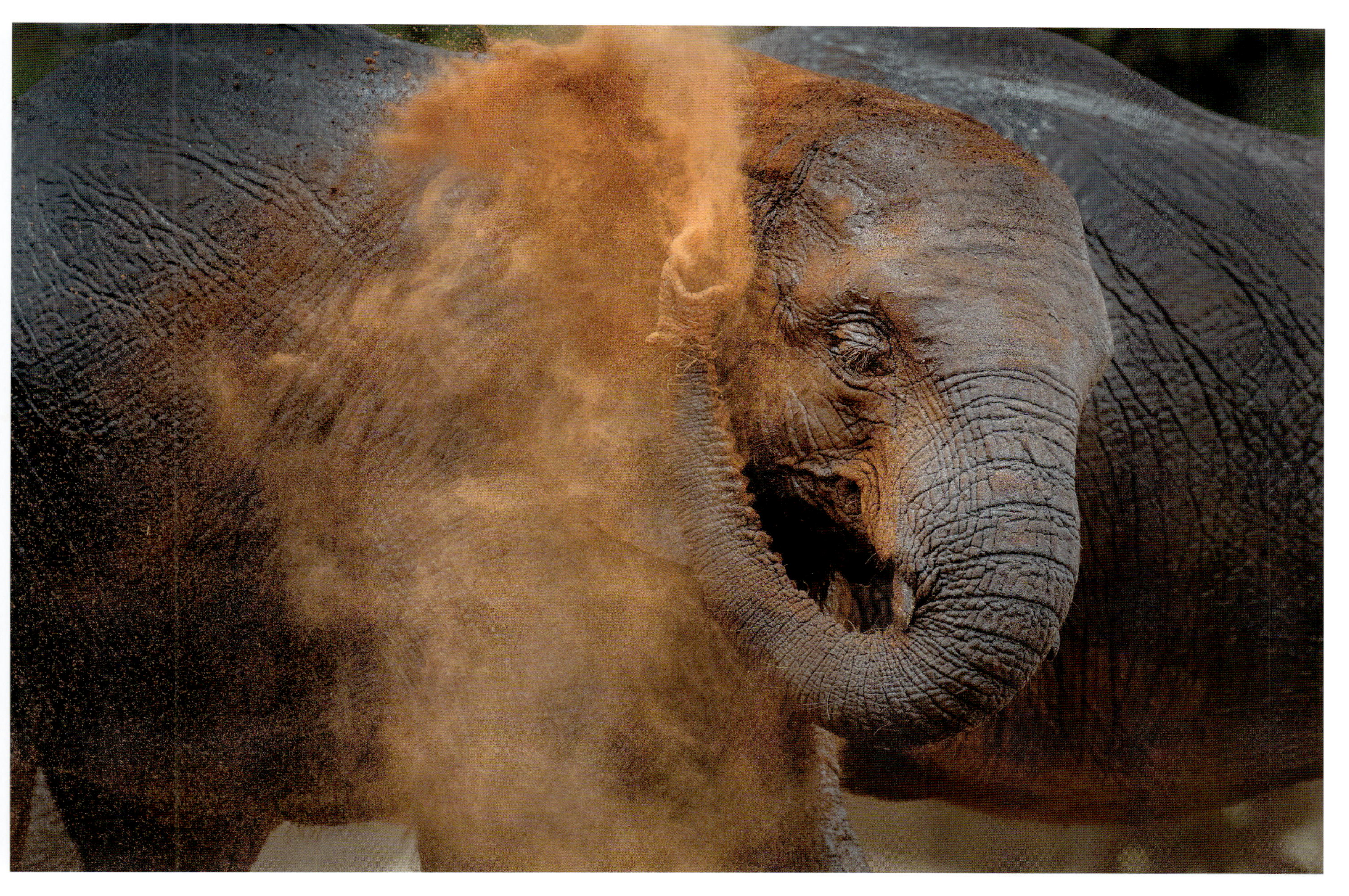

Piper Mackay
African Elephant
Tsavo West National Park, Kenya

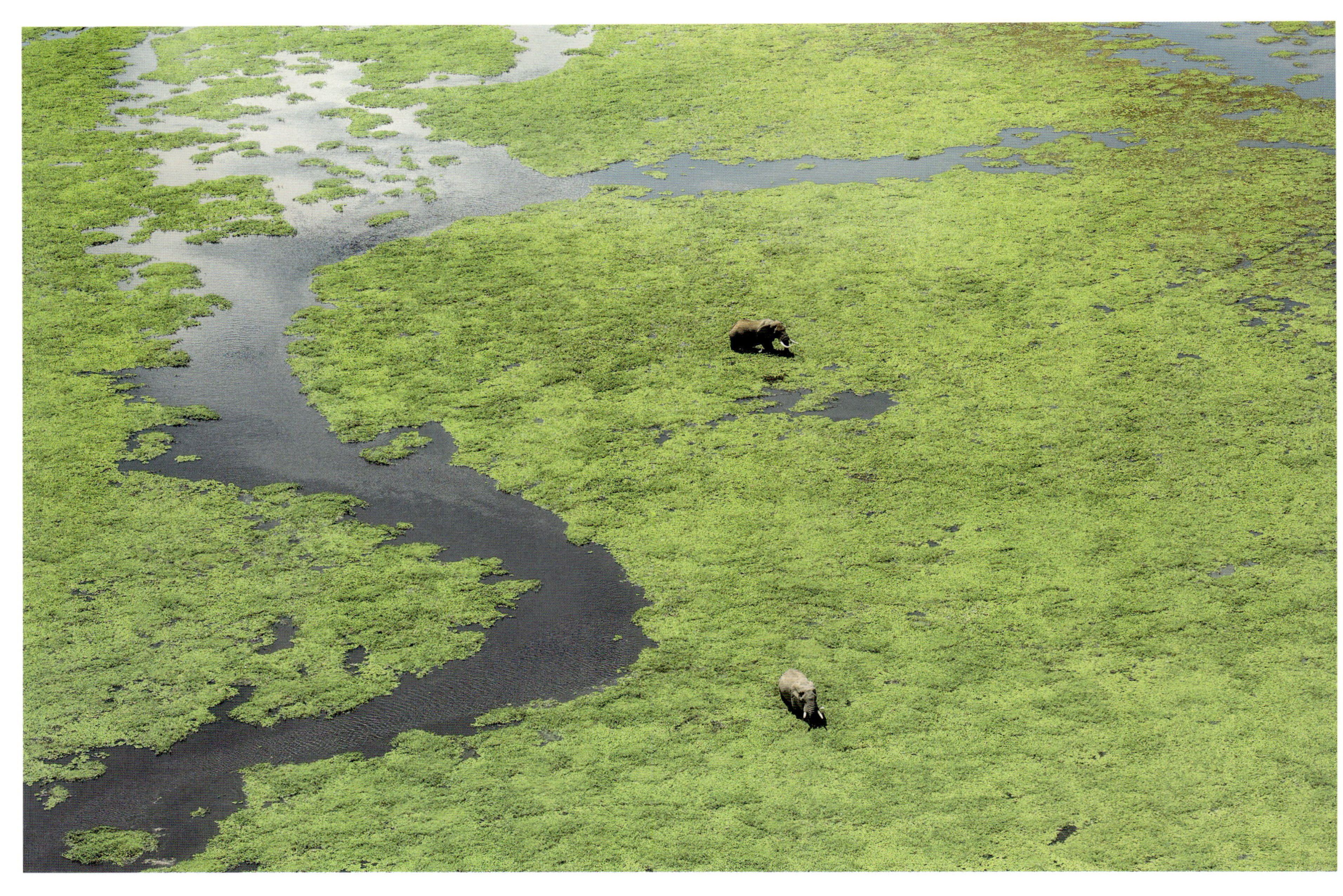

Joan de la Malla
African Elephants
Amboseli National Park, Kenya

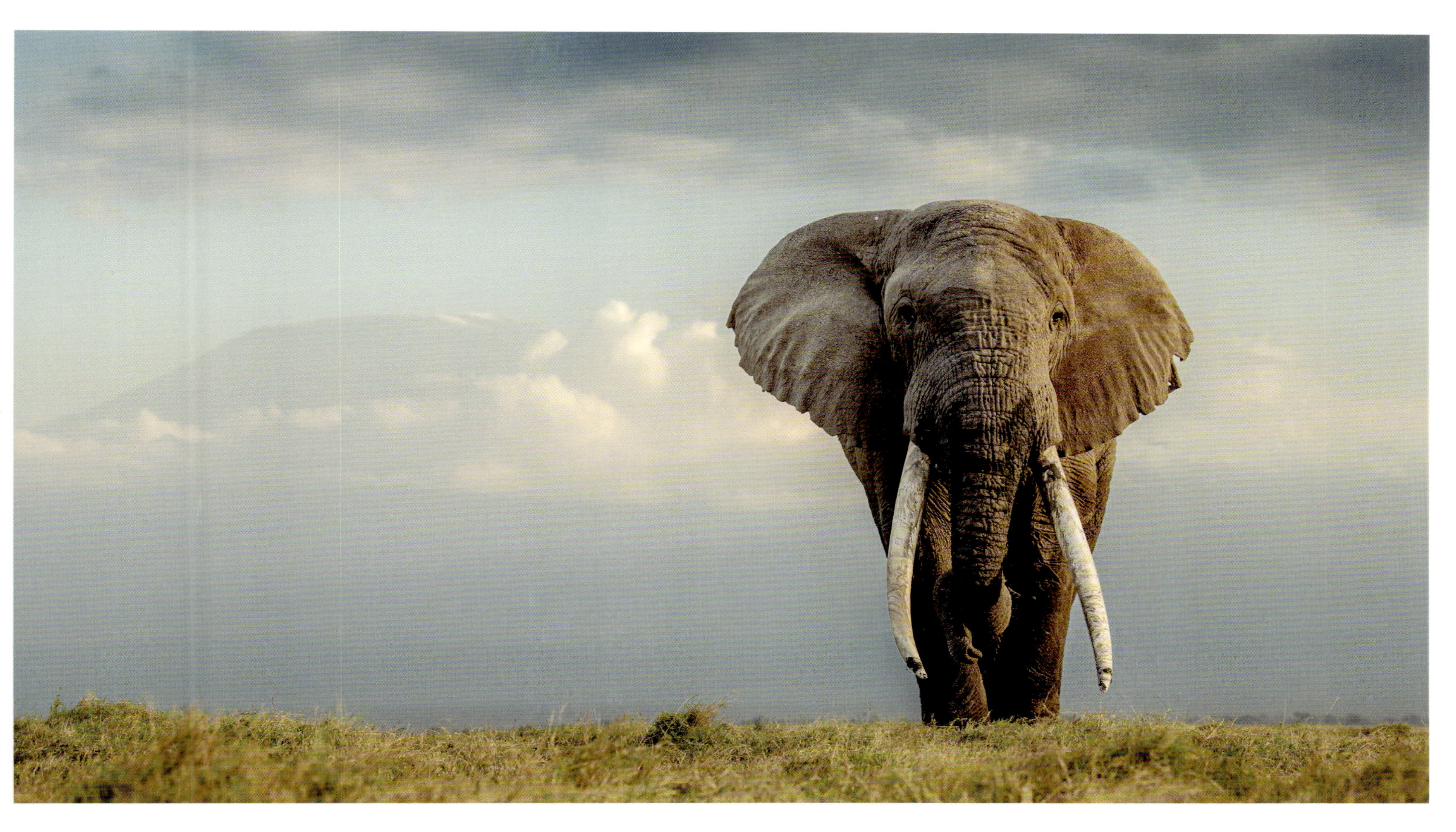

William Fortescue
African Elephant
Amboseli National Park, Kenya

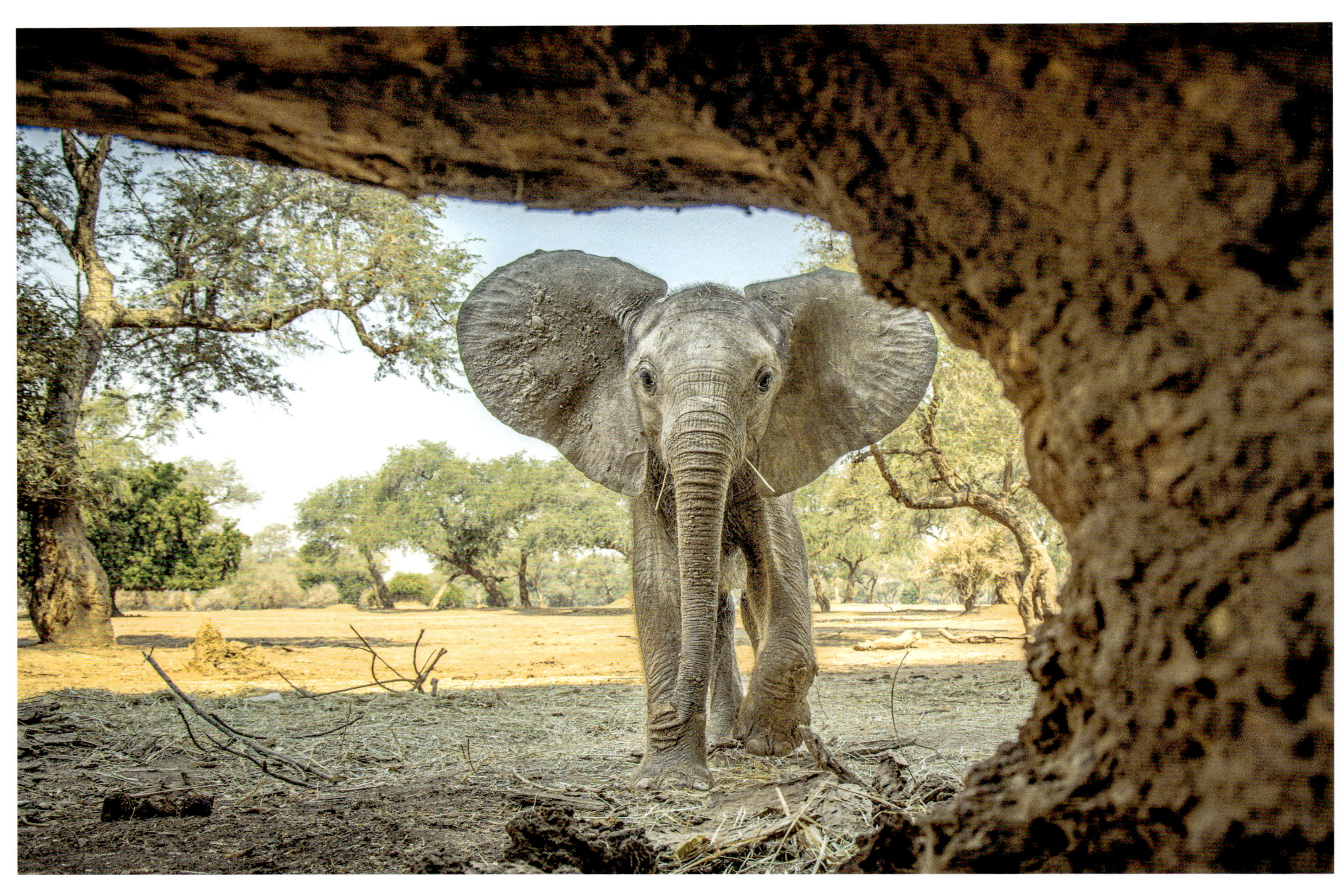

Tom Svensson
African Elephant
Mana Pools National Park, Zimbabwe

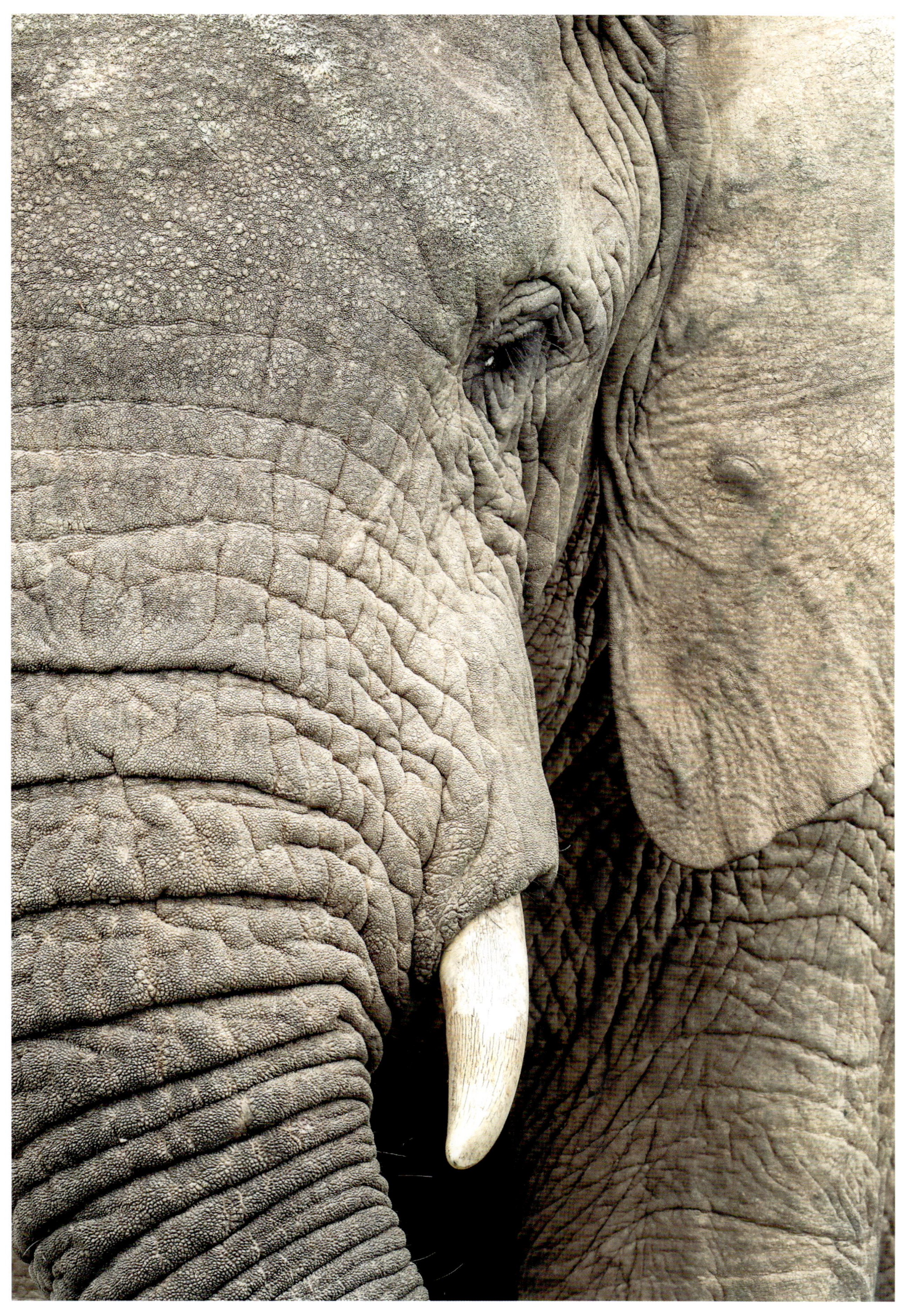

Graeme Green
African Elephant
Akagera National Park, Rwanda

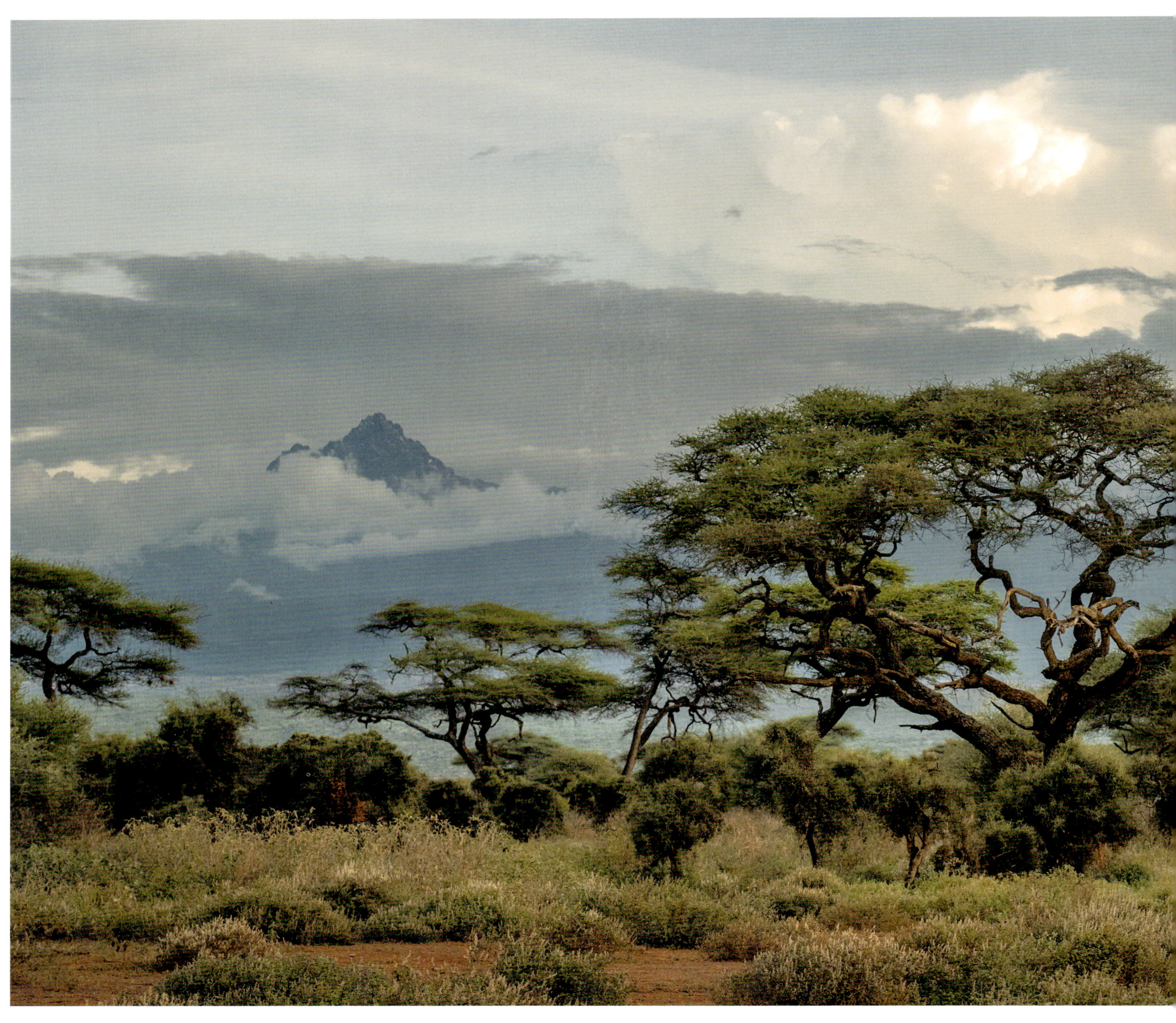

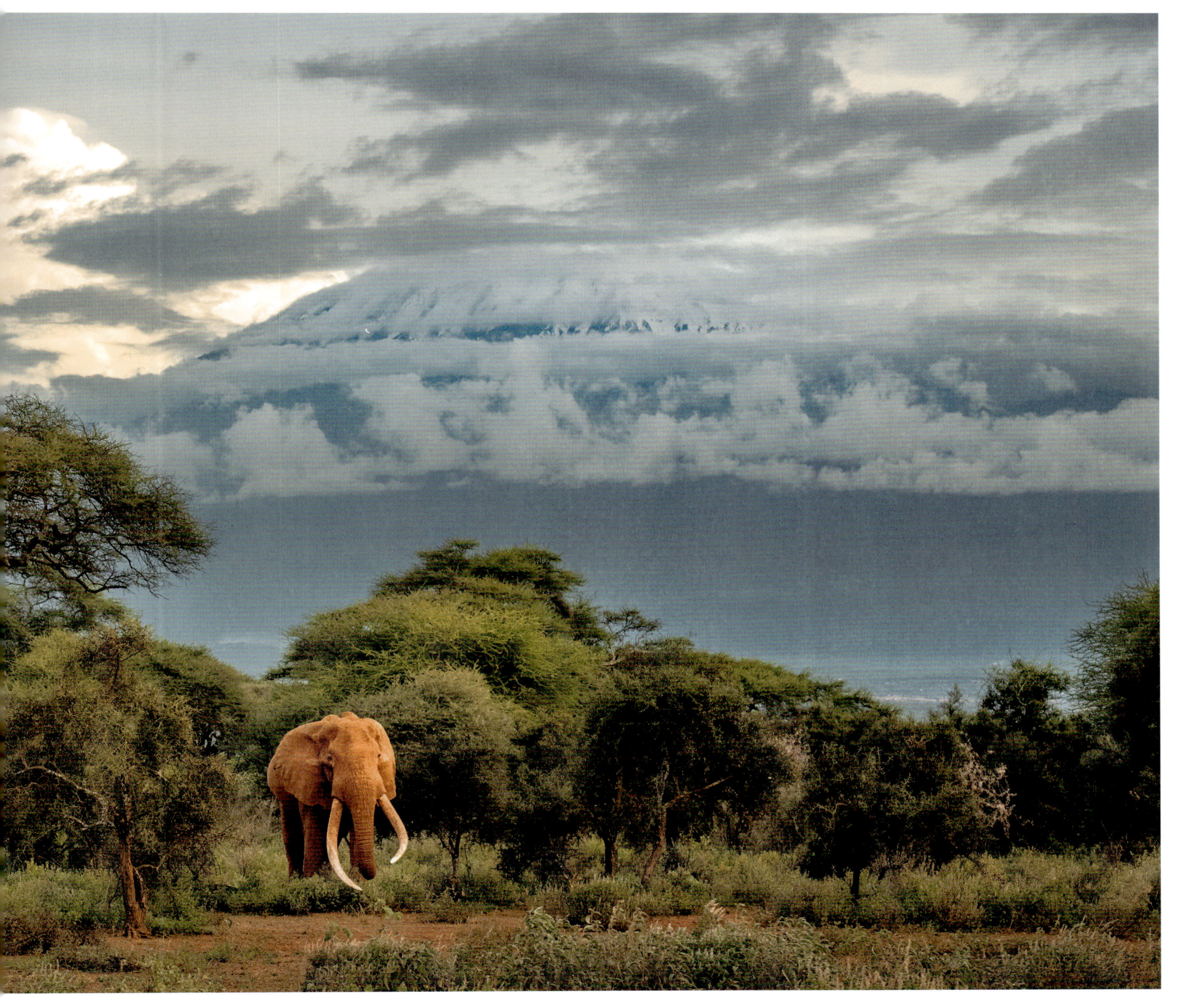

Federico Veronesi
African Elephant
Amboseli National Park, Kenya

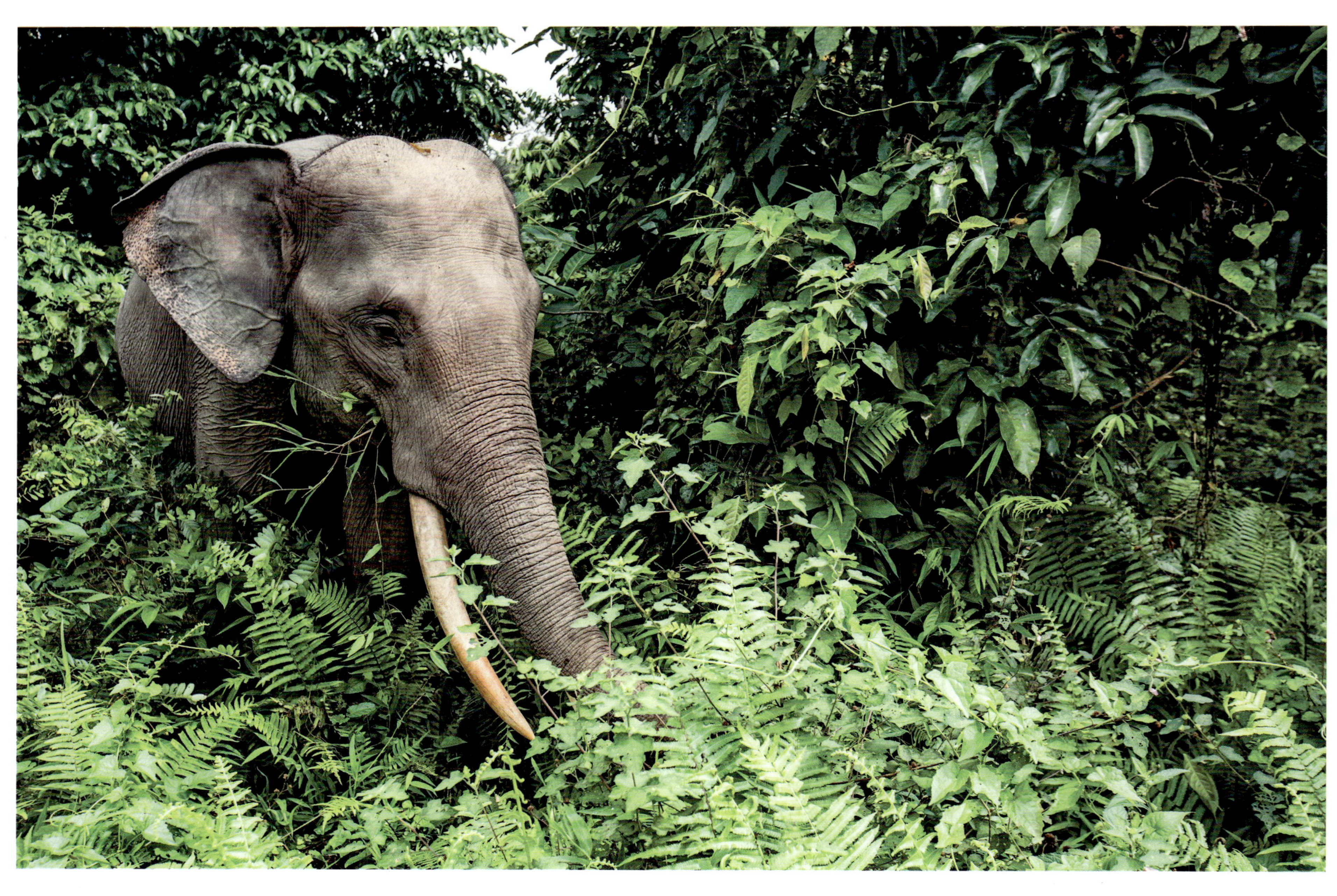

Paul Hilton
Sumatran Elephant
Leuser Ecosystem, Indonesia

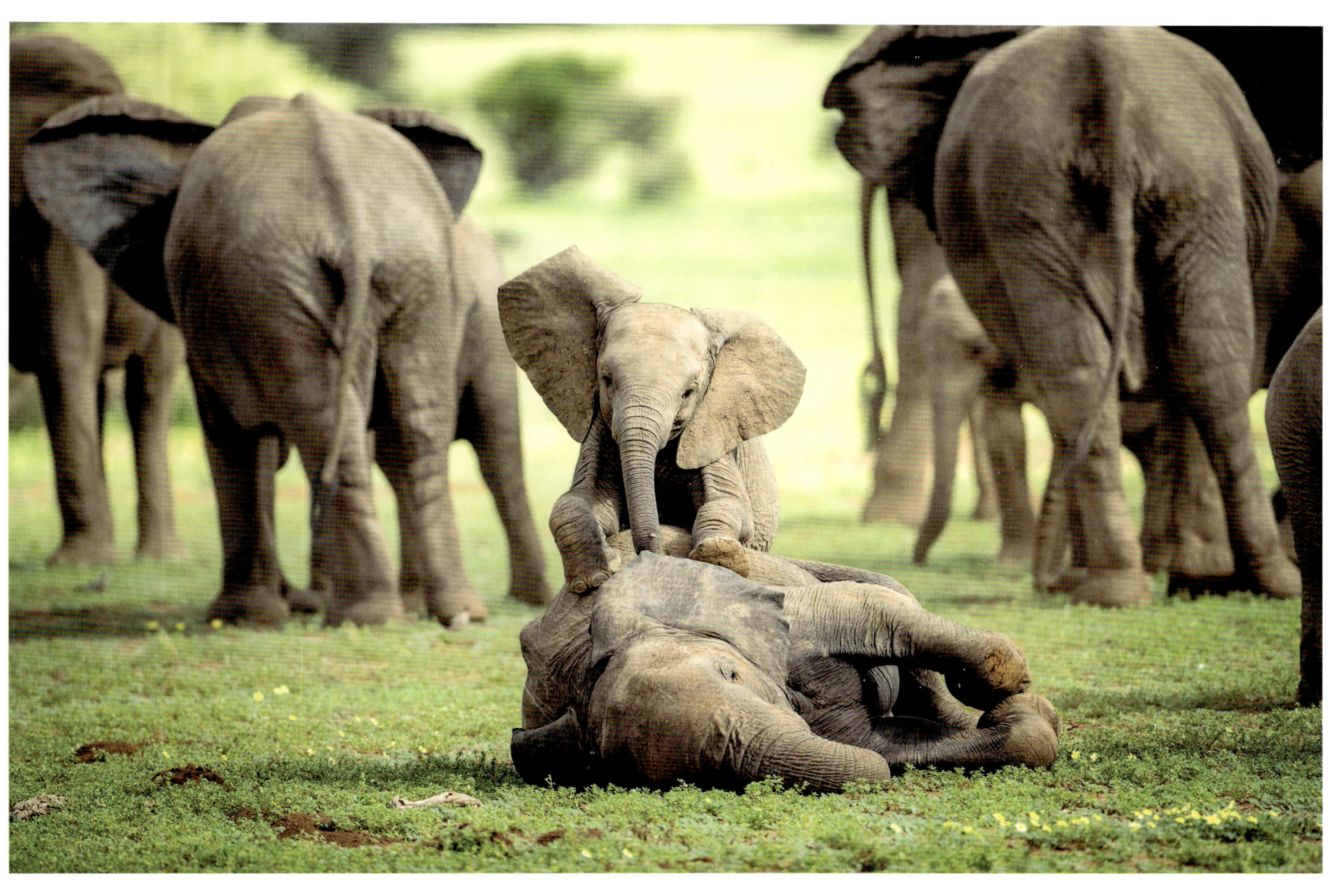

Lance van de Vyver
African Elephants
Mashatu Game Reserve, Botswana

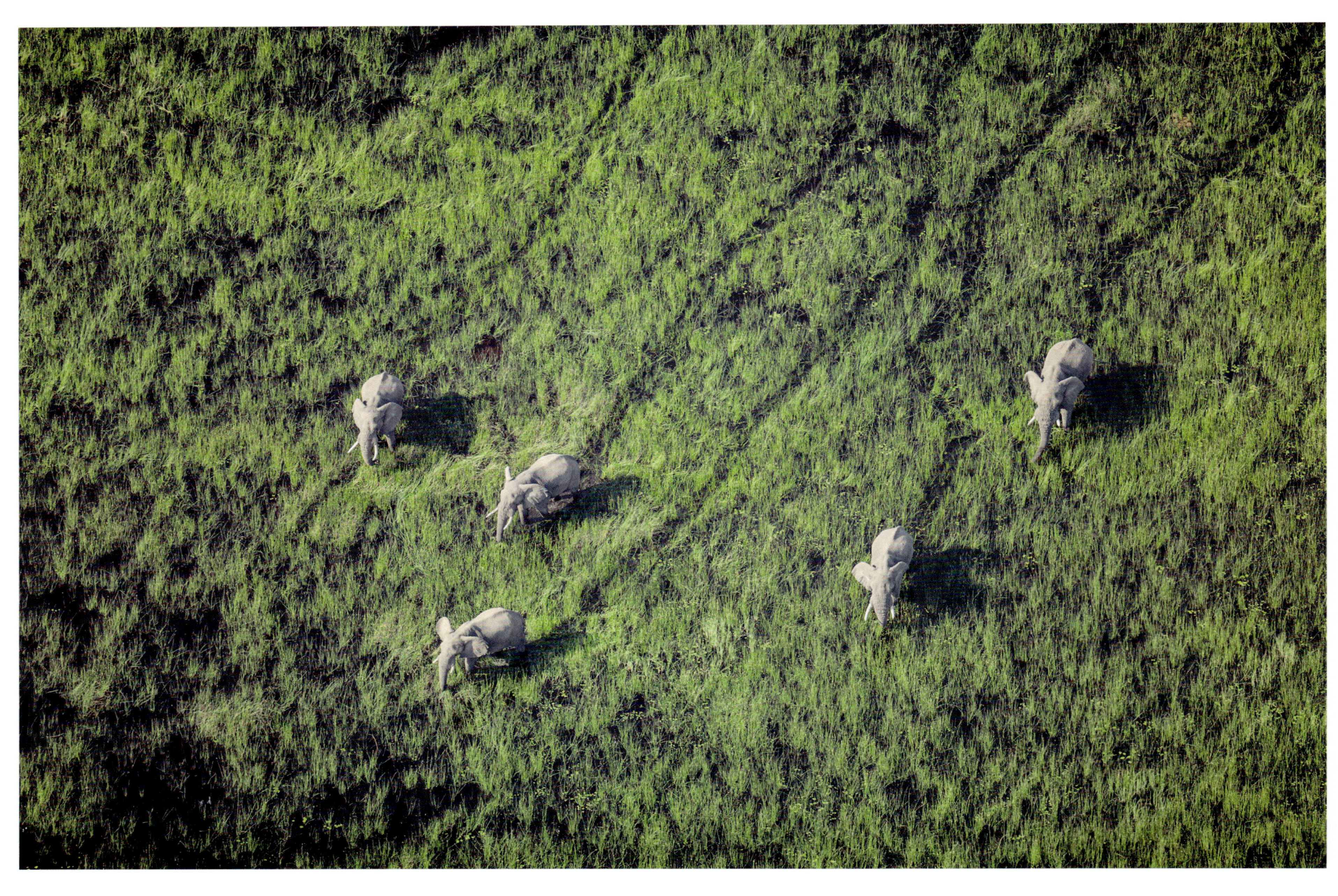

Jay Roode
African Elephants
Okavango Delta, Botswana

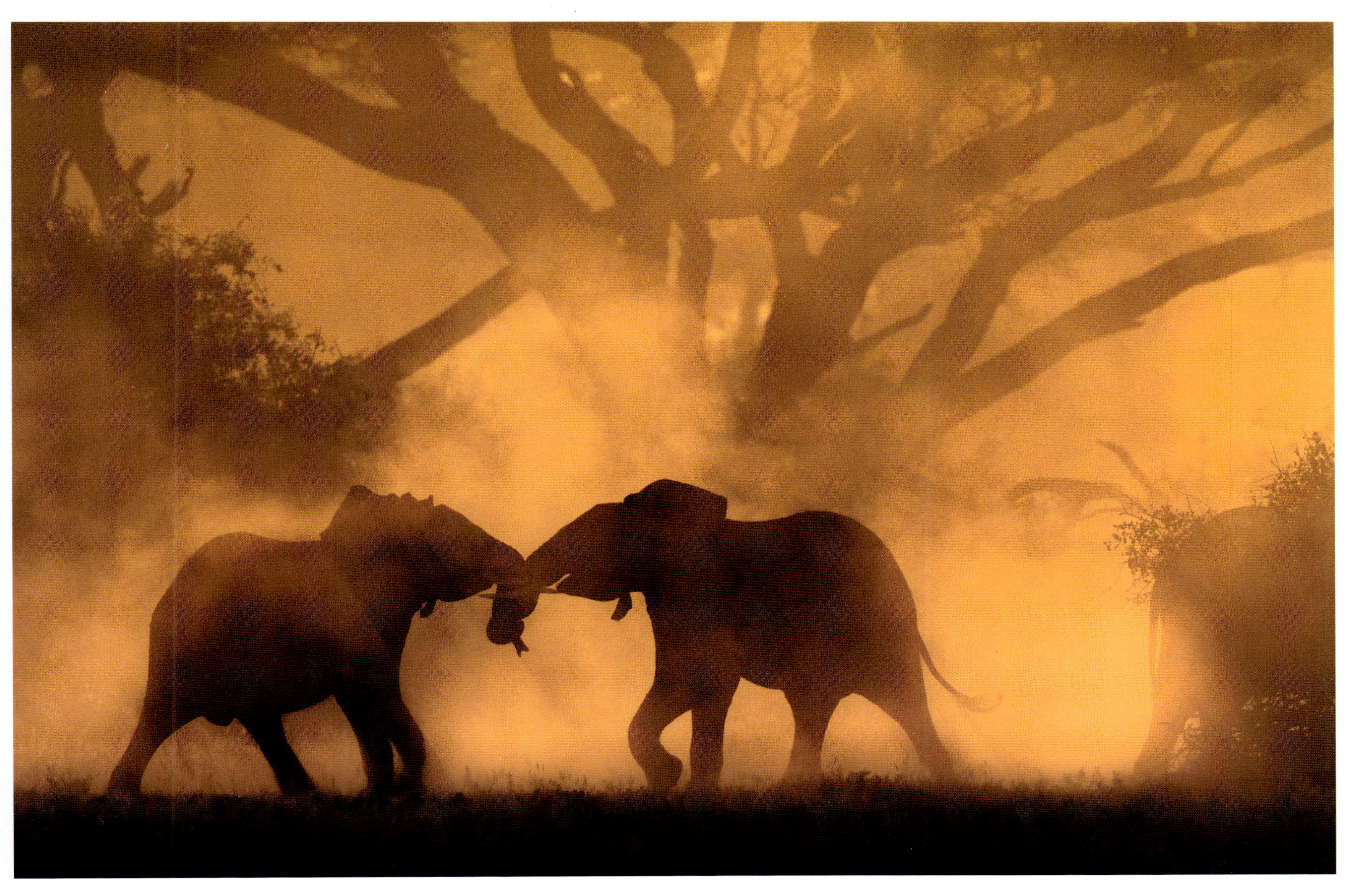

Rahul Sachdev
African Elephants
Amboseli National Park, Kenya

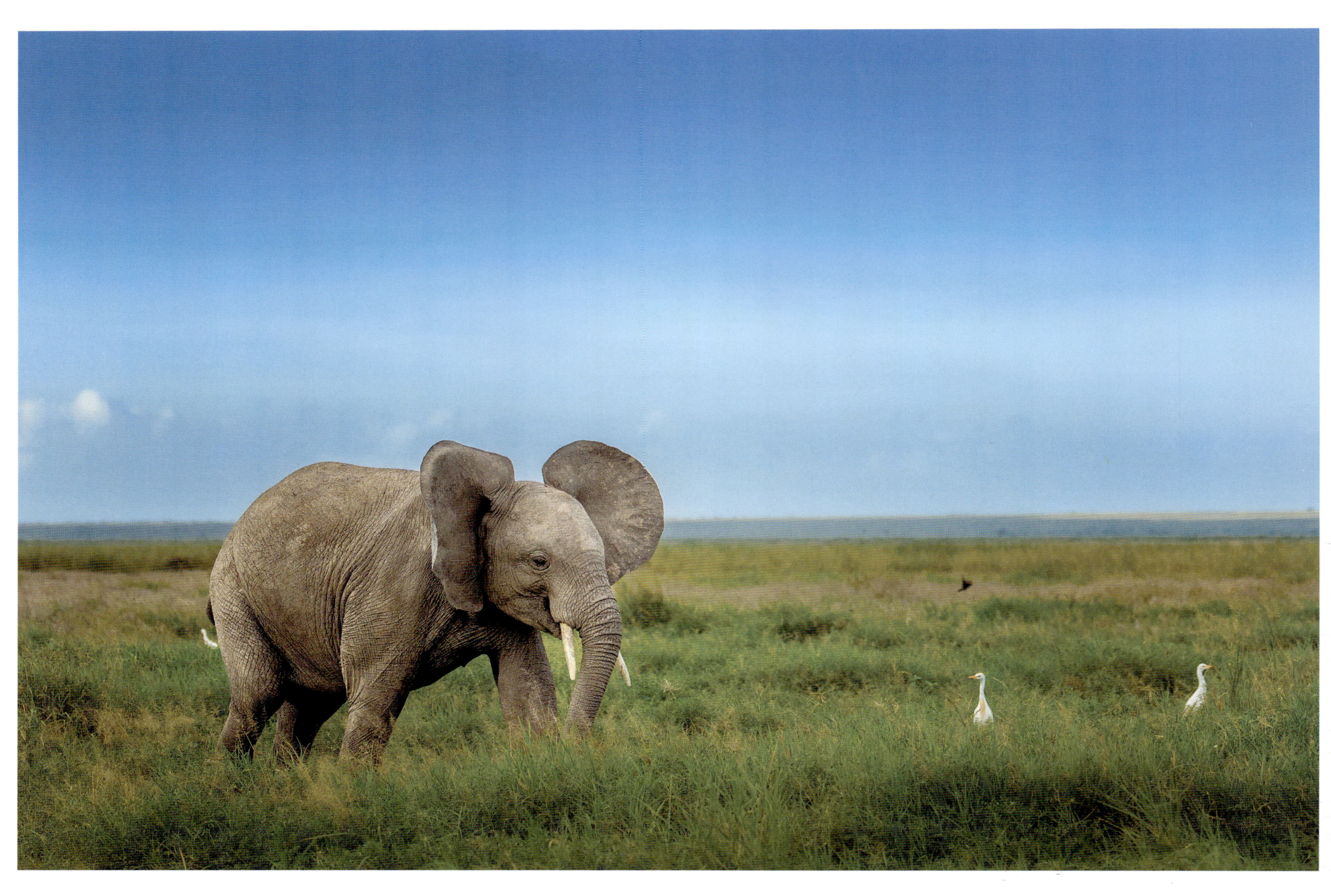

Rupayan Datta
African Elephant
Amboseli National Park, Kenya

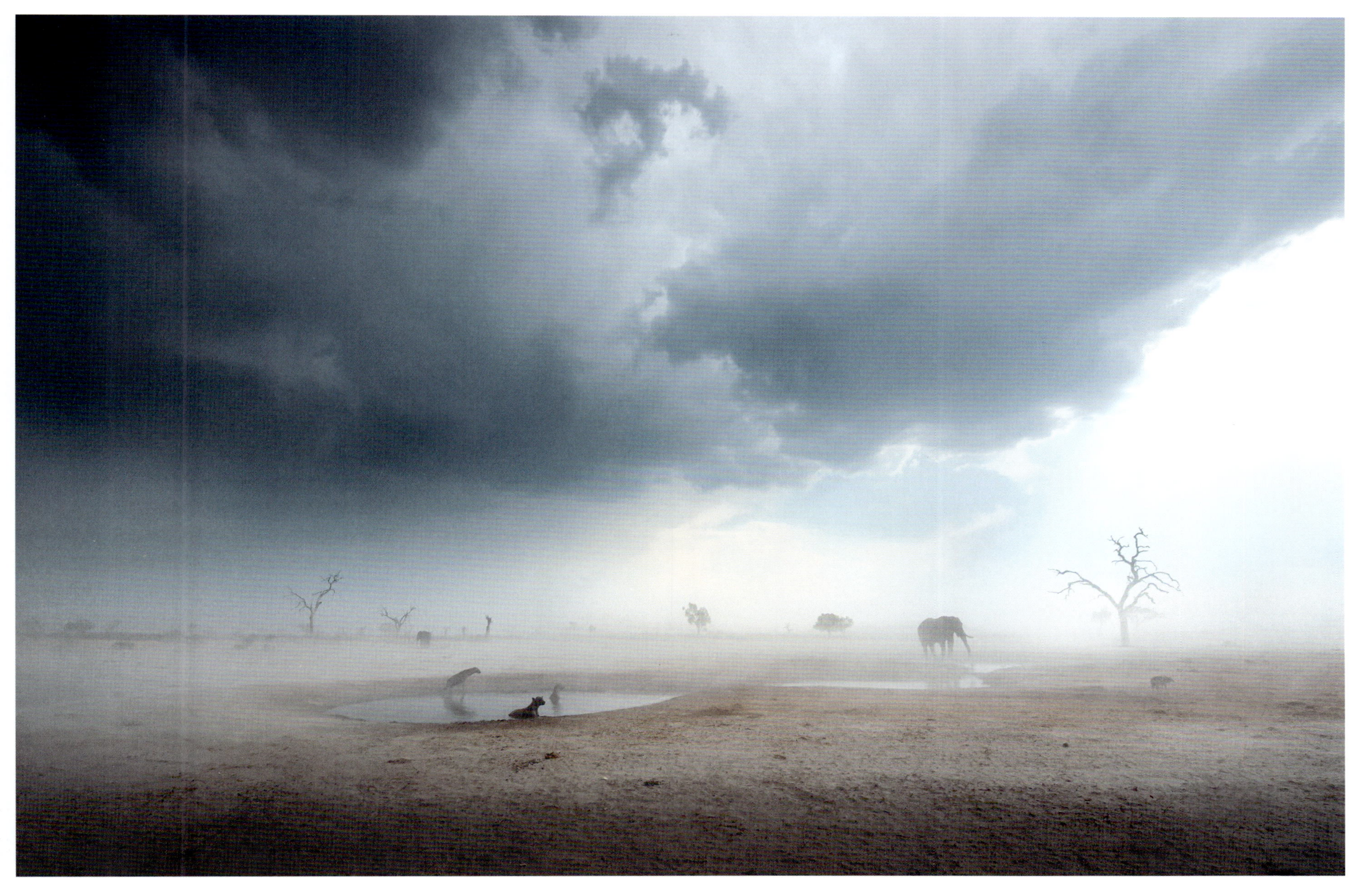

Hannes Lochner
African Elephant
Chobe National Park, Botswana

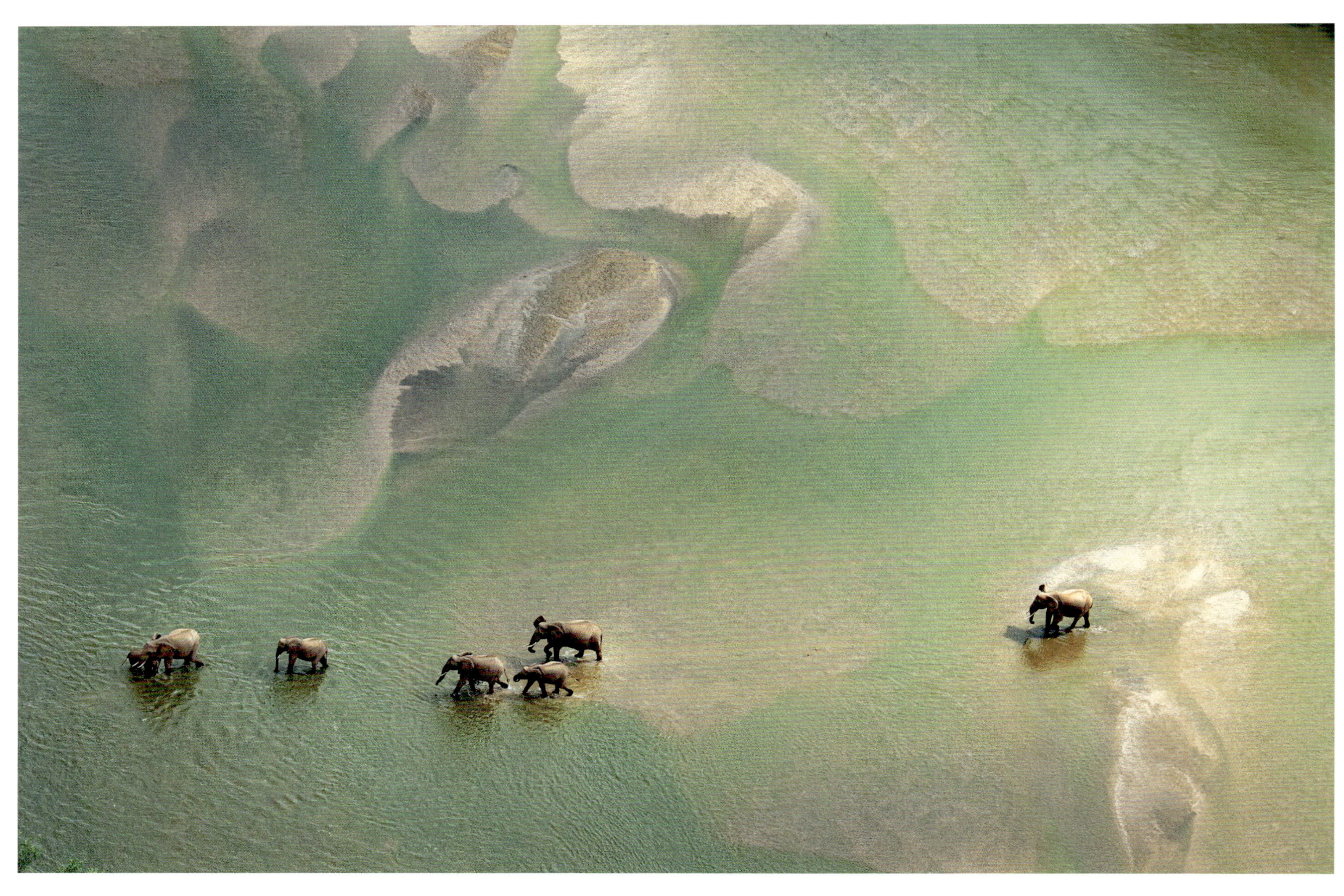

Mia Collis
African Elephants
Tsavo East National Park, Kenya

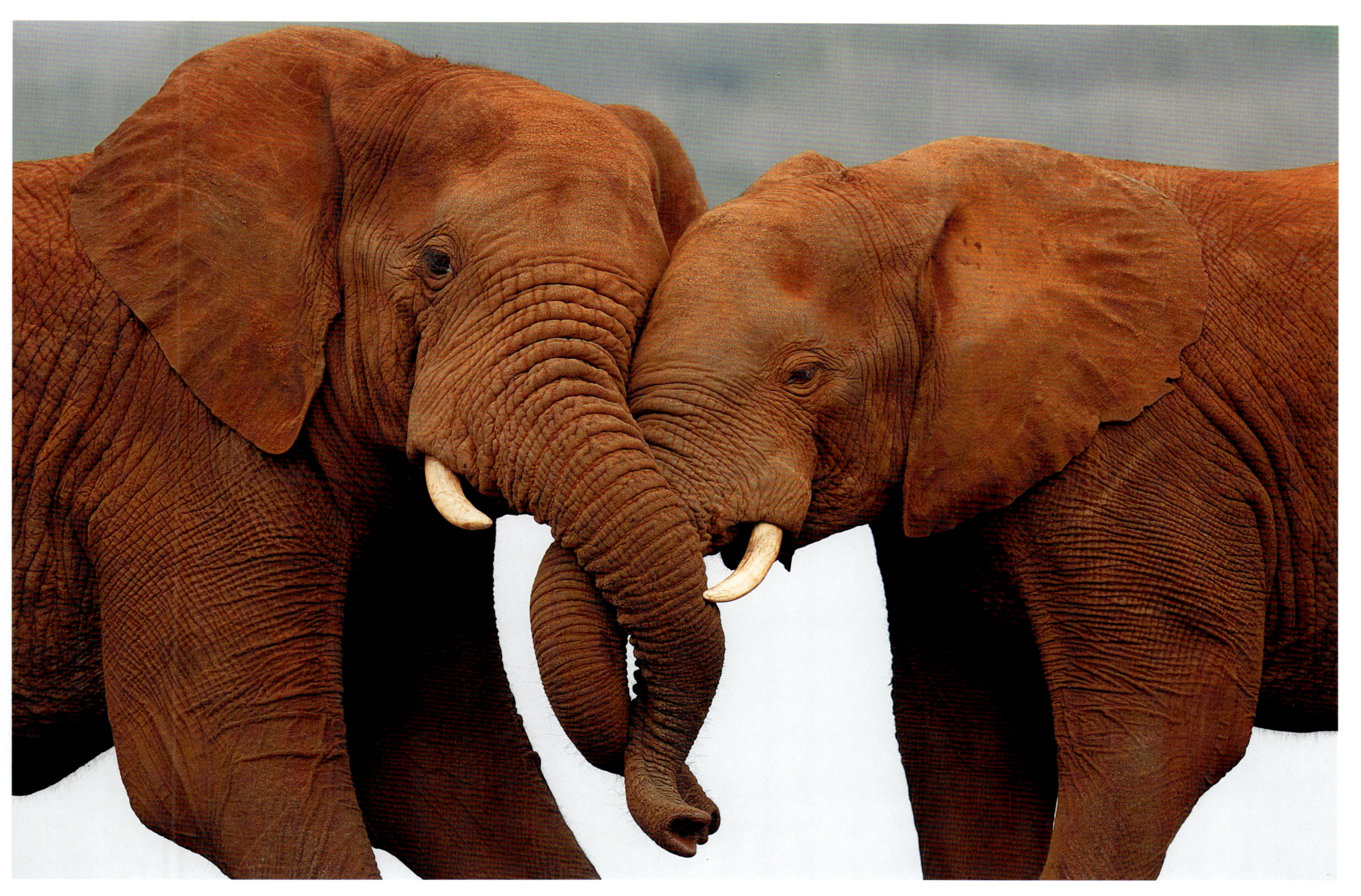

Staffan Widstrand
African Elephants
Zimanga Private Game Reserve, South Africa

63

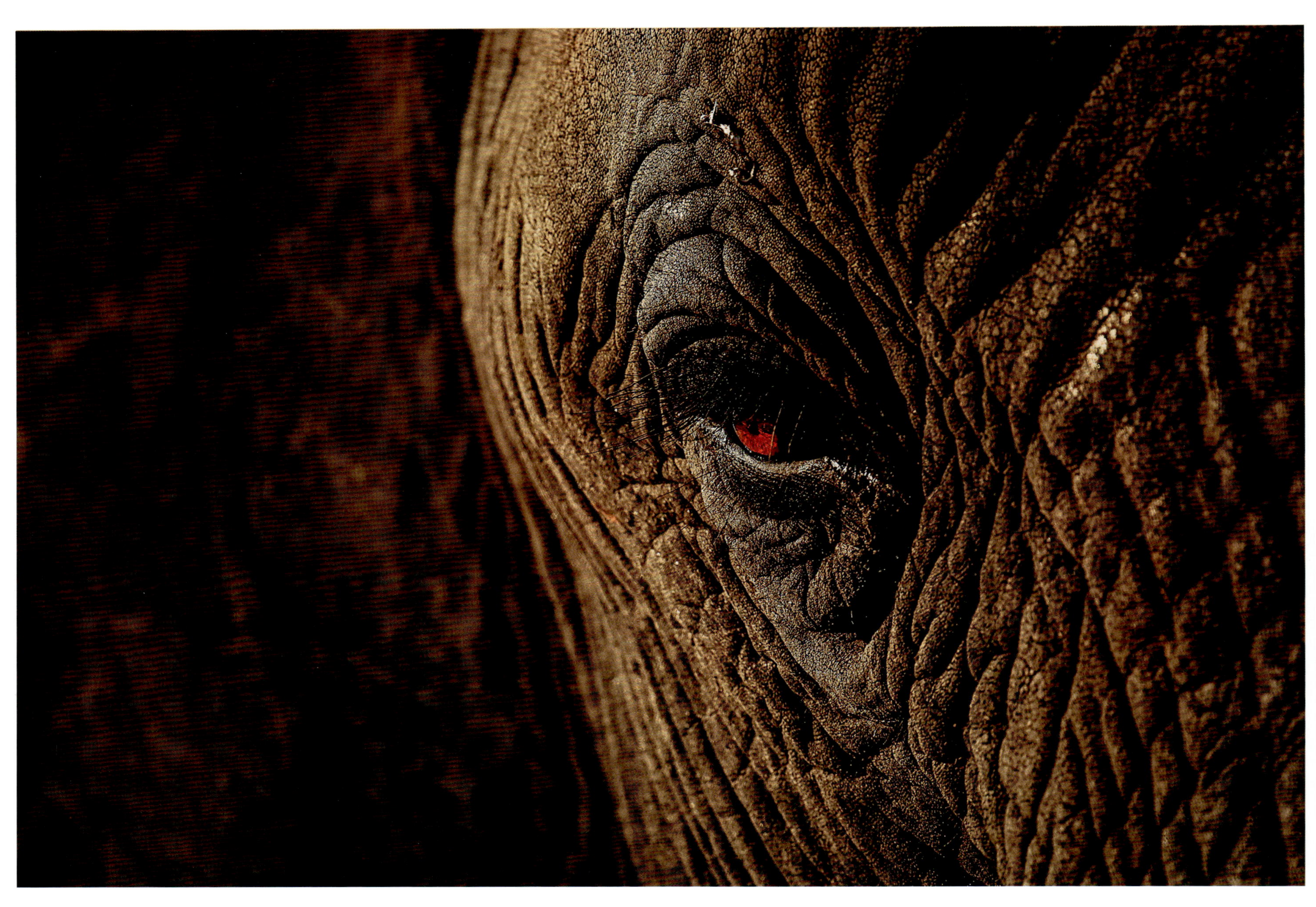

Karabo LeBronpeter Moilwa
African Elephant
Chobe National Park, Botswana

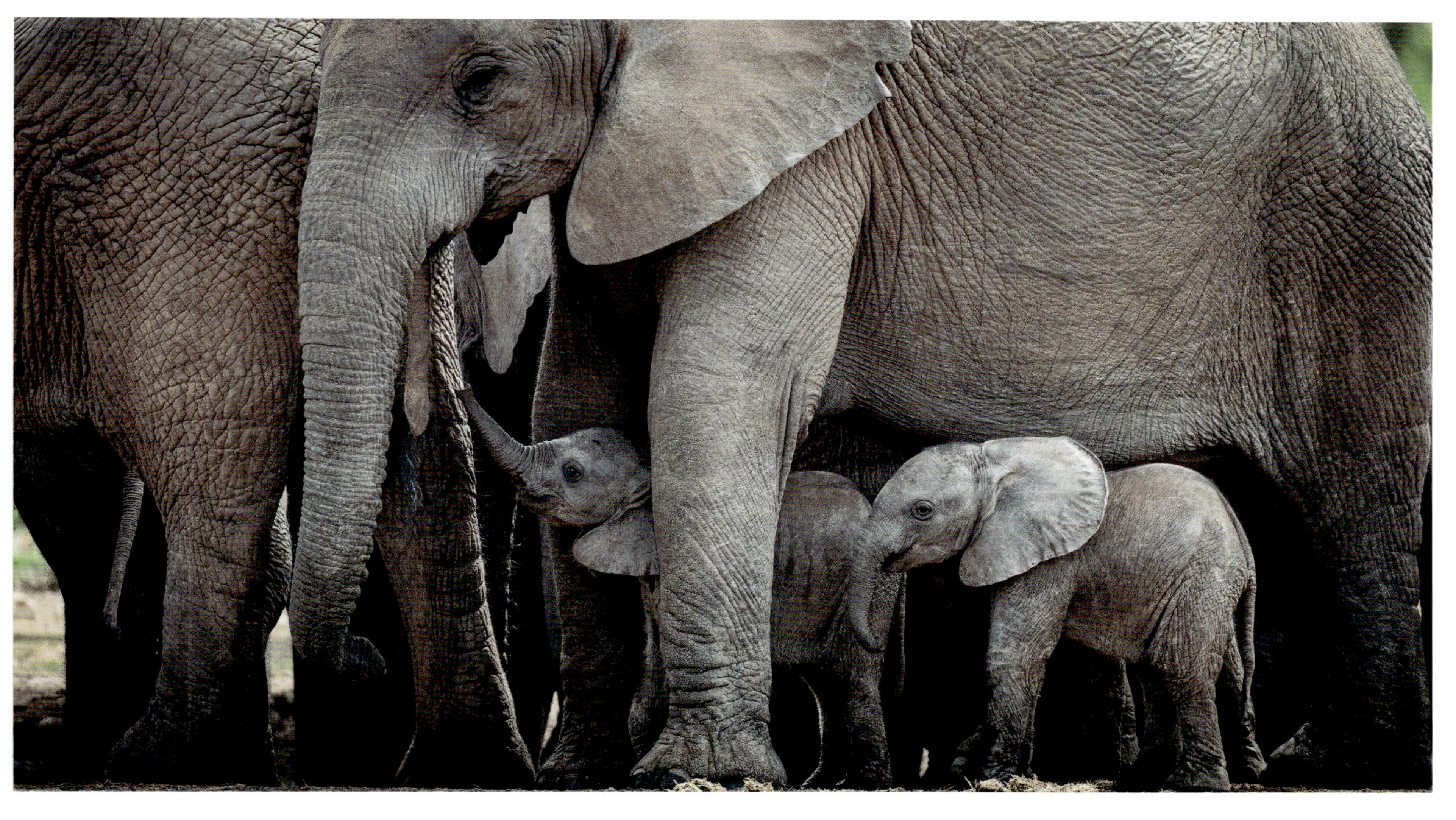

Stephanie-Emmy Klarmann
African Elephants
Addo Elephant National Park, South Africa

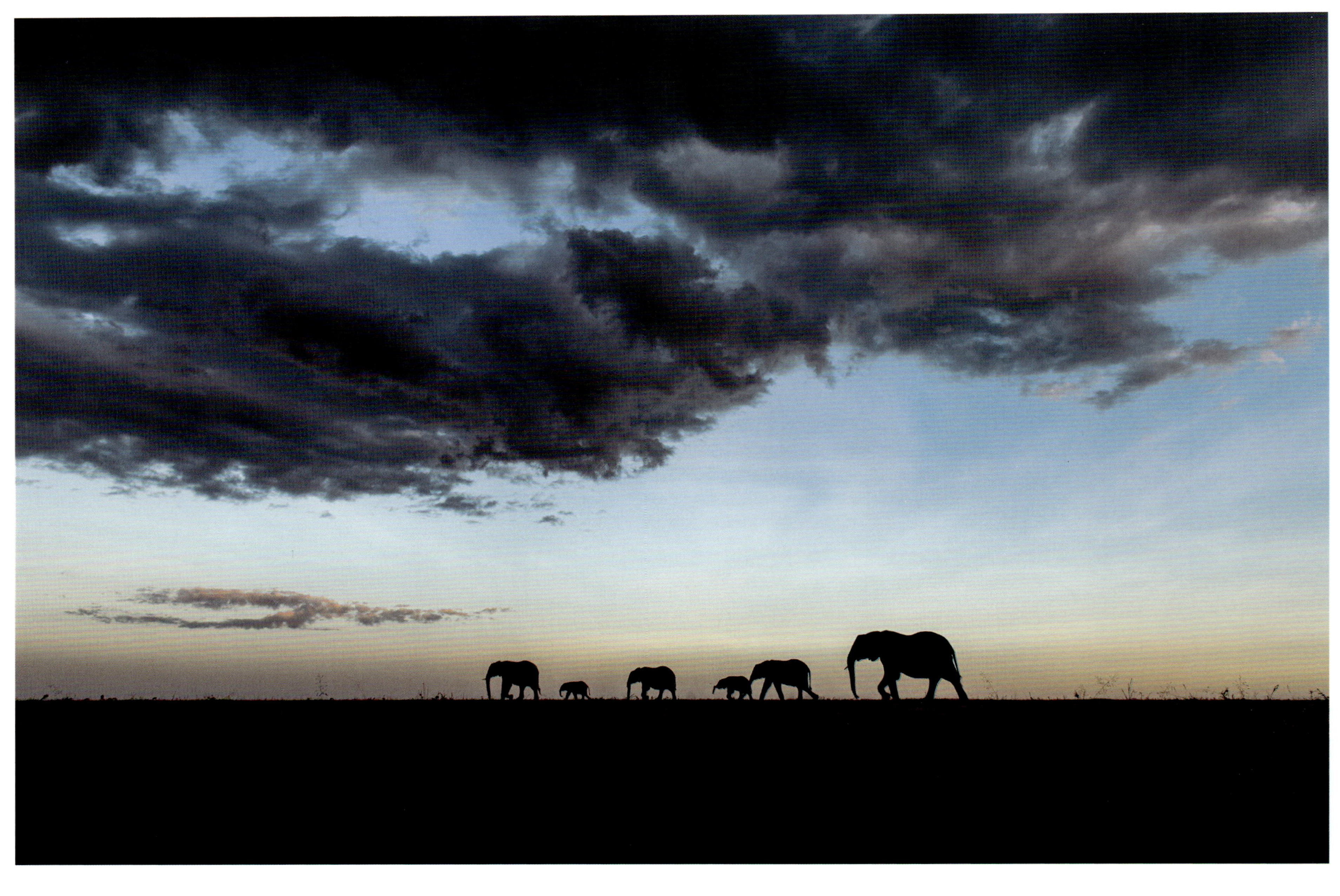

Gurcharan Roopra
African Elephants
Maasai Mara National Reserve, Kenya

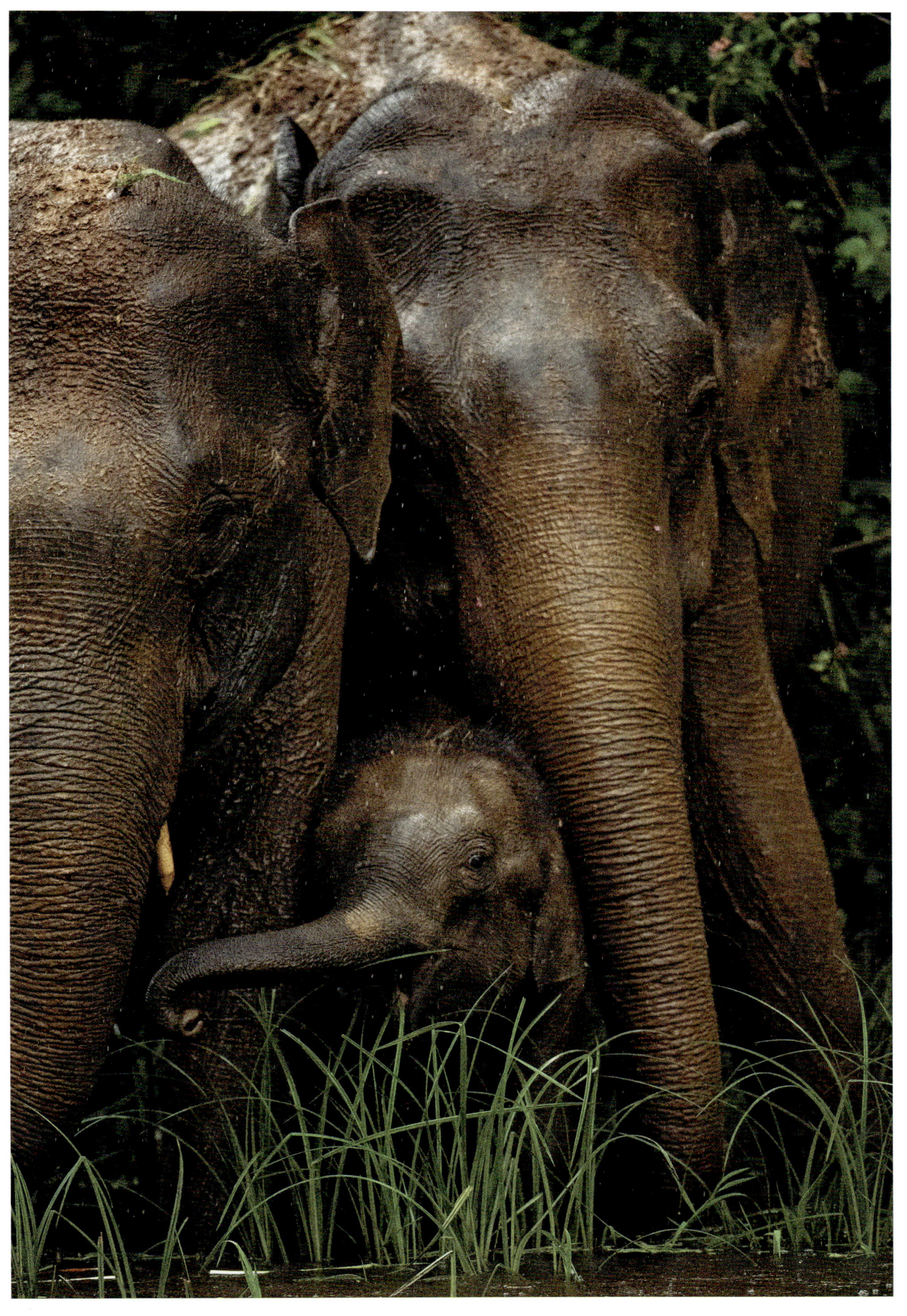

Sudhir Shivaram
Indian Elephant
Waynad Wildlife Sanctuary, India

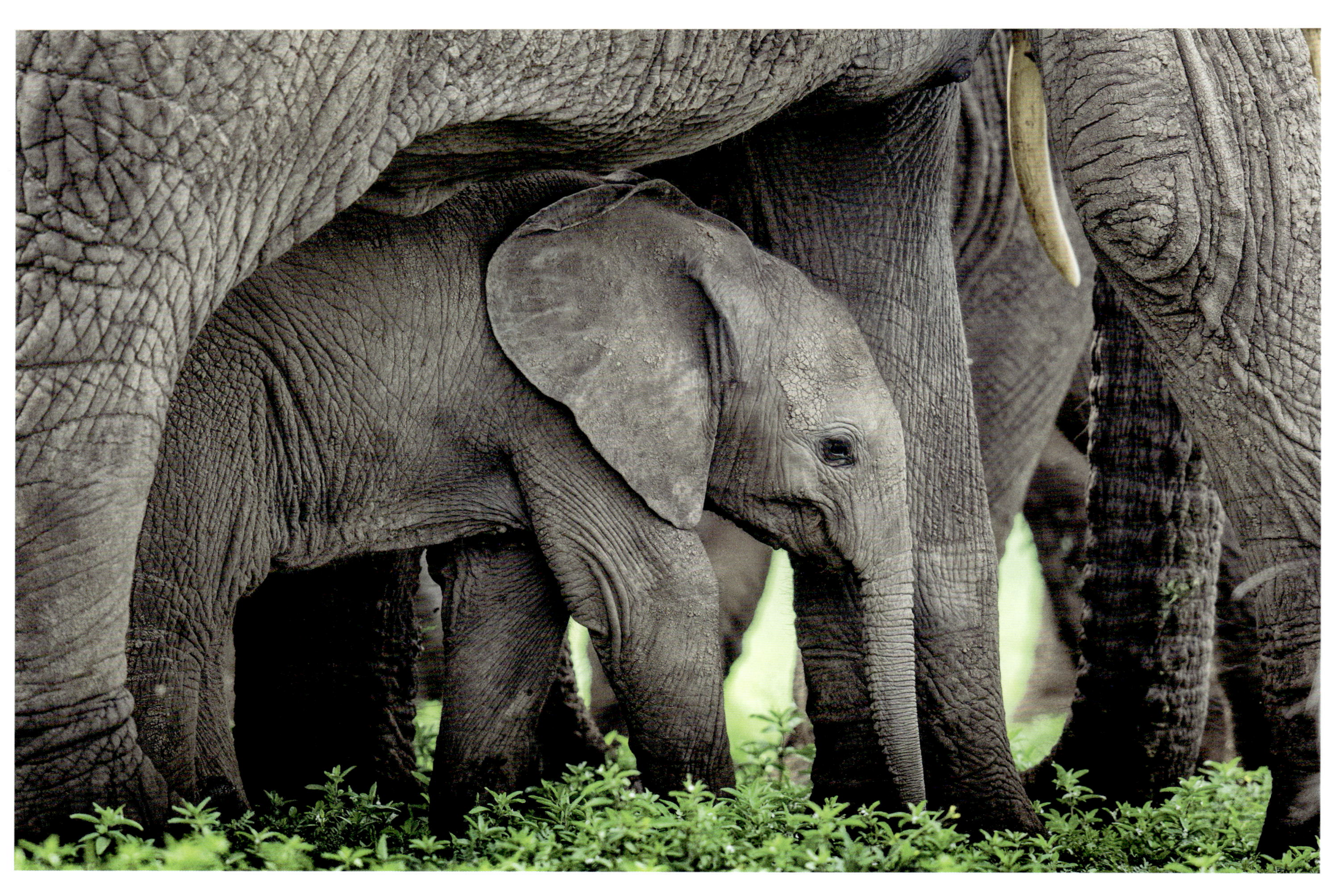

Karine Aigner
African Elephants
Ngorongoro Conservation Area, Tanzania

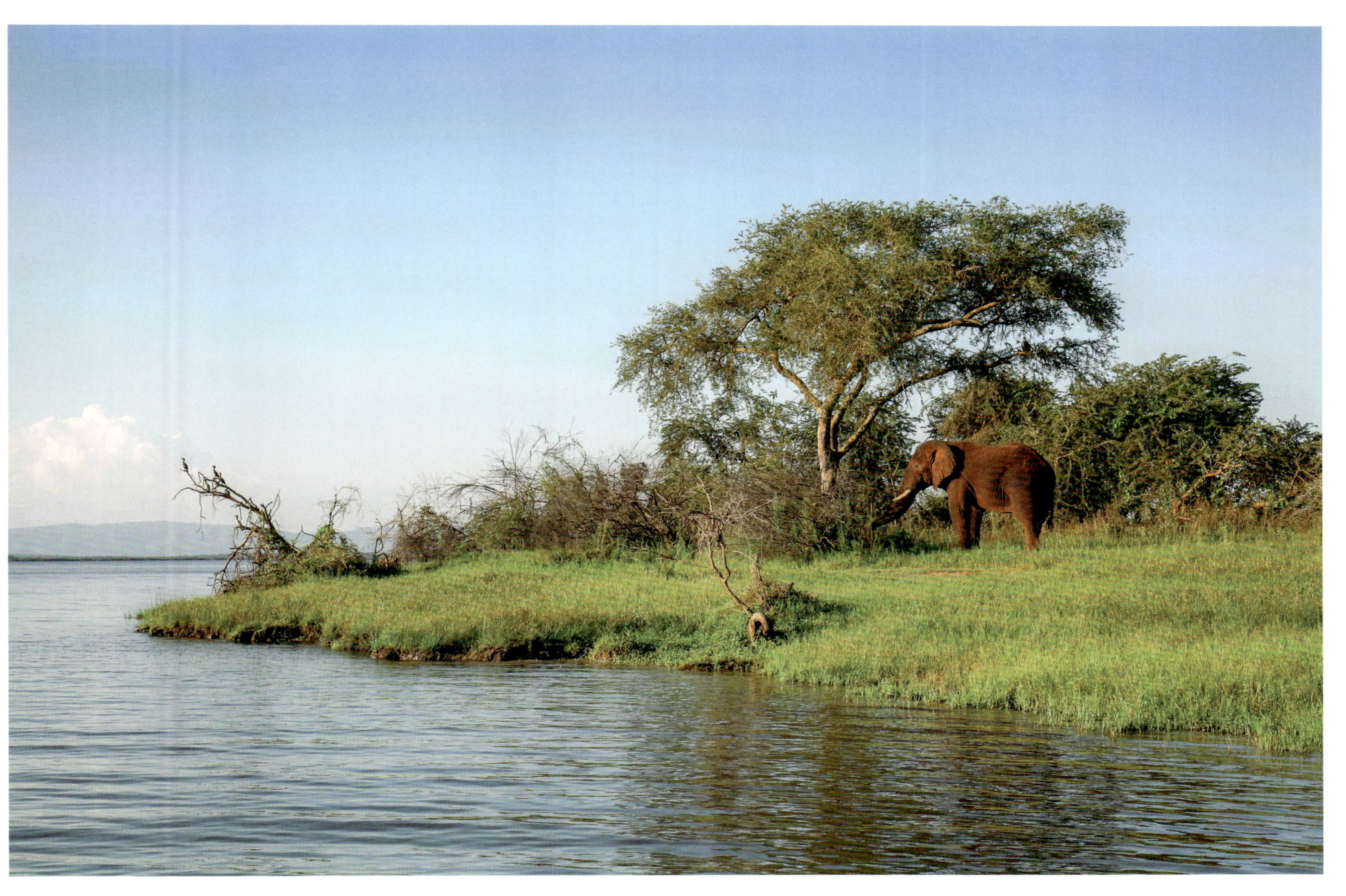

Graeme Green
African Elephant
Akagera National Park, Rwanda

POLAR BEARS

Polar Bears

Krista Wright

Executive Director, Polar Bears International

THE FIRST TIME I SAW A WILD POLAR BEAR, I was unprepared for just how big he was. It was a blustery day on the tundra, with blasts of wind rattling and shaking our Tundra Buggy. Cold seeped in through the floorboards and windows, and whiteout conditions all but erased the world outside. Suddenly a huge male polar bear appeared out of the swirling snow, heading directly toward our buggy with a slow, pigeon-toed gait. When he reached us, he stood on his hind legs and placed his massive paws below the windows, peering in at the people inside.

My heart thumped, and my first thought was, "This bear is enormous." My second thought was, "He has no fear." My third thought: "Despite his size and strength, he needs our help."

Ursus maritimus, the sea bear, is a marvel of nature, built for cold and Arctic conditions. Unlike his grizzly cousins, which make their living on land, the polar bear is beautifully adapted for a life hunting seals on the sea ice, wandering across frozen ocean waters in the subzero cold.

Polar bears' small ears and stubby tails are designed to prevent heat loss. Two layers of fur and a thick layer of blubber keep them warm, even when temperatures drop to −40°F (also −40°C.) Their huge paws are equipped with small bumps called papillae, which keep them from slipping on the ice. Small tufts of fur provide further traction. Their sharp, curved claws allow them to grab a seal that surfaces at its breathing hole in the ice and yank it out. Even polar bears' noses are specialized, making it possible for them to sniff out seals on the vastness of the sea ice, an ever-shifting, white-on-white world where slabs of ice creak and groan as northern lights twinkle overhead.

Many people think of frozen landscapes as empty, but polar bears are a reminder that these frozen landscapes are, in fact, teeming with life.

Every time I travel to the north and see polar bears, I'm struck by how connected they are to the Arctic ecosystem. They range in an amazing habitat with vast open spaces, a setting where the light, or the lack of light, lends the landscape a surreal quality. Even on the most overcast days, the subtle colors have a special beauty. The sun dogs, the mirages, and the northern lights all remind me that the polar bears' home is a world apart. Being there gives me a sense of the world as it was before people. It's as close as anywhere to being pristine.

I must wear special gear to survive in Arctic conditions, but polar bears are completely at ease in extreme cold, not only able to survive, but able to thrive. Therein lies the problem for them. As mighty as they are, human-caused climate warming is disrupting the world they've known for hundreds of thousands of years, with changes taking place at a pace too fast for them to adapt.

A polar bear's life is tied to the sea ice. Sea ice is to the ocean what soil is to a forest. It forms the base of the Arctic food chain. Tiny channels in the ice filter light, creating an environment where algae grows, which feeds what some of our friends in the science community like to call the "little squiggly creatures." These in turn feed the fish, which feed the blubber-rich seals and whales, which feed the polar bears. Polar bears are unlike any other bear on Earth, in that the frozen ocean is quite literally essential to their survival.

Polar bears are at the top of the Arctic food chain, preying primarily on ringed and bearded seals. They rely on the ice to hunt, breed, roam, and sometimes den. But climate change is melting the sea ice polar bears require. Already in parts of the Arctic, longer ice-free seasons and longer fasting periods, where the bears are forced ashore away from their seal prey, have led to troubling declines in some polar bear populations.

In Canada's Western Hudson Bay, for example, where I saw my first polar bear, the population has dropped by 30 percent since the 1980s, a decline directly linked to longer ice-free seasons. Polar bear cubs especially are having a hard time, with fewer surviving to adulthood in regions that have experienced dramatic sea ice loss. Because of their vulnerability, cubs are the ones that really tug at my heart. Prolonged fasts make it difficult for nursing mothers to produce enough milk to nourish their cubs.

In 2021, the Western Hudson Bay polar bears were off their sea ice hunting grounds for about 170 days due to a delayed freeze-up. According to scientists, that's more than fifty days beyond the point at which cub survival rapidly declines. While there is likely to be variation in the duration of ice-free periods, this extreme is a harbinger of what's to come.

Unless we greatly reduce carbon emissions and keep temperature rises below the 3.6°F (2°C) set at the Paris Climate Accords, we could lose all but a few polar bears by the end of this century. With that would come the loss of an achingly beautiful ecosystem, including a food chain that begins with algae and other tiny creatures in the sea ice and ends with Arctic cod, seals, and polar bears.

Standing on that ice and feeling it move and shift beneath my feet always reminds me of the incredible journey polar bears' ancestors took as they ventured from shore, leaving their terrestrial lives behind some 500,000 years ago. Trying to picture an Arctic that is ice-free is like trying to picture a rain forest without trees or an ocean without water.

But climate change is not just about polar bears and the fragile Arctic ecosystem. It's about all other wildlife around the globe, and people, too. As top predators, polar bears are an indicator species. The impacts on polar bears due to melting sea ice almost certainly mean all other species that depend on Arctic Sea ice are being impacted in some way as well. Yet many of these species live under the ice, where it can be challenging to study them.

As a conservationist, I firmly believe our decisions should always be focused on future generations. What kind of world do we want to leave behind? The science on climate change couldn't be clearer. We know what we need to do to solve the climate crisis, and we still have a window of time to act to save polar bears and to avoid the worst impacts. But that window is closing with each passing day.

It's time for our leaders to act with a tremendous sense of urgency to end our dependence on fossil fuels, with a goal of limiting temperature rise to well below 3.6°F (2°C), preferably no more than 2.7°F (1.5°C).

It's also up to us as citizens to move our leaders to act, from talking about climate change—making it a kitchen-table issue—to following a conservation ethic in our own lives, voicing our support for climate-friendly policies, and getting involved with community projects.

In addition to addressing the overarching threat of climate change, we must also work to ensure healthy populations. This includes protecting polar bear mothers and cubs during the vulnerable denning period and working to reduce conflict with people, which is a growing problem, as polar bears are increasingly spending more time ashore in more places due to melting sea ice.

We know what we need to do to ensure a future for polar bears. If we act swiftly, use the tools and resources available to us, and meet the goals set in the Paris Agreement, we can ensure polar bears remain in most of their current range indefinitely. The sad reality is that if we don't act swiftly to address climate warming and face a future without polar bears, polar bears will be the least of our concerns, as climate impacts on a global scale will threaten our most basic needs for survival, such as clean air, clean water, and food availability. The good news is that if we work together and come together across communities, we can protect our shared future and ensure polar bears roam the Arctic sea ice for generations to come.

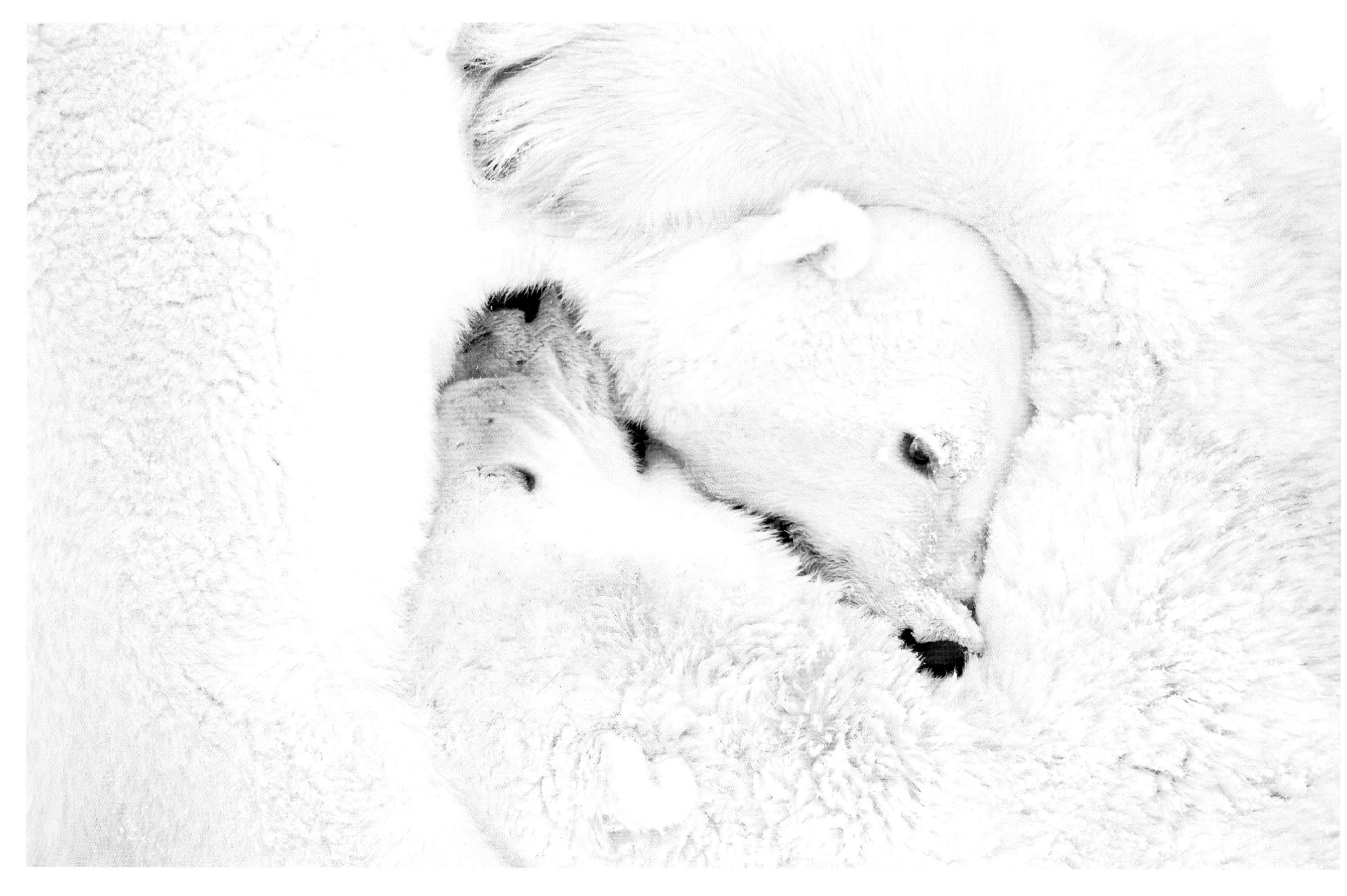

Daisy Gilardini
Wapusk National Park, Manitoba, Canada

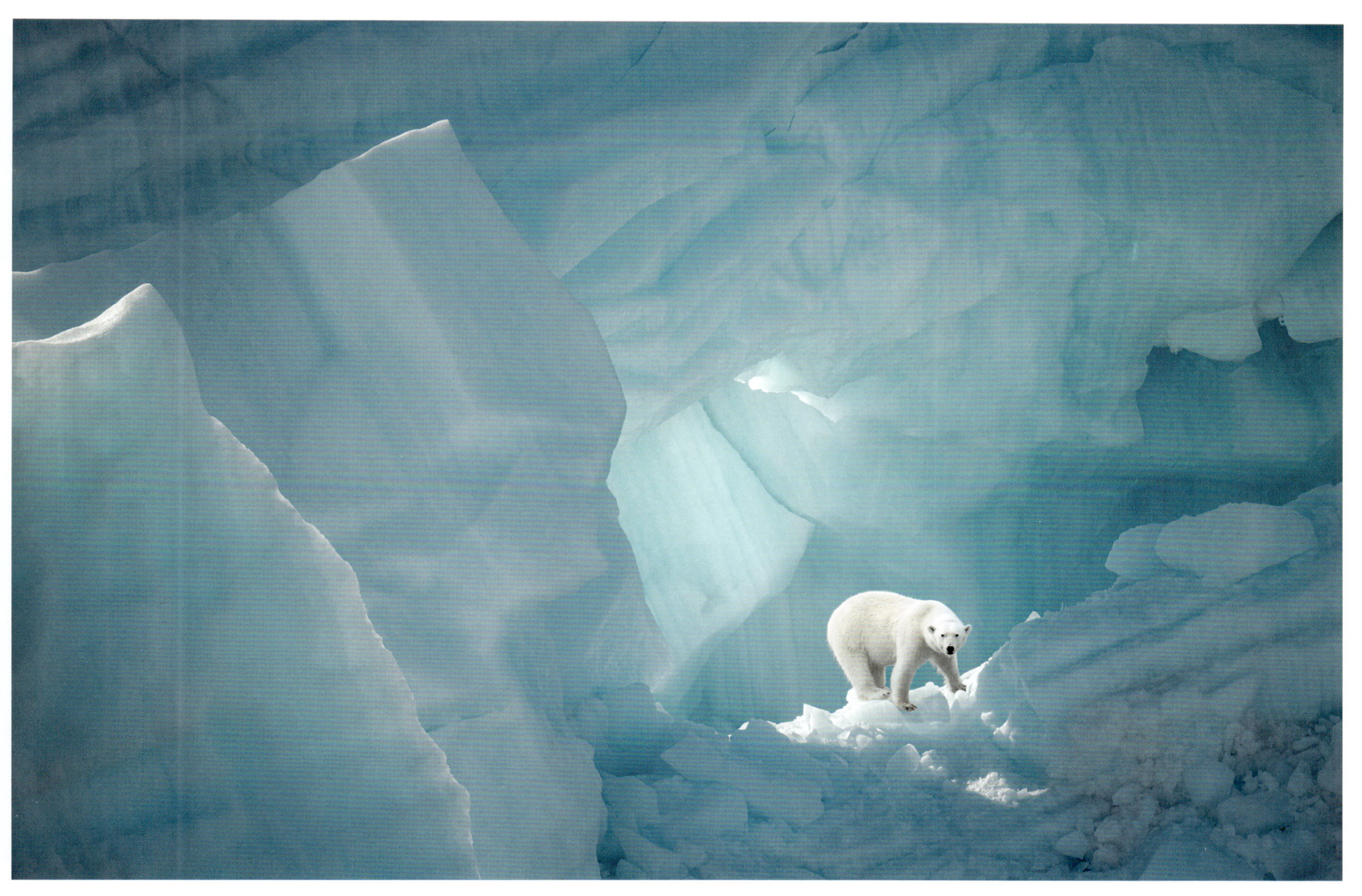

Marsel van Oosten
Barents Sea, Svalbard, Norway

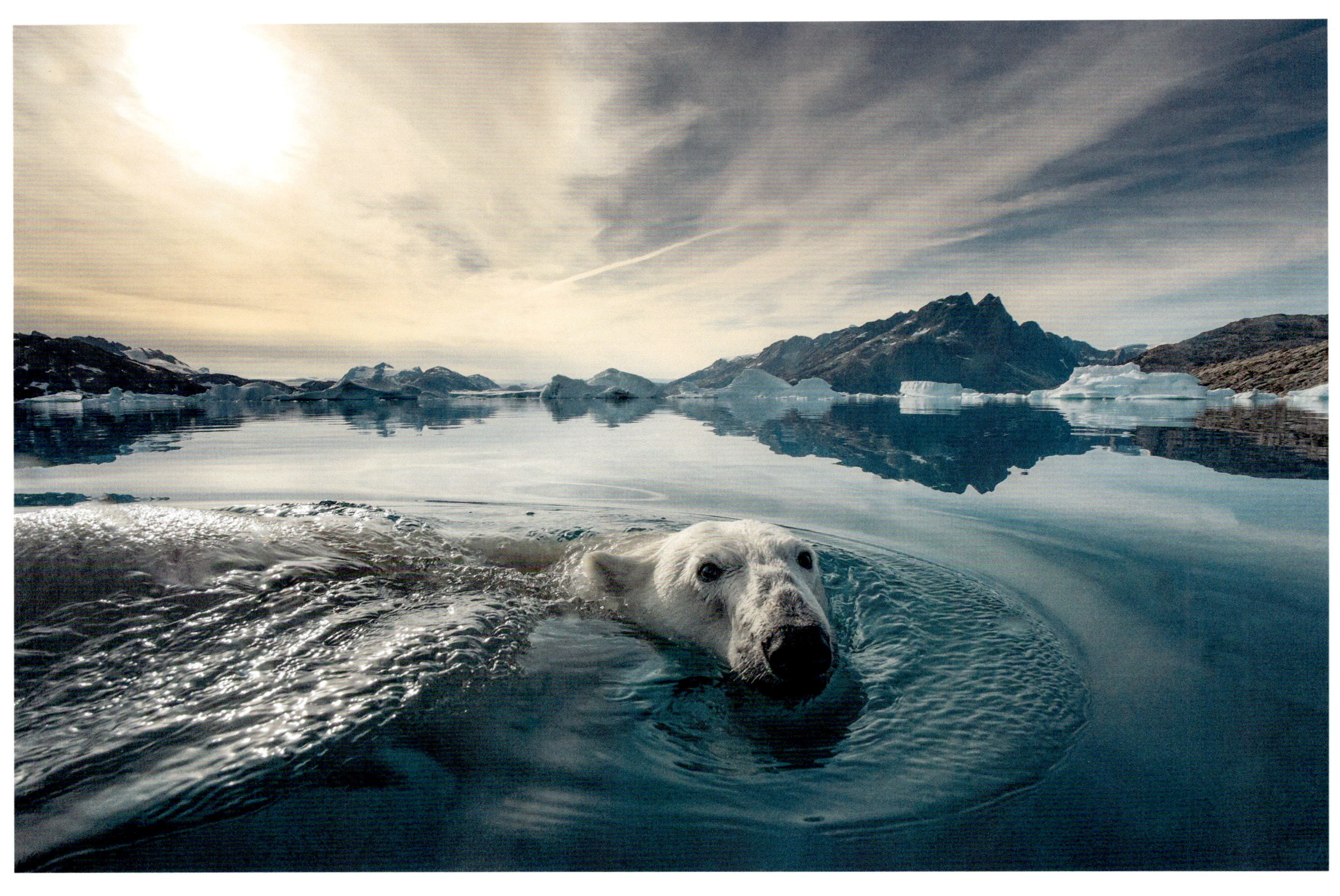

Andy Mann
Thorland Peninsula, Greenland

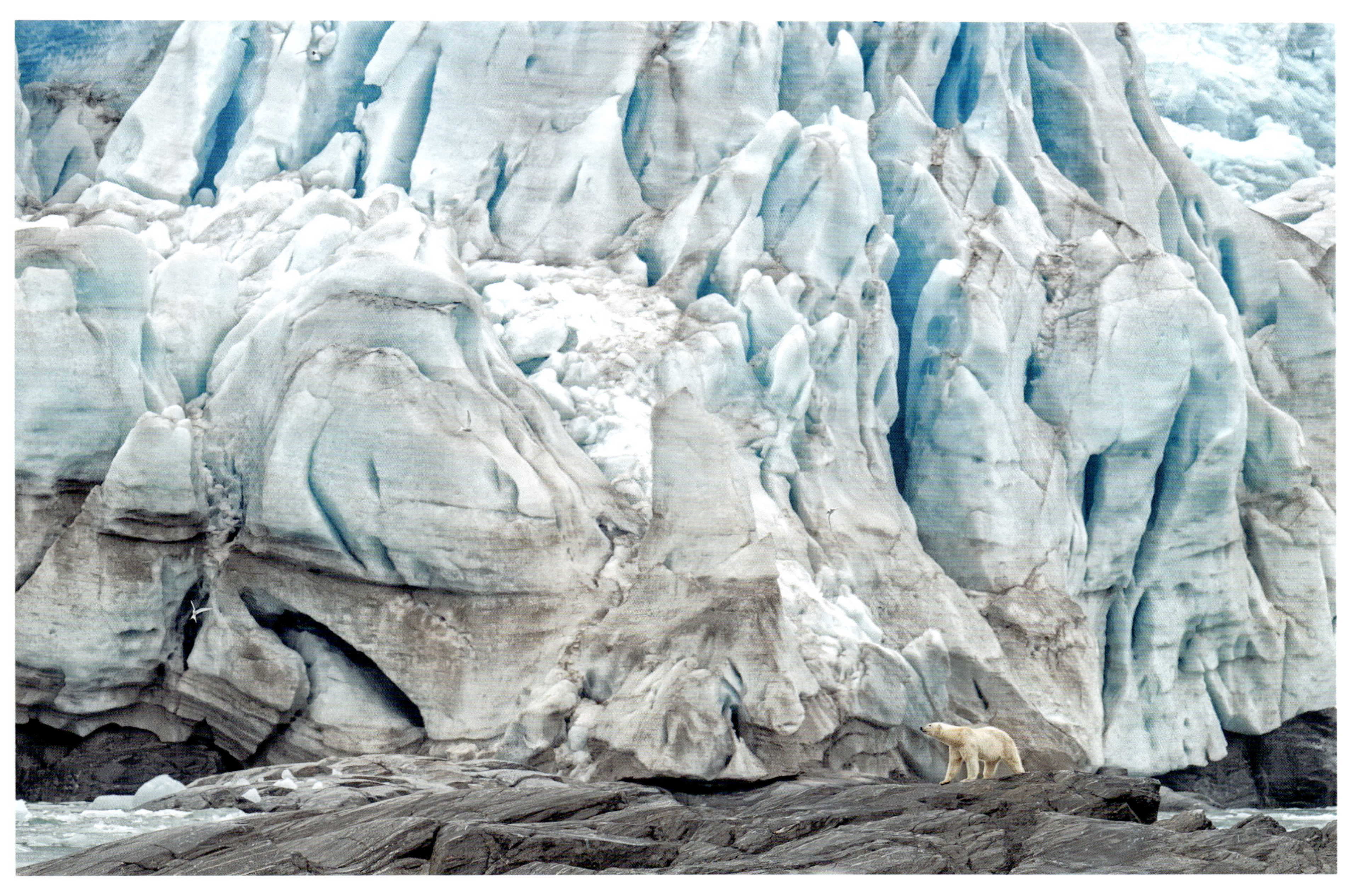

Anette Mossbacher
Nordenskiöldbreen Glacier, Svalbard, Norway

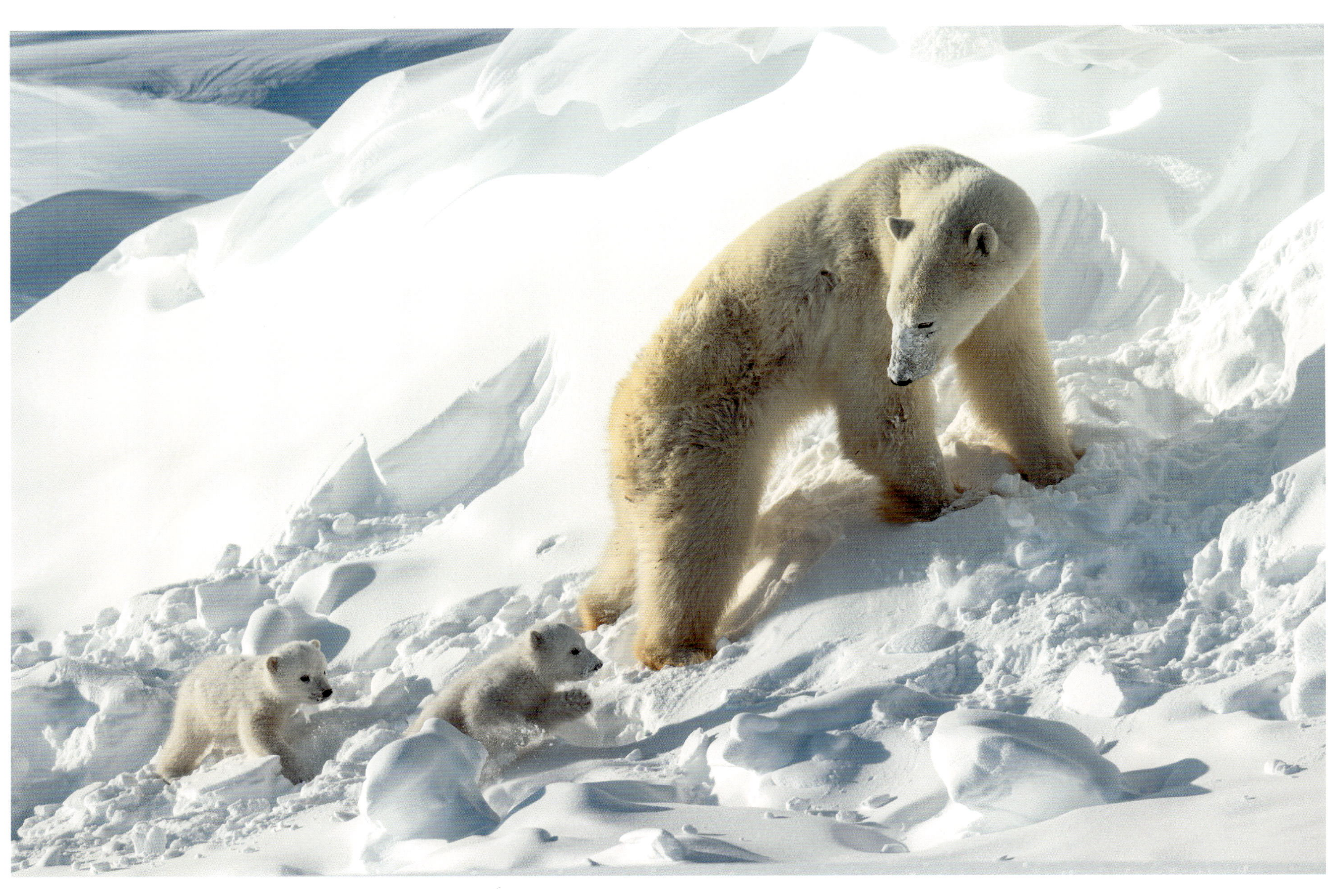

Hao Jiang
Wapusk National Park, Manitoba, Canada

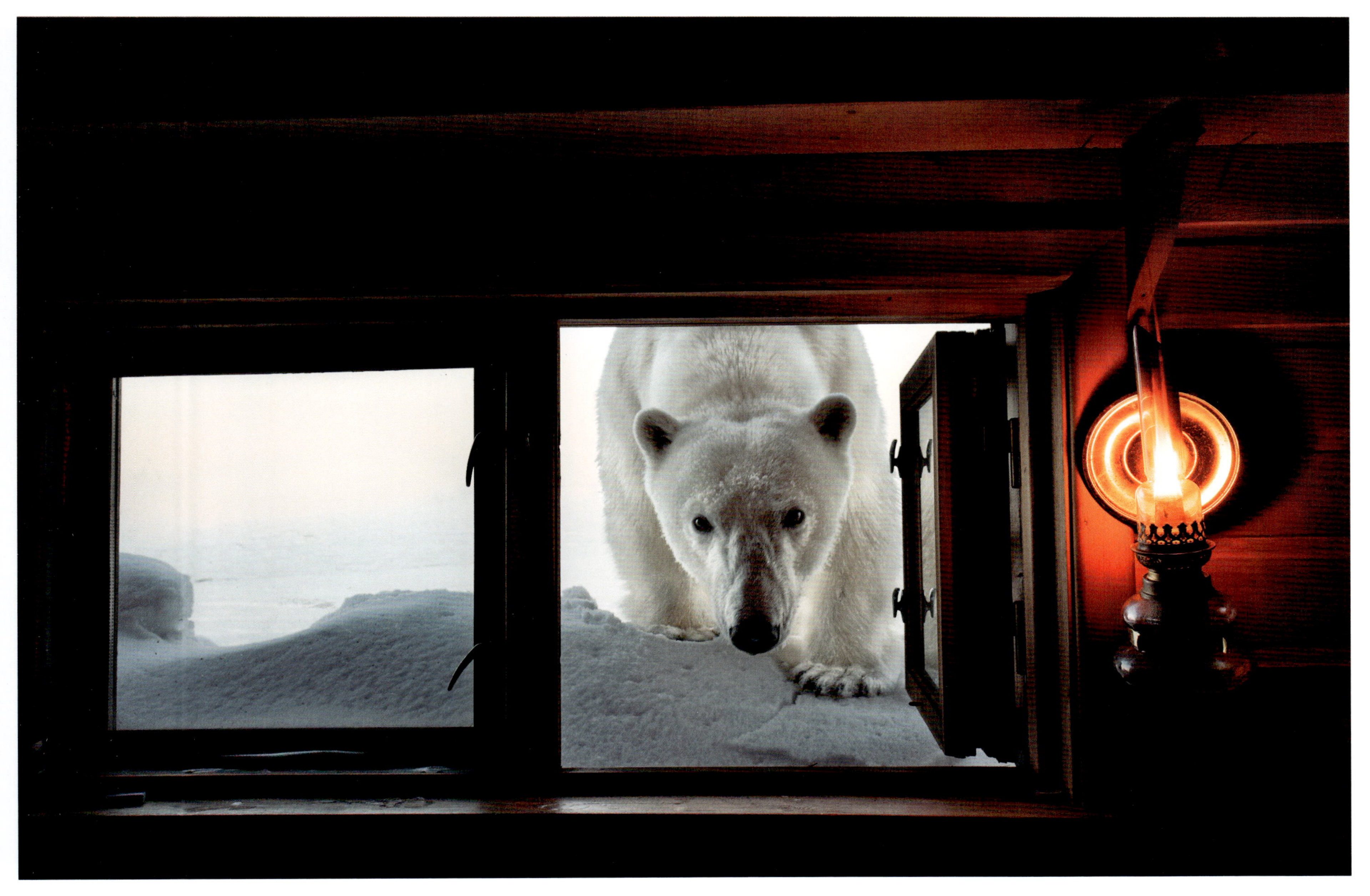

Paul Nicklen
Svalbard, Norway

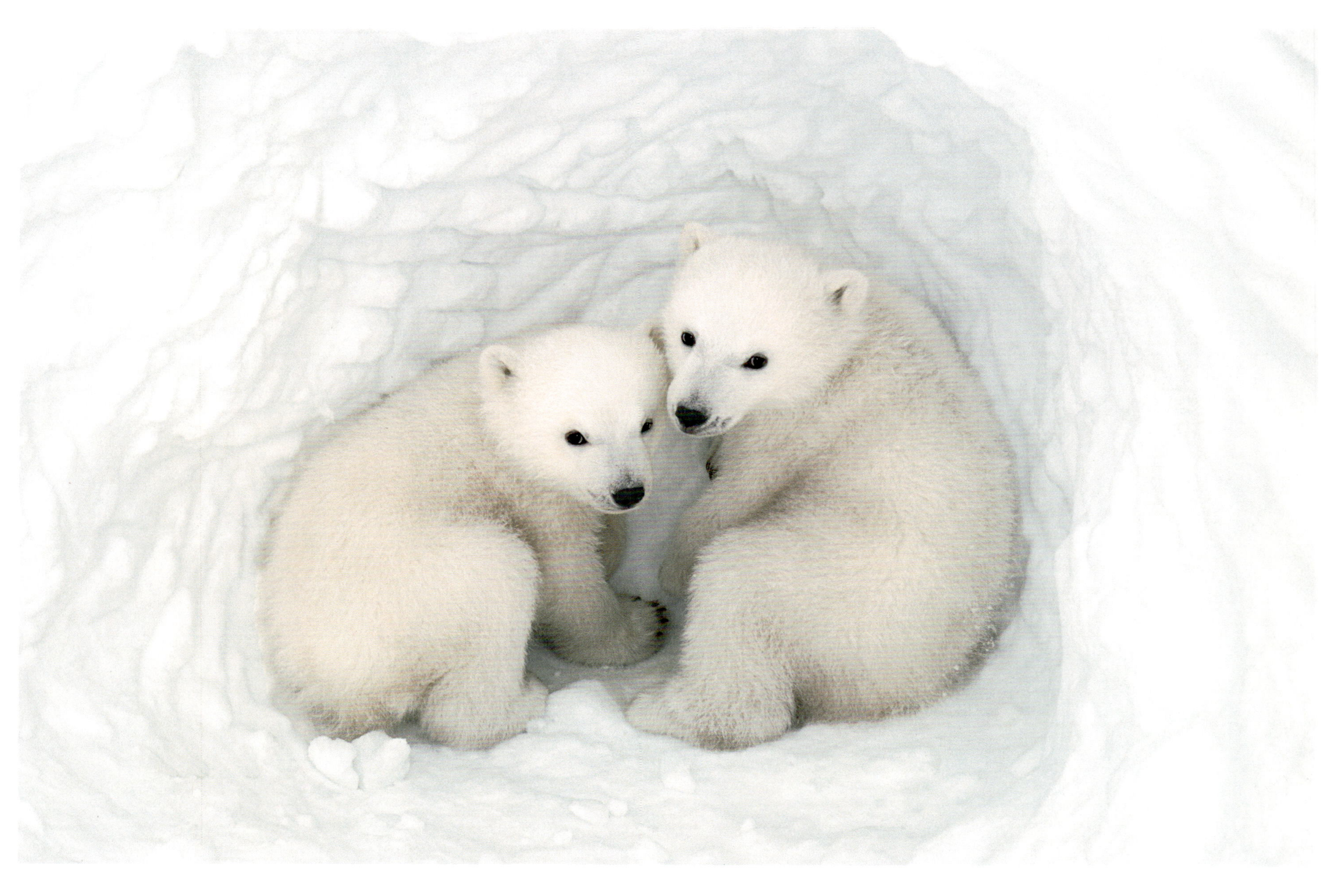

Jenny E. Ross
Wapusk National Park, Manitoba, Canada

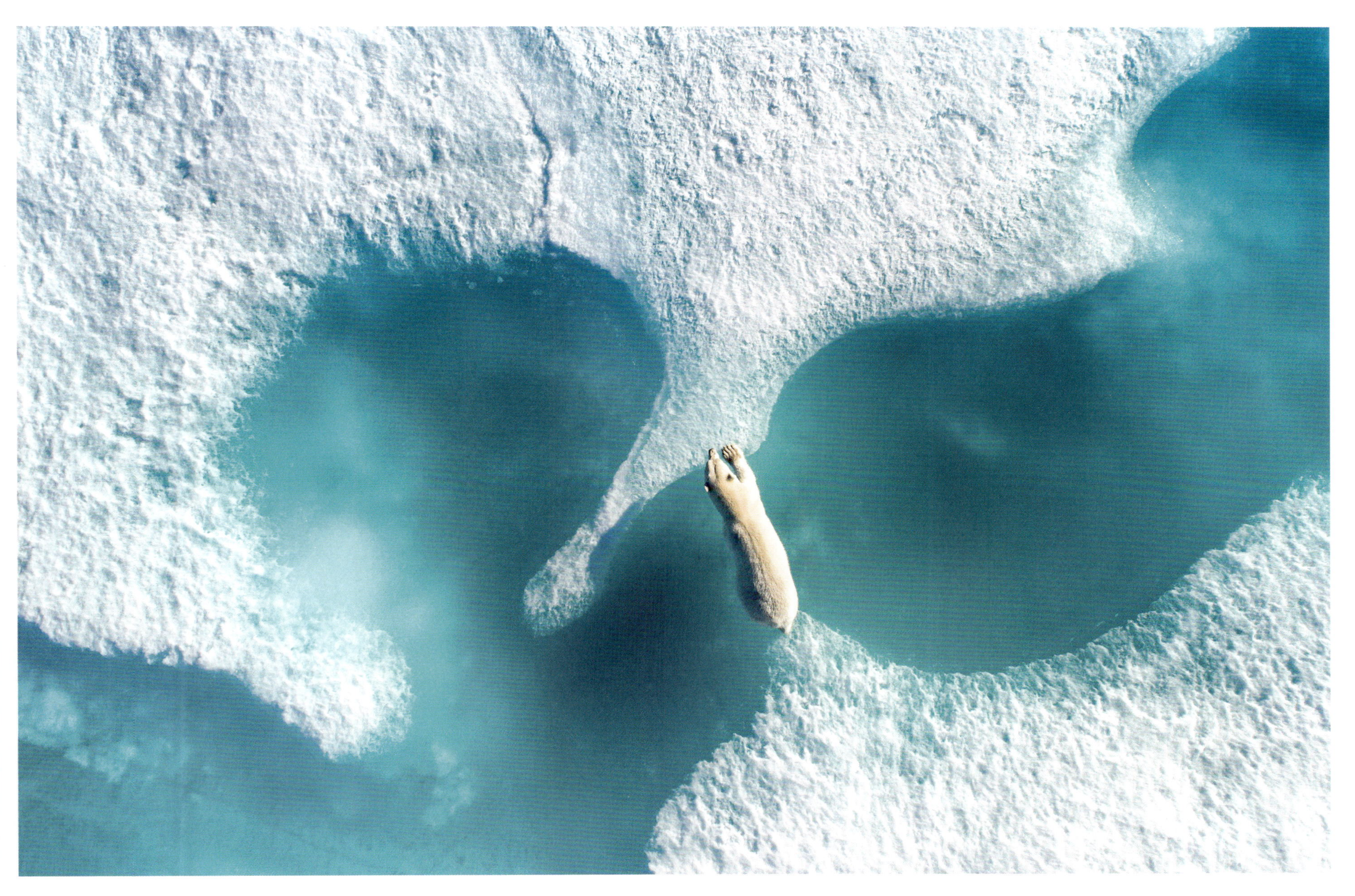

Florian Ledoux
Baffin Island, Nunavut, Canada

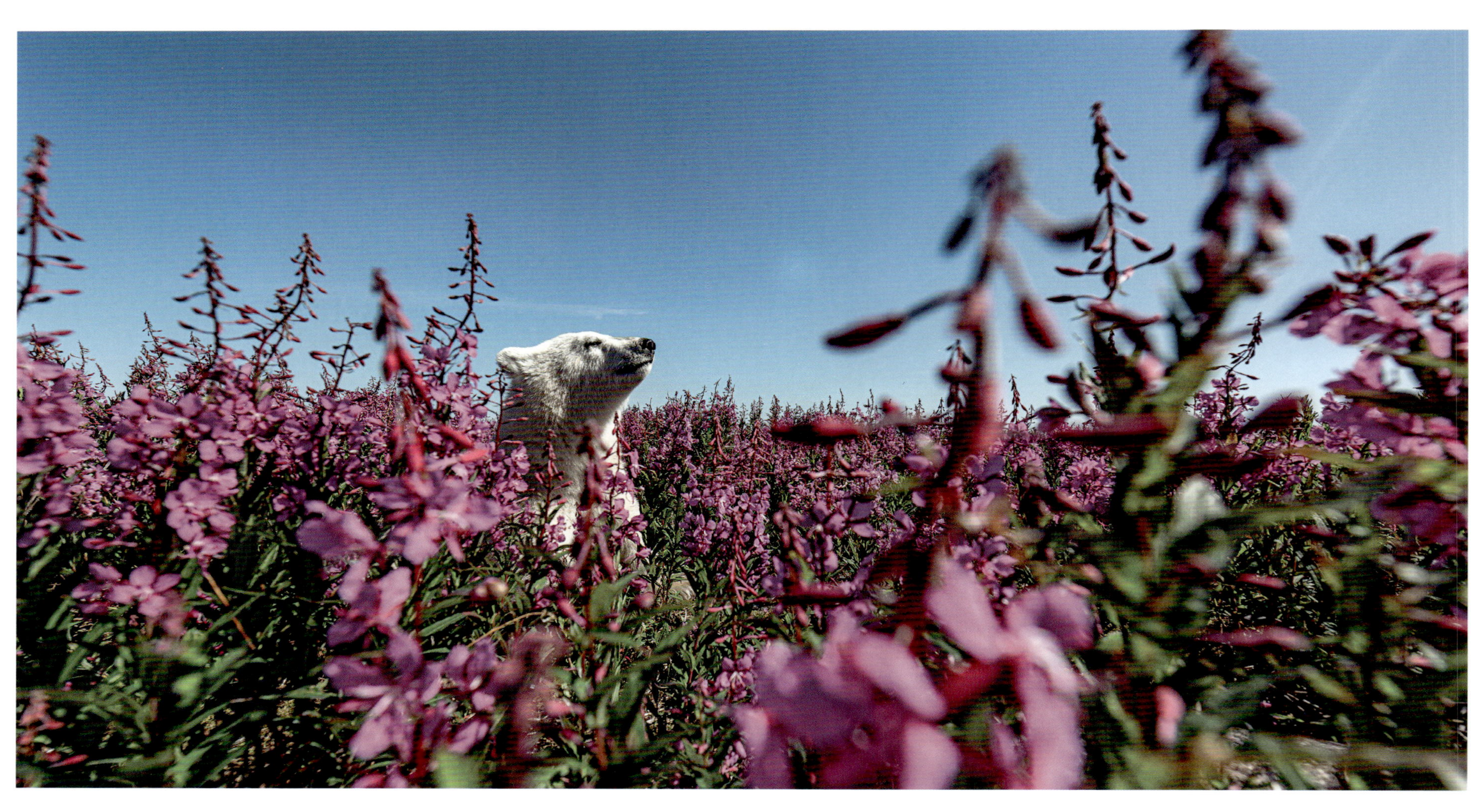

Martin Gregus
Hudson Bay, Manitoba, Canada

Françoise Gervais
Baffin Island, Nunavut, Canada

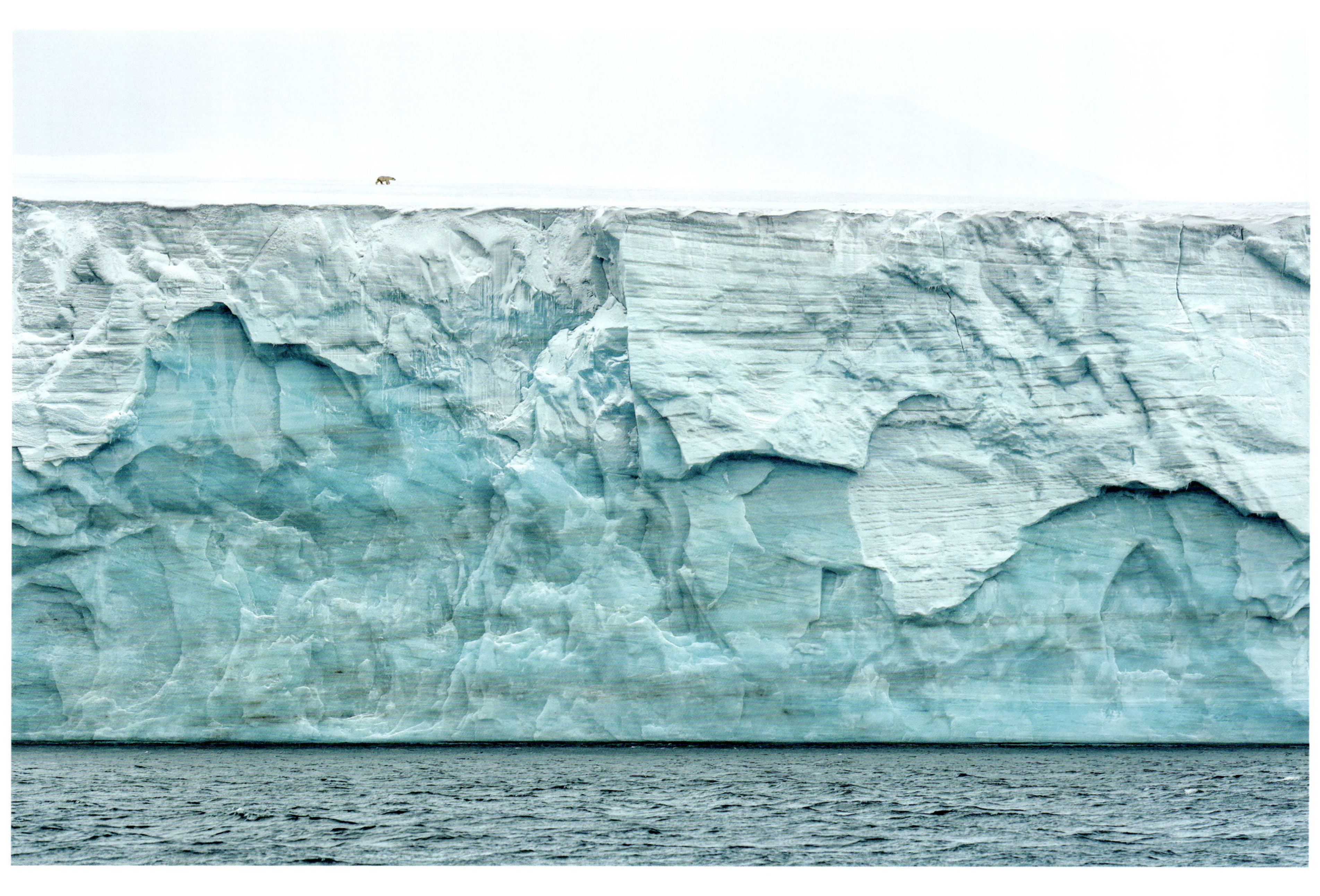

Sergey Gorshkov
Russian Arctic National Park, Russia

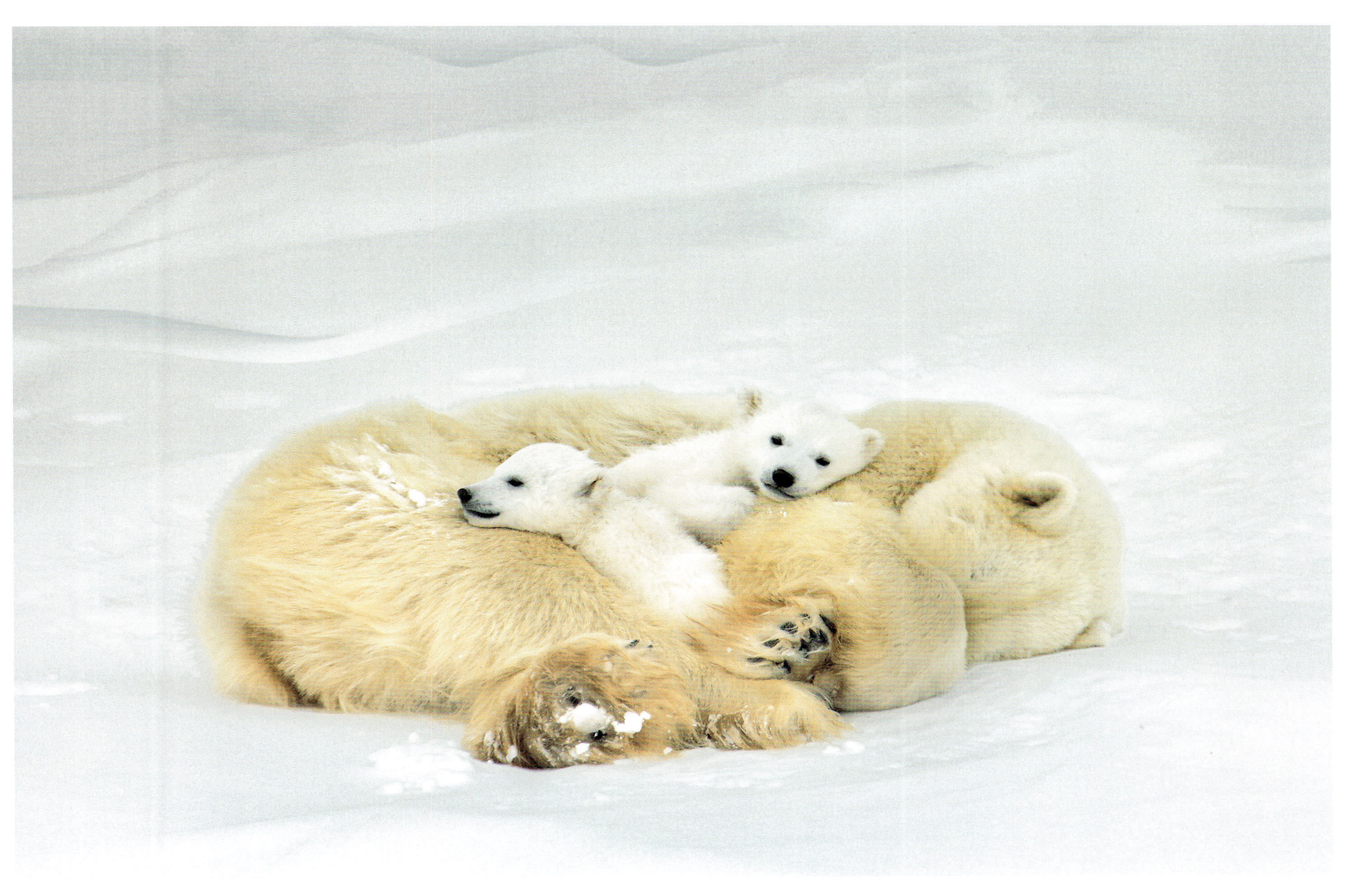

Michelle Valberg
Wapusk National Park, Manitoba, Canada

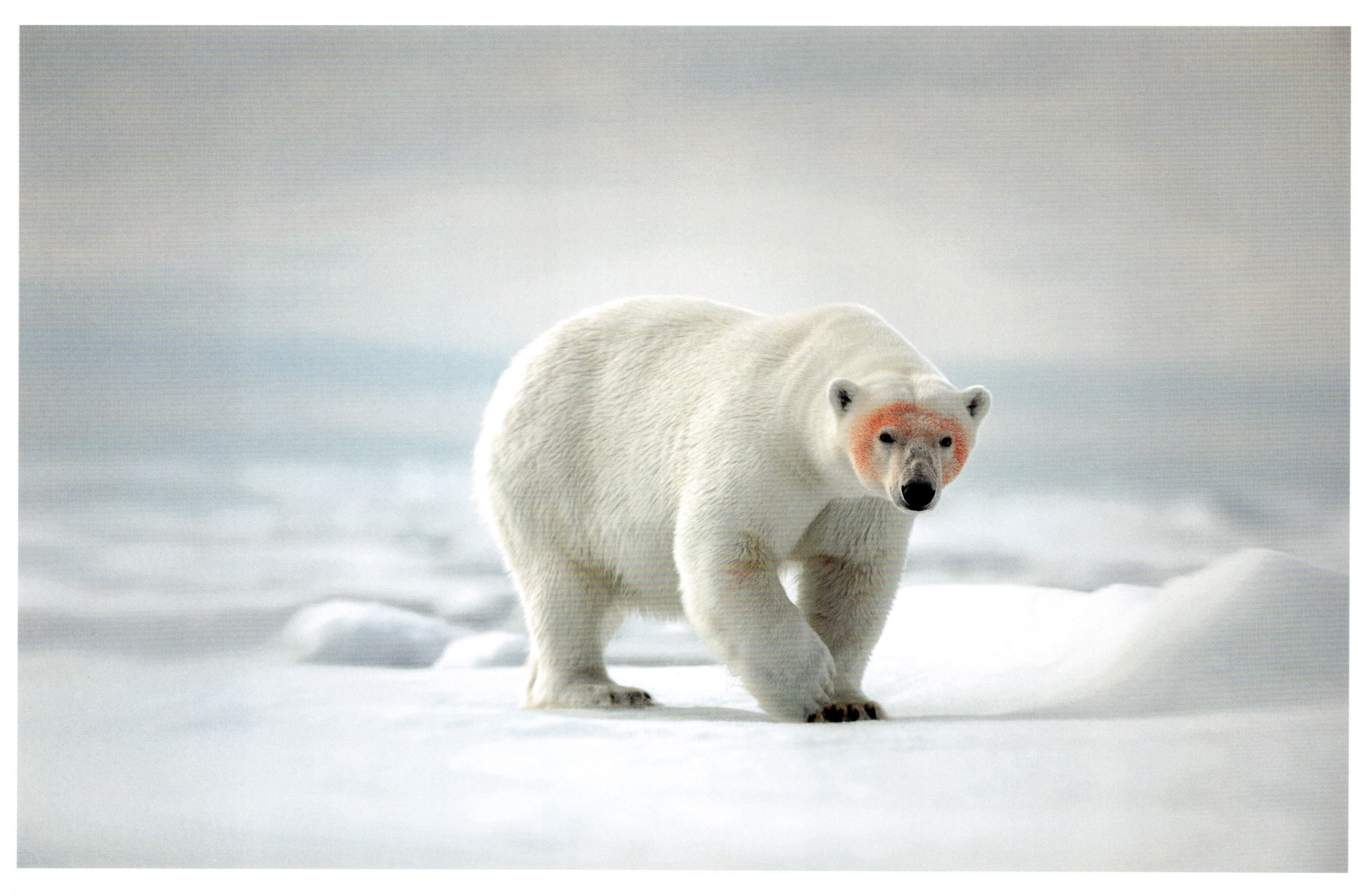

Joshua Holko
Arctic Ocean, Svalbard, Norway

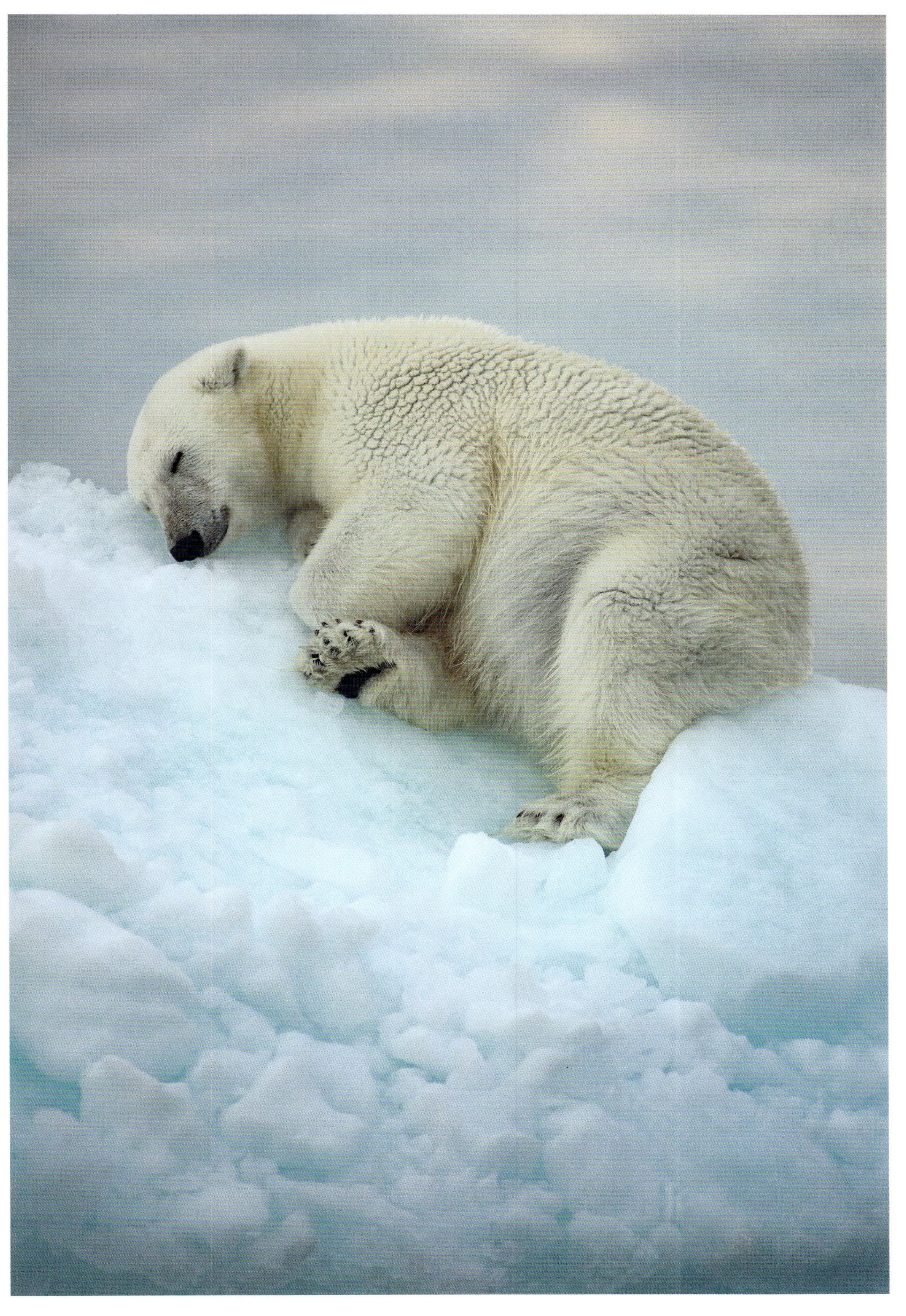

Irene Amiet
Barents Sea, Svalbard, Norway

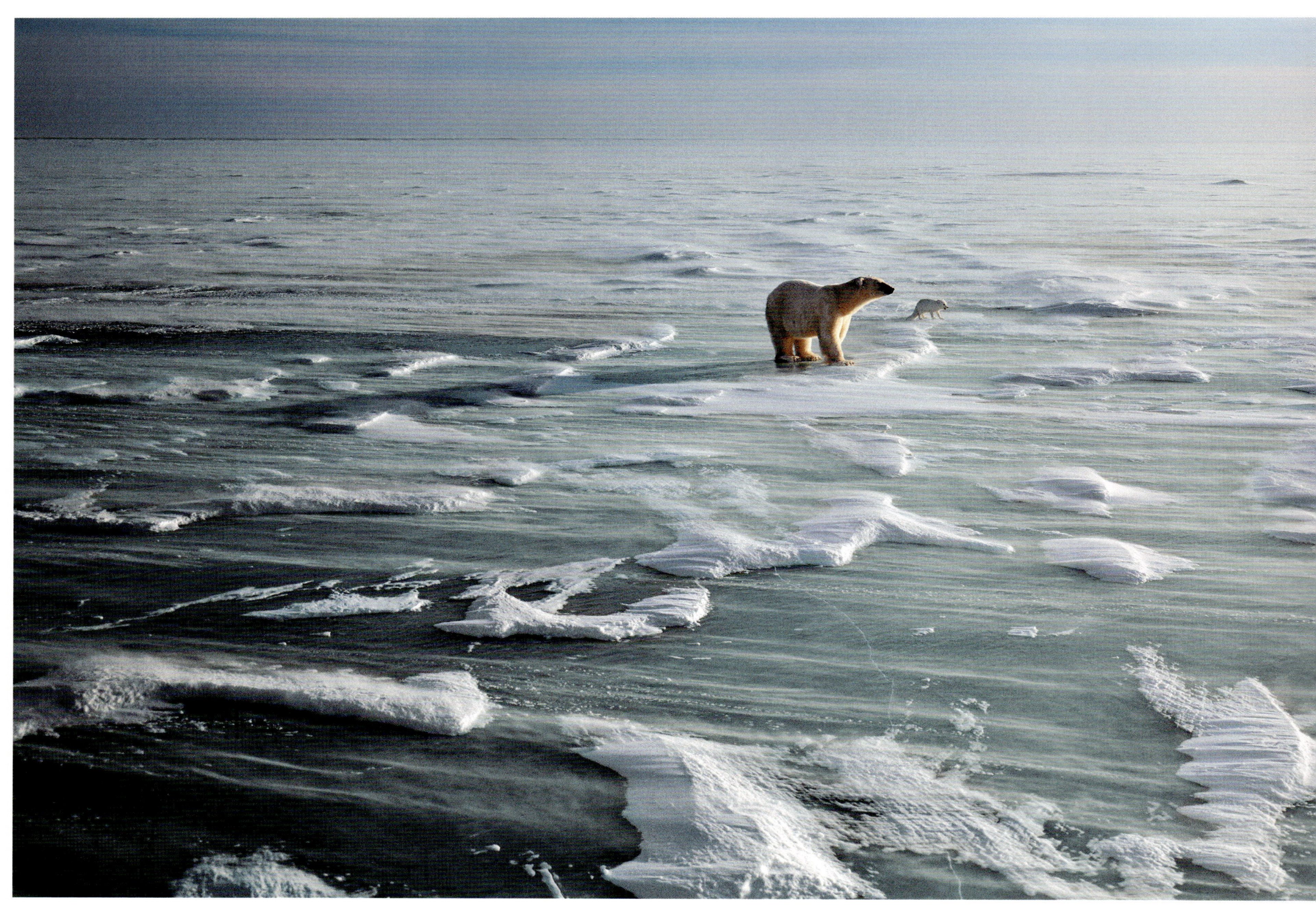

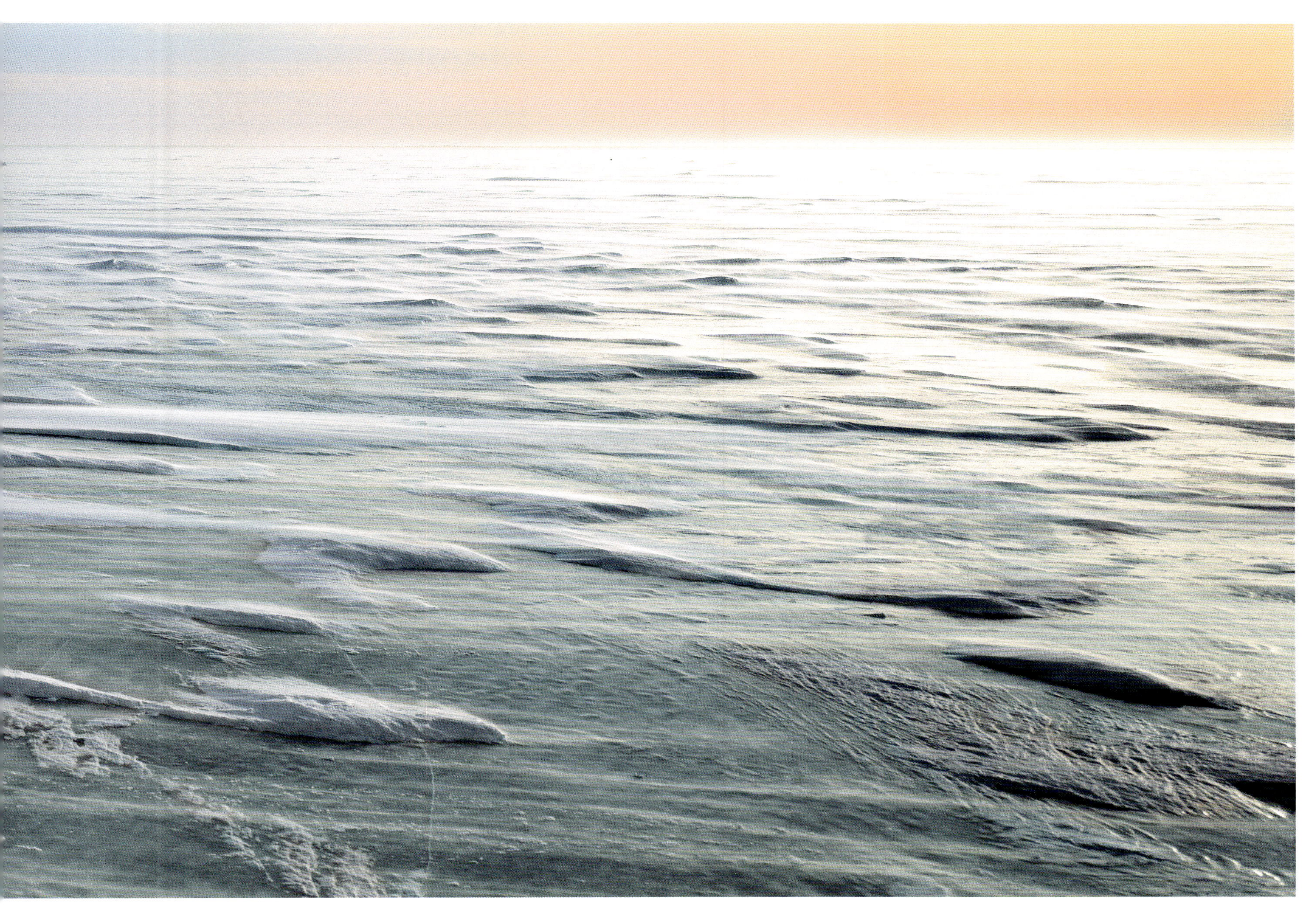

Thomas D. Mangelsen
Hudson Bay, Manitoba, Canada

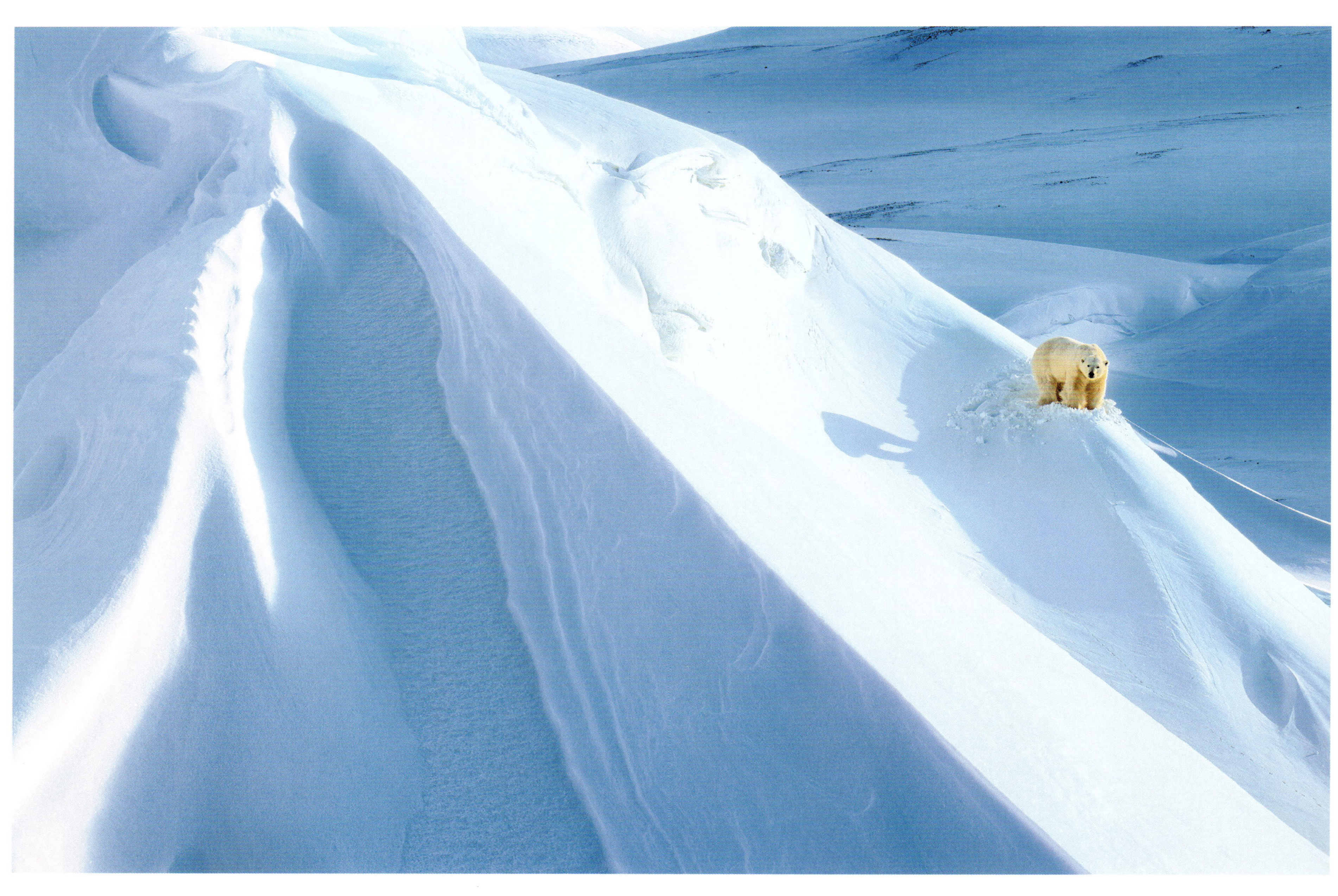

Jasper Doest
Spitsbergen Island, Svalbard, Norway

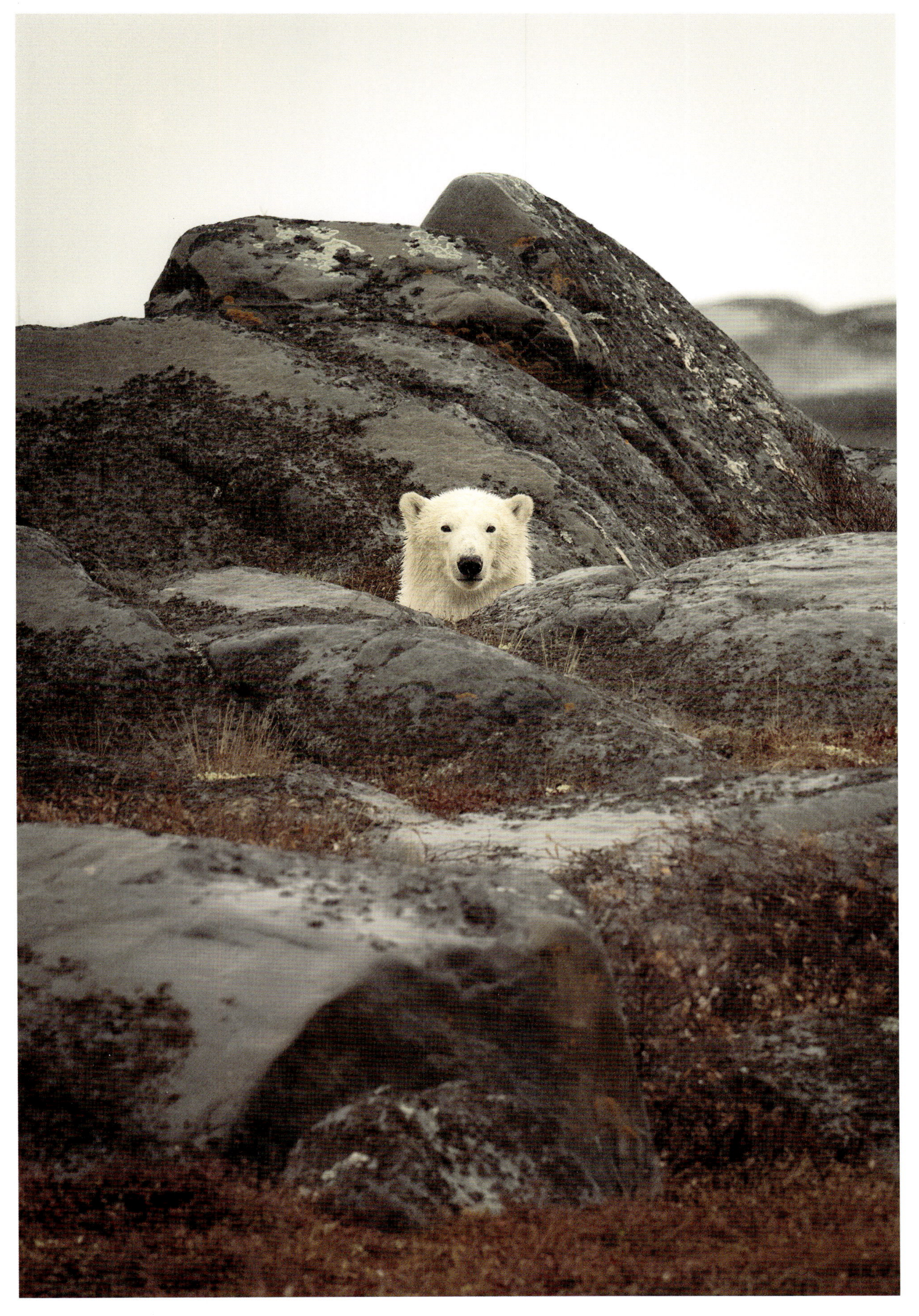

Drew Hamilton
Hudson Bay, Manitoba, Canada

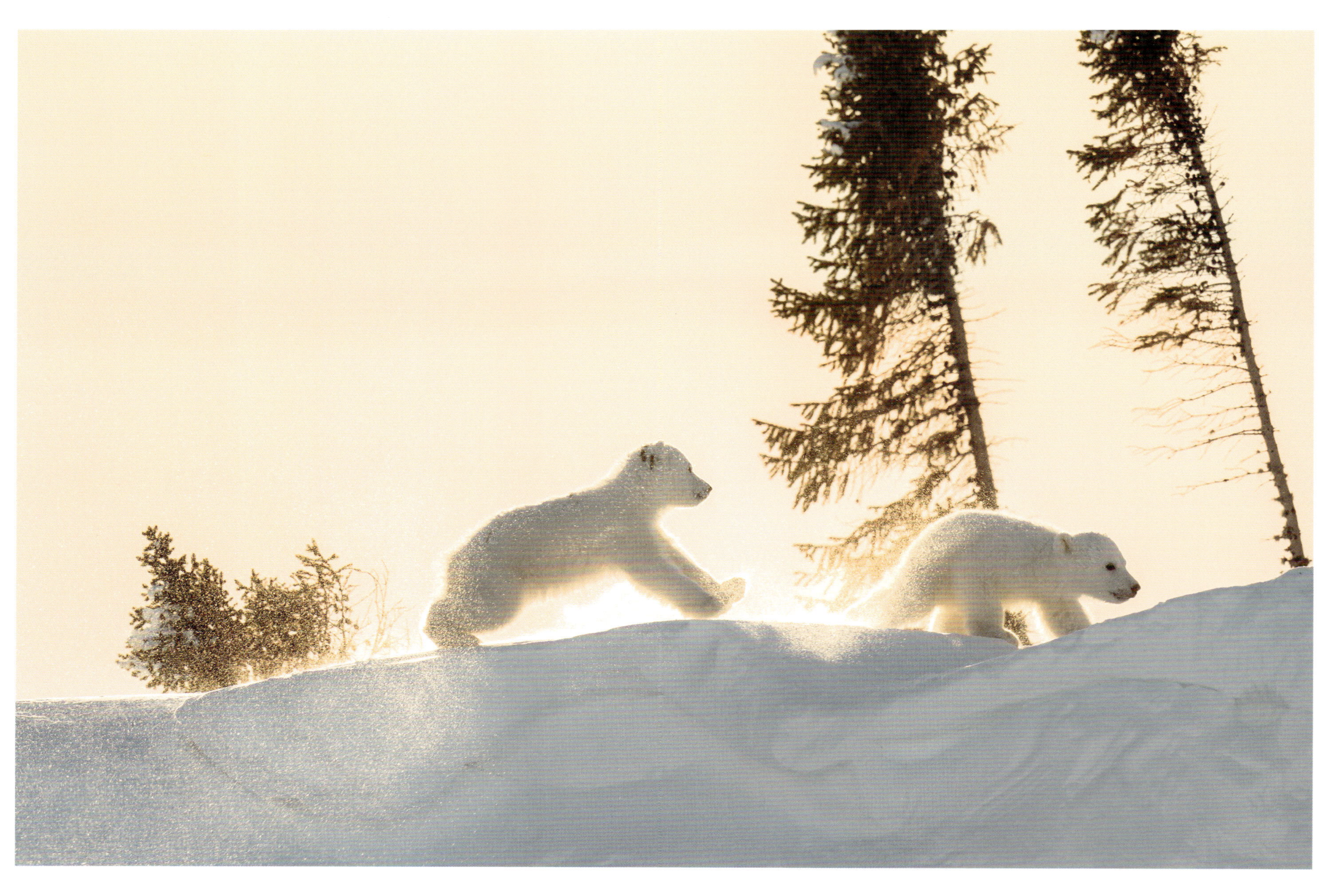

Daisy Gilardini
Wapusk National Park, Manitoba, Canada

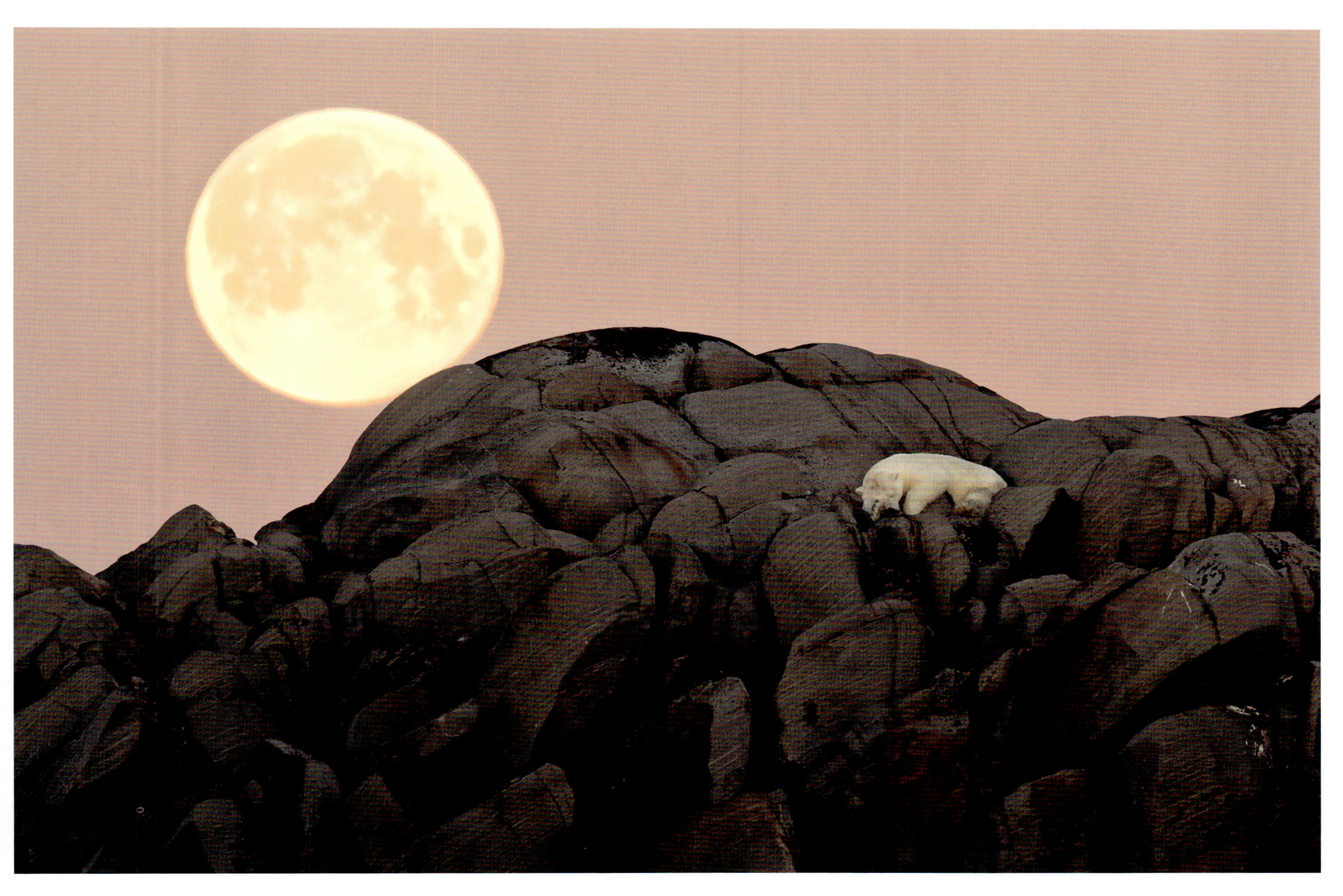

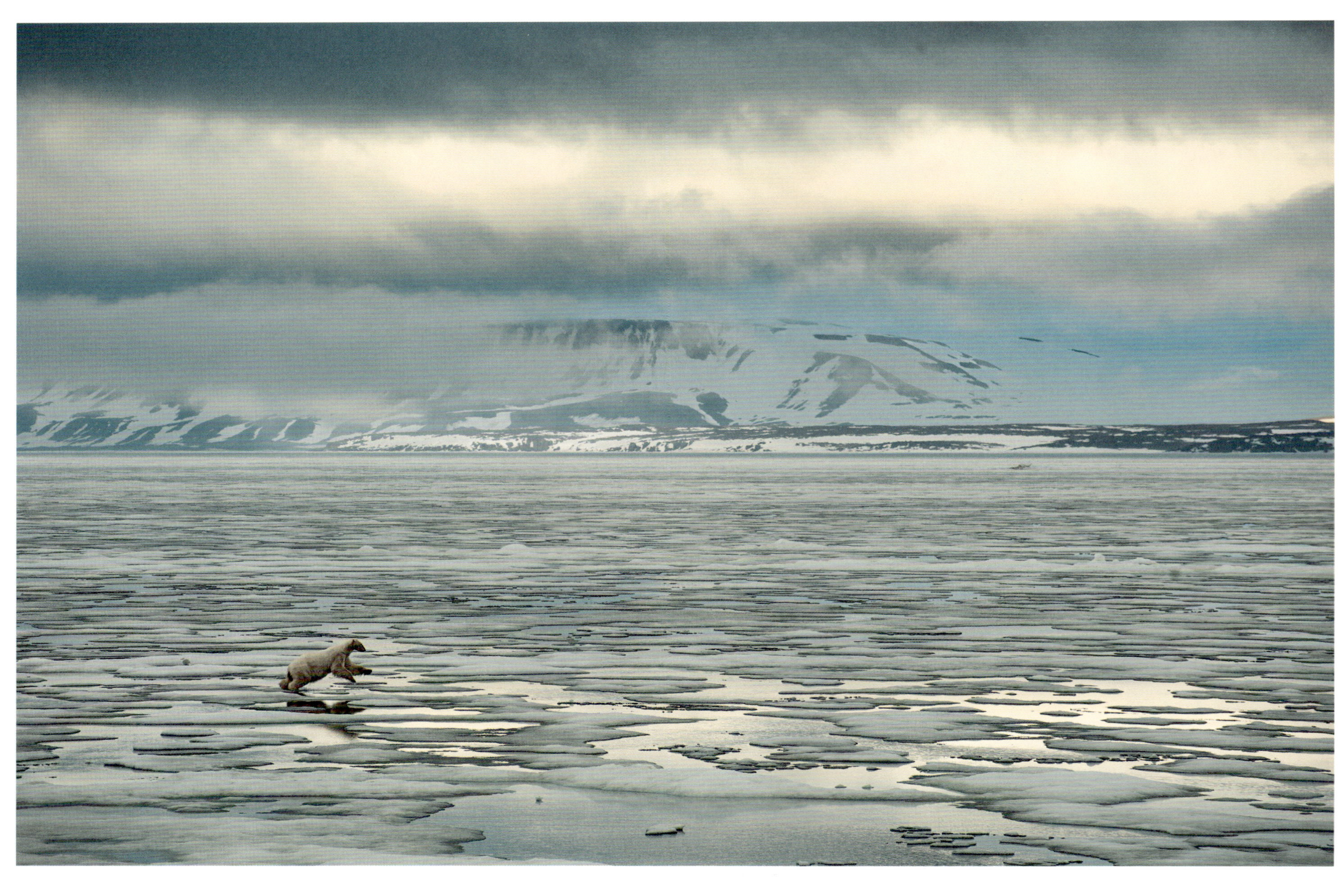

Jim Richardson
Svalbard, Norway

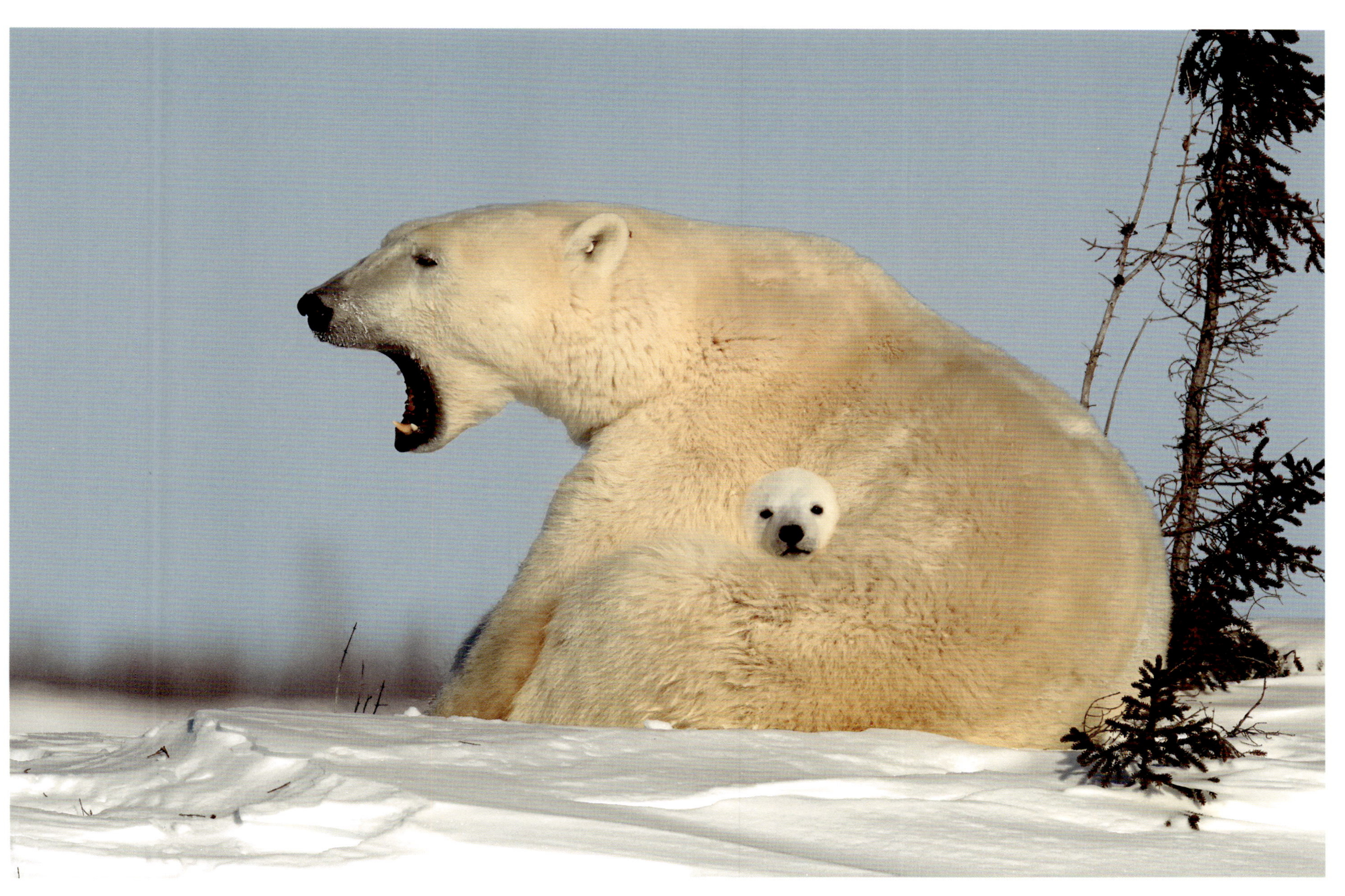

Shogo Asao
Wapusk National Park, Manitoba, Canada

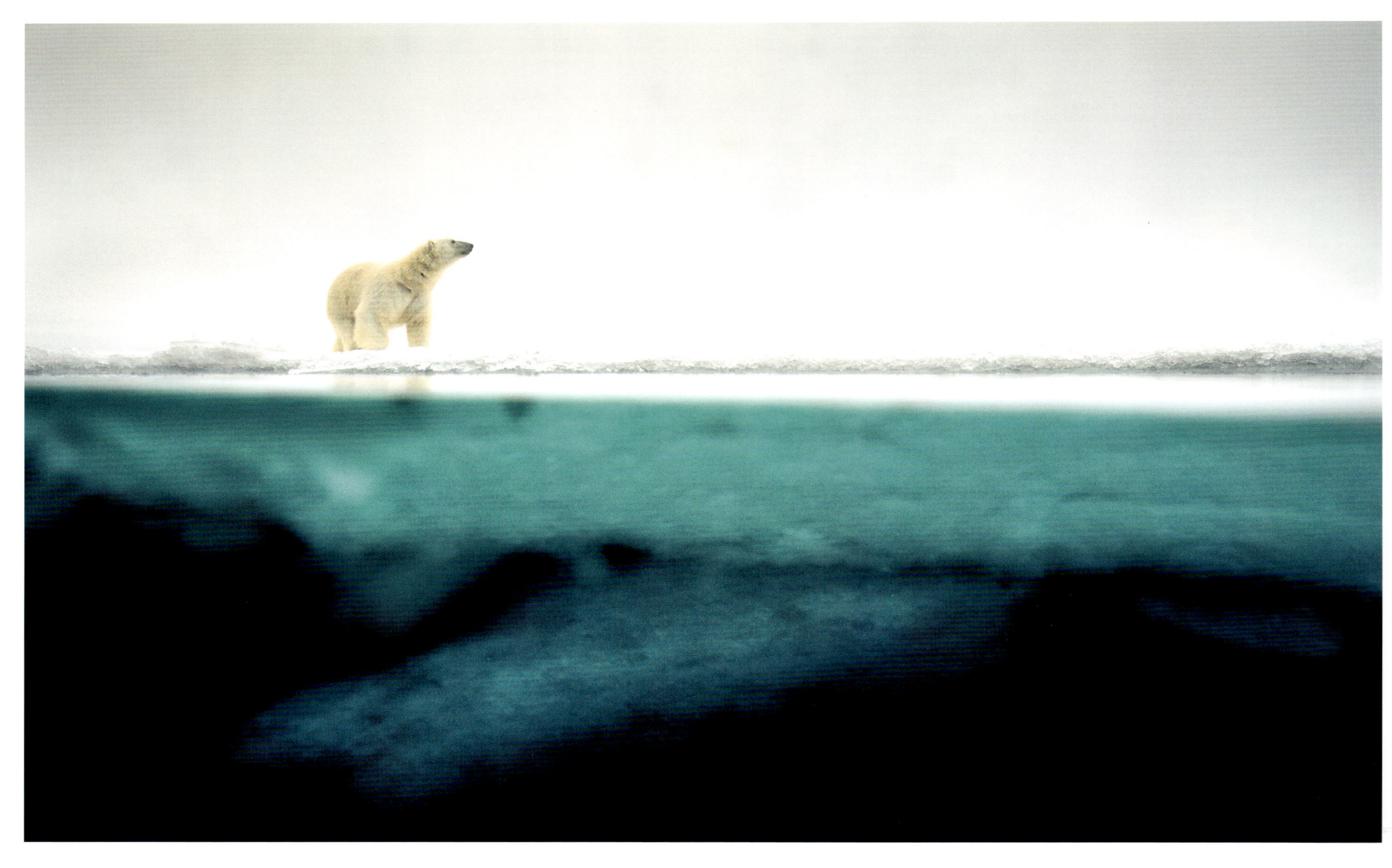

Ole J. Liodden
Svalbard, Norway

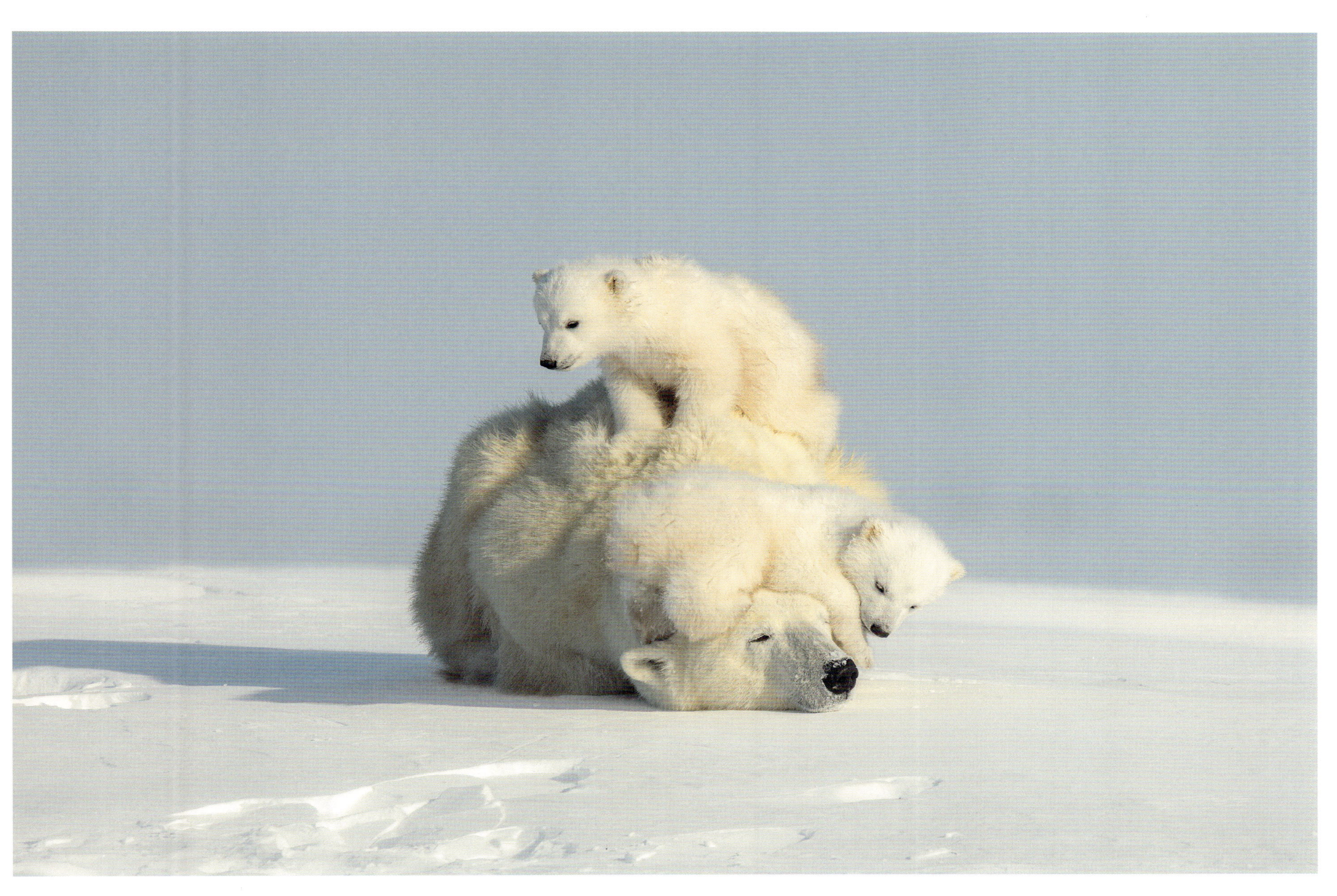

Hao Jiang
Wapusk National Park, Manitoba, Canada

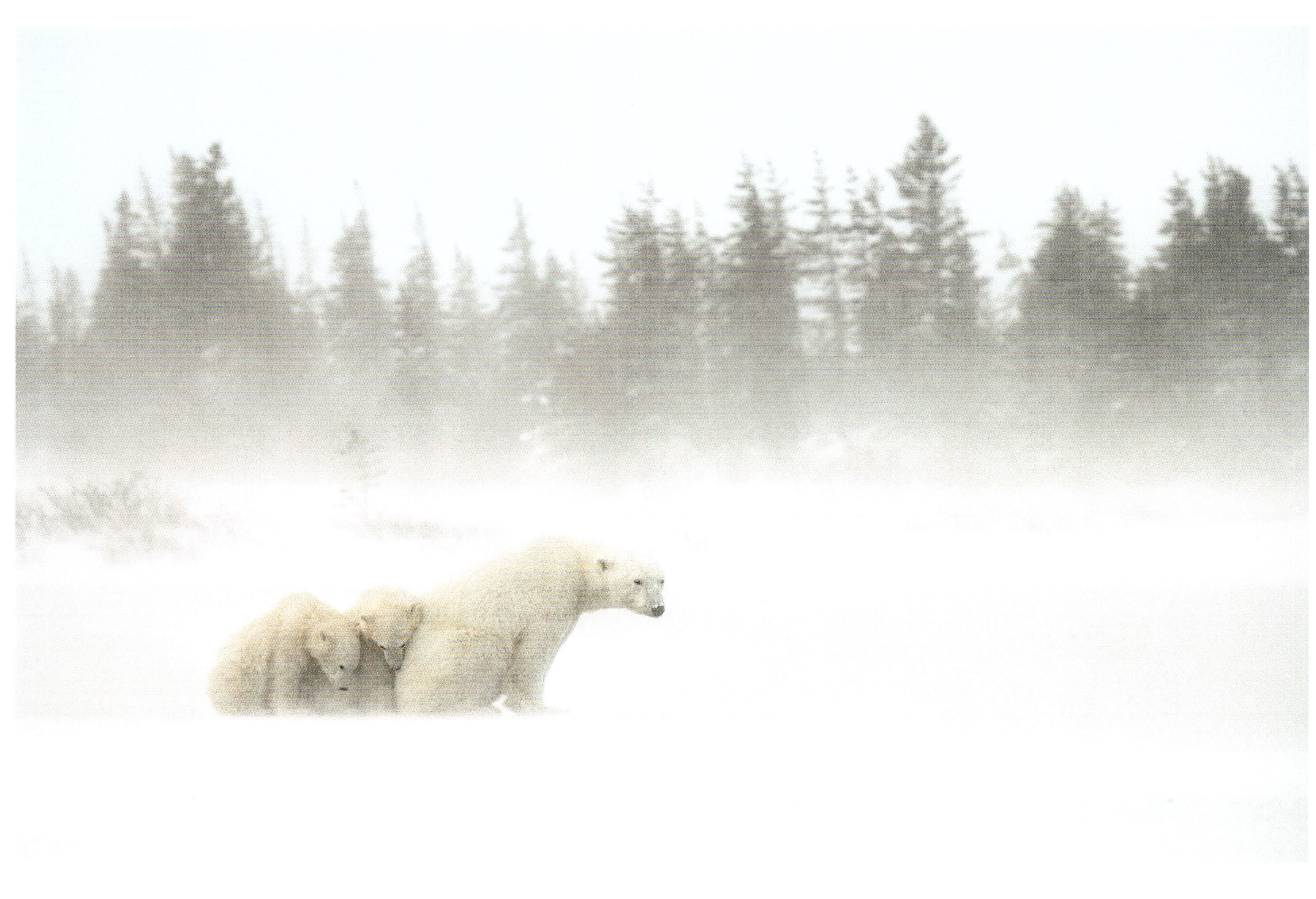

Marco Ronconi
Hudson Bay, Manitoba, Canada

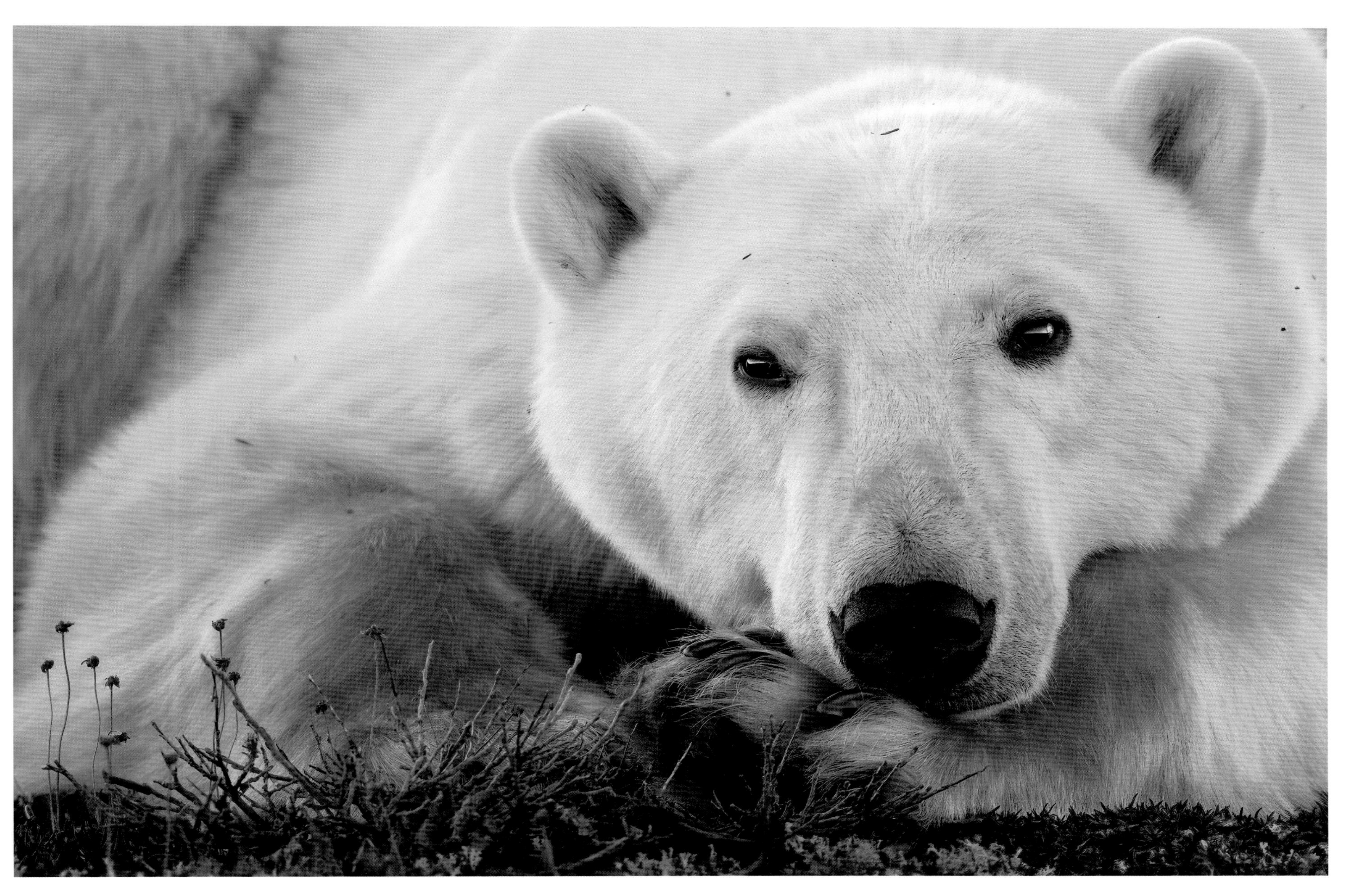

Dave Sandford
Hudson Bay, Manitoba, Canada

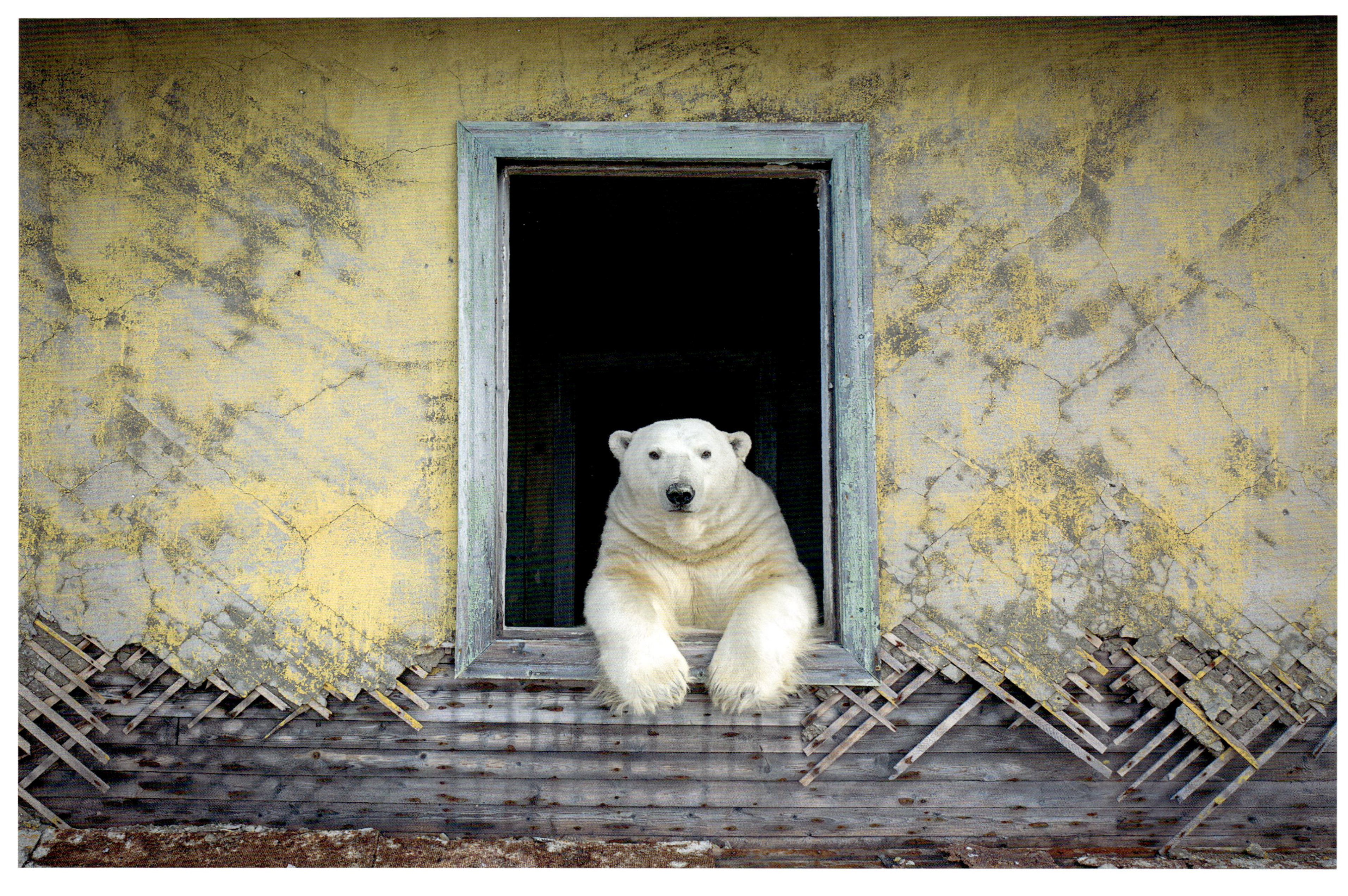

Dmitry Kokh
Kolyuchin Island, Russia

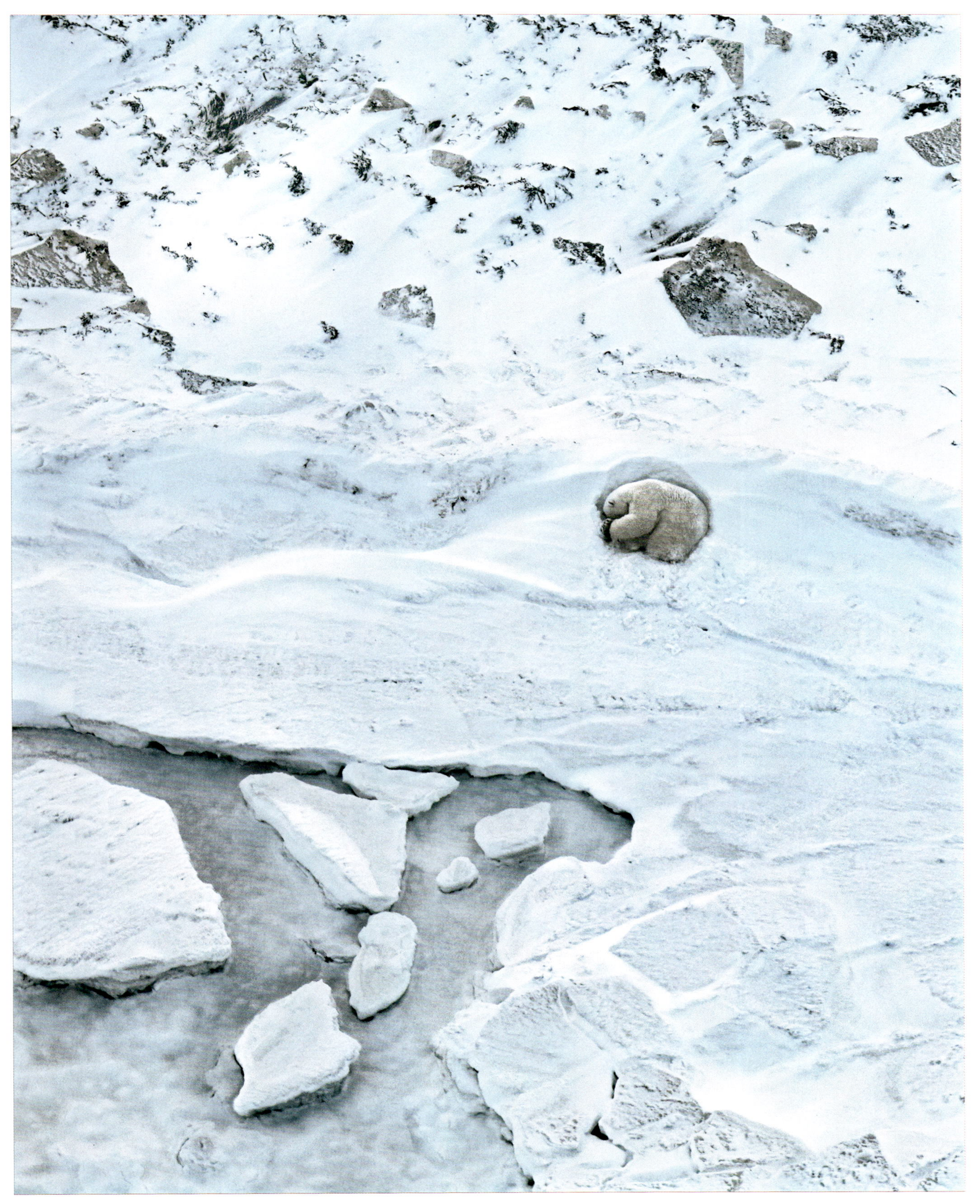

Tim Flach
Hudson Bay, Manitoba, Canada

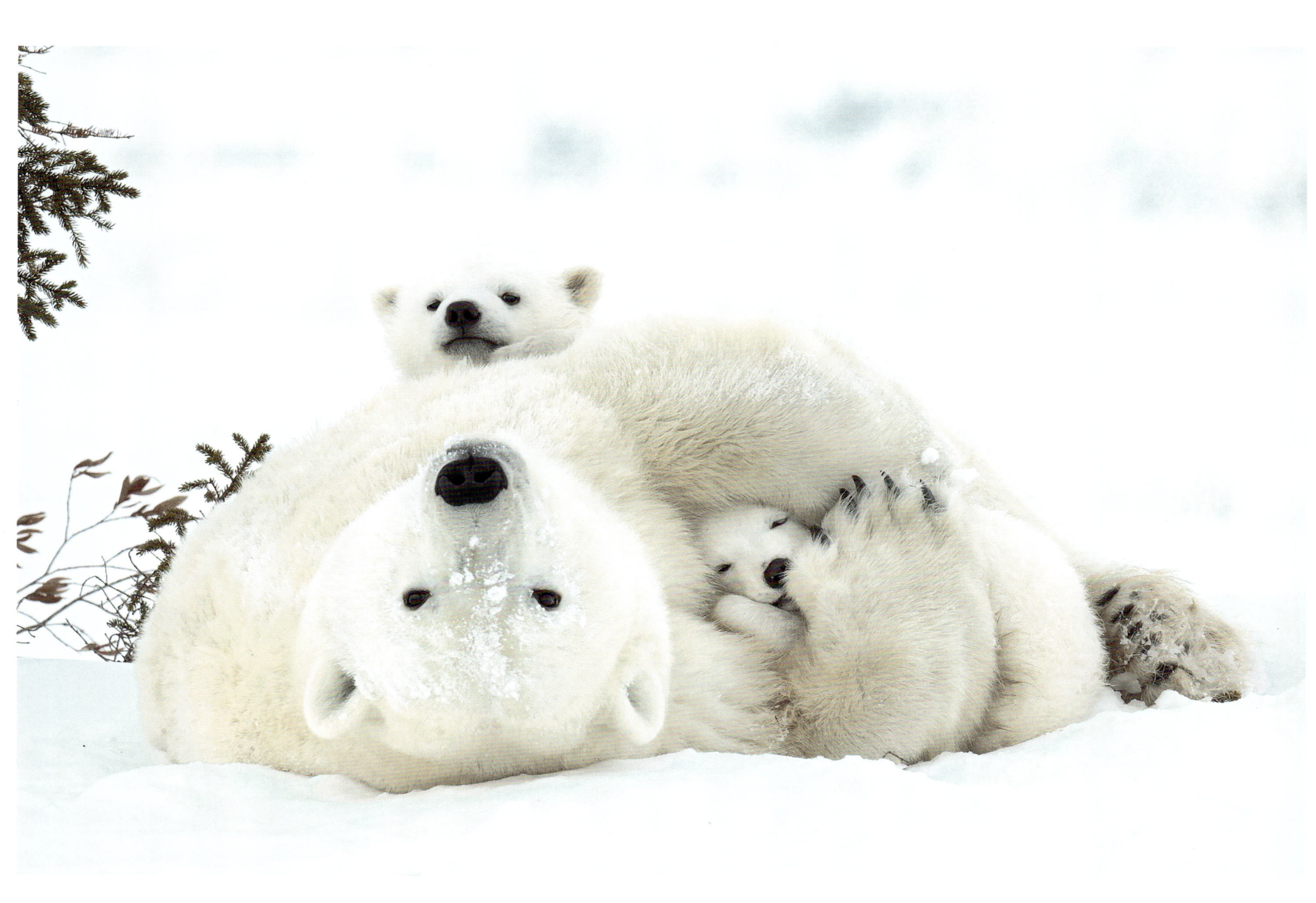

Daisy Gilardini
Wapusk National Park, Manitoba, Canada

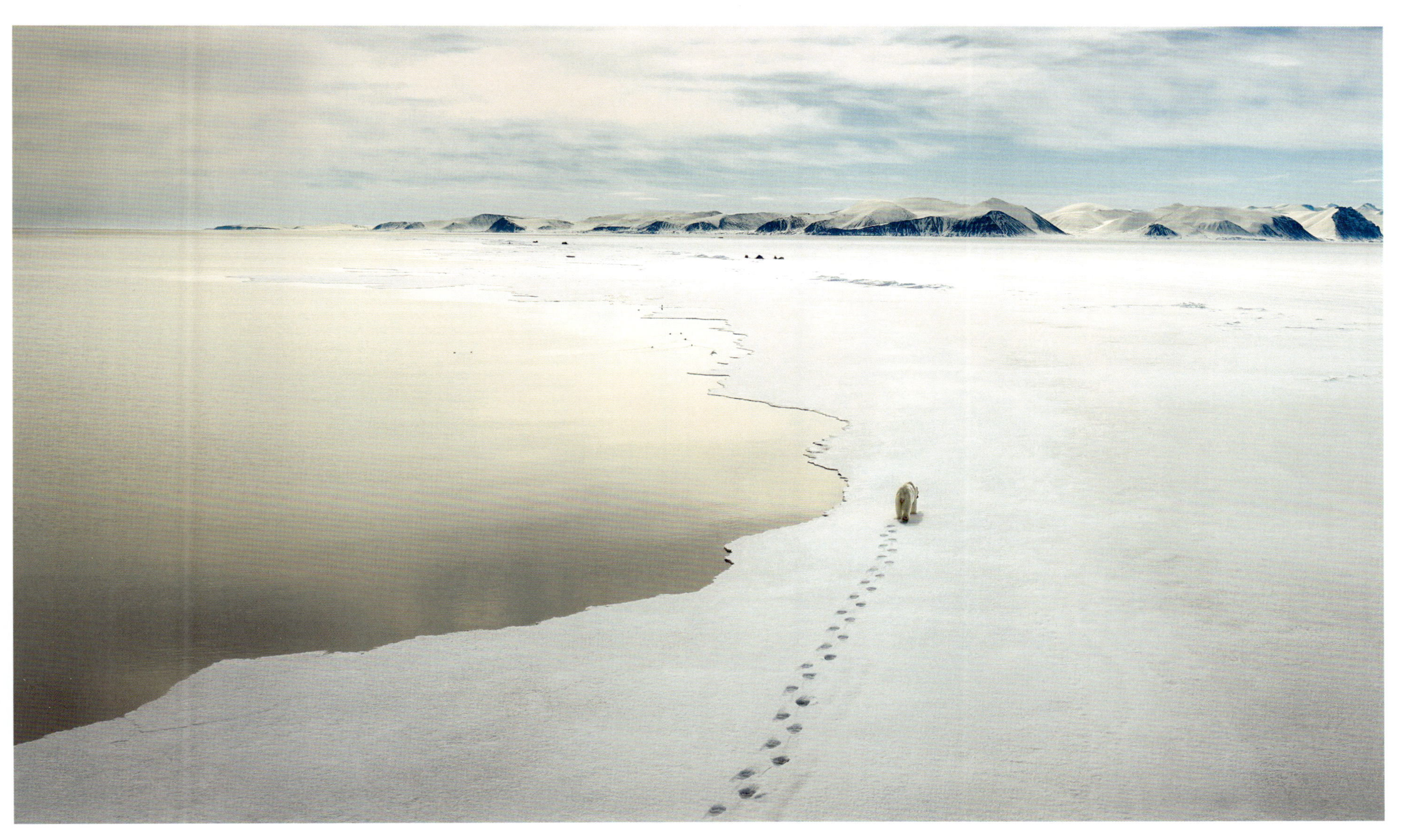

Jenny Wong
Baffin Island, Nunavut, Canada

LIONS

Lions

Dr. Moreangels Mbizah

Founder and Executive Director, Wildlife Conservation Action

LIONS ARE SO SPECIAL TO ME. From the first time I saw lions in the Savé Valley Conservancy in Zimbabwe, I felt a deep connection to these animals. There is something remarkable about lions, an aura that you don't find in any other animals.

The fusion-fission dynamics of lions, in which the size and makeup of their social groups change over time, is something that fascinates me. They maintain very strong bonds between members of their pride, but they also often split into smaller subgroups and then come together to form a larger group from time to time. All of this is often dependent on prevailing ecological conditions. These smaller subgroups tend to kill smaller-sized prey, compared to the larger-sized prey, like buffalo and sometimes baby elephants, that are killed by larger prides.

A few days after I had joined the Lion Research Project in Hwange National Park in Zimbabwe, I went out with other researchers to look for lions so we could put a GPS radio collar on one of them to study it. We drove around the wildlife area just outside the park for hours looking for these lions, and finally found them hiding in the bush and feeding on an old elephant carcass. It was my first time seeing lions in Hwange. We managed to get very close to them, as we needed to dart one of them. When the lion we'd darted was immobilized, we carefully approached it and managed to put on the collar. This was an experience that will always stay etched in my heart. Touching the lion and watching its tummy heave as it breathed was magical.

Lions are an important and iconic part of African culture, and a symbol for strength, courage, pride, wisdom, authority, and protection. The lion is considered the king of the jungle, despite the fact that lions don't spend their time in the jungle, but instead prefer the savanna. They have also had a huge influence in literature, film, and art, and they're a very popular and cool source of imagery. Many companies from around the world use lions in their logos.

In most Bantu cultures, a lion is a totem that symbolizes strength, courage, and personal power. Those people with the lion totem have the responsibility to protect the lion. In the Zimbabwean Shona culture, a lion is called "mhondoro." It's believed that mhondoro spirits reside in the bodies of maneless lions until they have a human host to possess, and that the person who is possessed will give advice based on the communication from the spirit. Losing the African lion would mean losing a part of who we are as an African people, a part of our culture and heritage.

There are fewer than 20,000 lions remaining in the wild. In Africa, they currently inhabit less than 8 percent of their former range. Although lions also previously existed in many other countries, outside of Africa, lions can only be found today in the wild in one location: Gir National Park in India.

Lions are currently facing complex threats. Unfortunately, many of these threats are caused by humans. Habitat loss is one of the major challenges. Their habitat is shrinking and becoming more disconnected due to the increase in human populations and increased demand for agricultural land. Human-wildlife conflict is another huge threat. Humans and large predators, like lions, have been coexisting together in the same spaces for hundreds of years. However, the interactions between humans and lions are now increasing, due to the encroachment of humans into wildlife areas. Local communities that live around wildlife areas often come into contact with lions, and many times these interactions are negative, with lions killing livestock and injuring or killing people. As a result, these communities retaliate by killing the lions.

Lions are also facing a decline in their prey, due to illegal bushmeat poaching of prey species. Some lions, too, may be caught and killed in the snares intended for herbivores. Lions are also being targeted for body parts for the illegal, international wildlife trade, including as substitutes for highly prized tiger bones, as well as being used for traditional customs in parts of Africa.

Our best chance of saving lions is by involving everyone in conservation efforts. The communities that live with the lions are the ones best positioned to help lions the most. Coexistence can be promoted by reducing interactions between humans and lions and preventing human-lion conflict from happening. This can be done through the strengthening of traditional livestock kraals, or pens, and the provision of mobile predator-proof livestock bomas, which protect livestock from predation by lions.

Local people should be at the forefront of the solutions to the challenges facing lions and other wildlife species. They can play a huge role in protecting habitats and increasing connectivity between fragmented wildlife habitats. We must create more opportunities for local and Indigenous conservationists and offer them the support that they need to contribute to lion conservation and lead conservation efforts in their countries.

In the past, conservation has just been about protecting wildlife species and habitats, and very little concern was given to the people that live around these areas. Conservation should be about both nature and people and should aim to reduce the costs local communities face from living with and protecting wildlife, as well as increasing the benefits. If local communities don't have a direct connection or benefit from protecting lions, they have no reason to want to do so. Local communities should be involved in every stage of each conservation project, from planning to implementation. It's also important to train them and give them skills, such as project management. They should be able to make decisions, and their voices need to be heard. If communities feel left out or feel that an outsider is telling them what to do, they might resist. Some signs of resistance could include poaching, vandalizing property, or just influencing other people not to cooperate or get involved in conservation activities. If local communities don't protect these lions, then no amount of outside intervention will work.

When you protect lions, you protect the entire ecosystem. If lions disappear, then the prey populations of herbivores will balloon, and the herbivores will overgraze the grass and plants. The savanna would become a sandy desert and we would end up losing a lot of species. This is why we need to invest more in protecting lions across their range, protecting their habitat, and connecting lion landscapes.

We need to find holistic solutions to conservation challenges that address the needs of both people and wildlife. We must actively dismantle the hurdles we have created, which are leaving local people and Indigenous populations out of conservation efforts. We need a new conservation model that is built upon the empowerment of local people and their involvement in conservation decision-making, one that also addresses their socioeconomic challenges.

I remain optimistic about the future of wildlife and conservation. Although there are many depressing stories and losses that we have encountered in our fight to protect biodiversity, there are also vital wins and triumphs that we should celebrate. These wins give me hope that we will succeed in protecting the planet and making it a safer and more beautiful place for future generations.

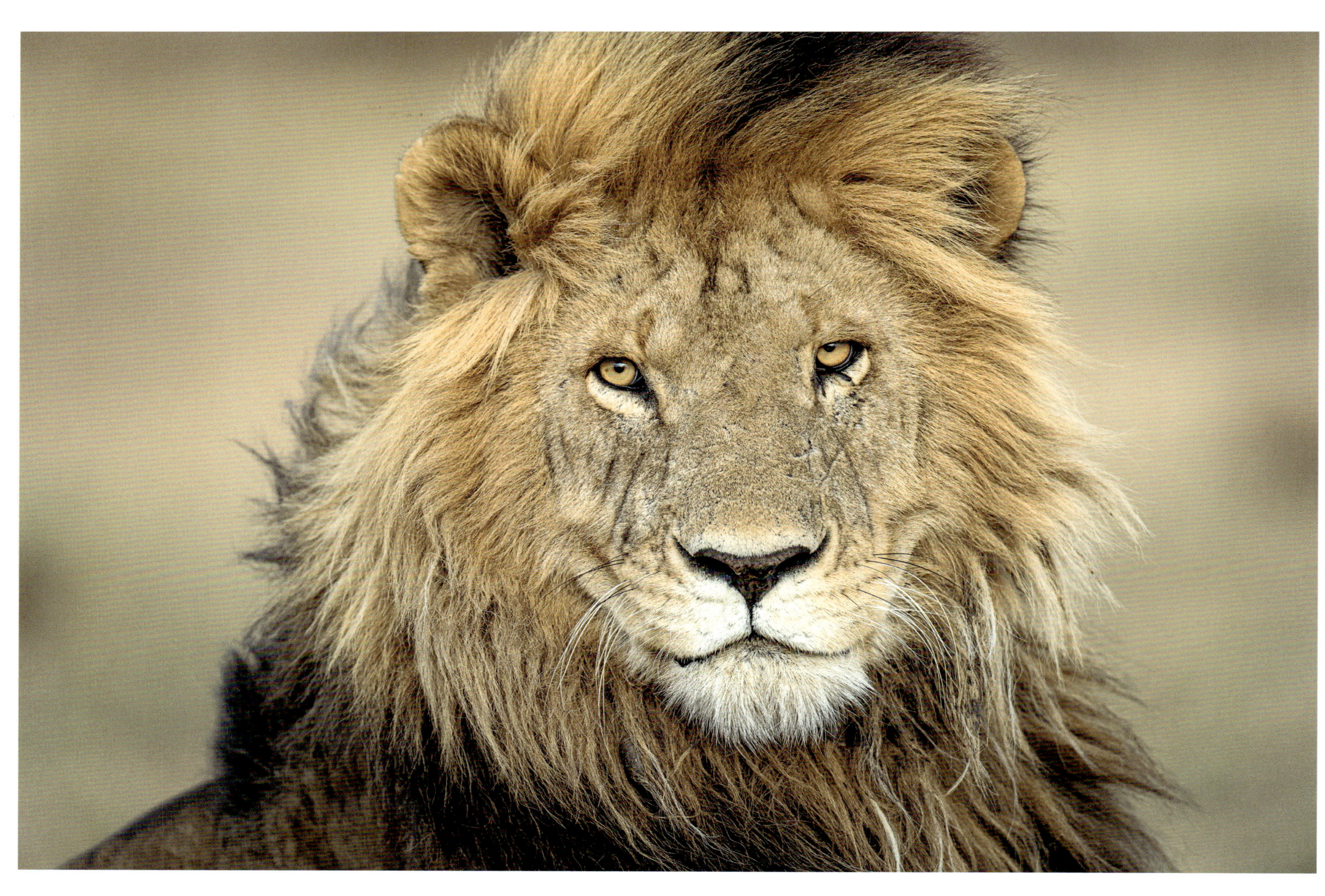

Richard Peters
African Lion
Maasai Mara National Reserve, Kenya

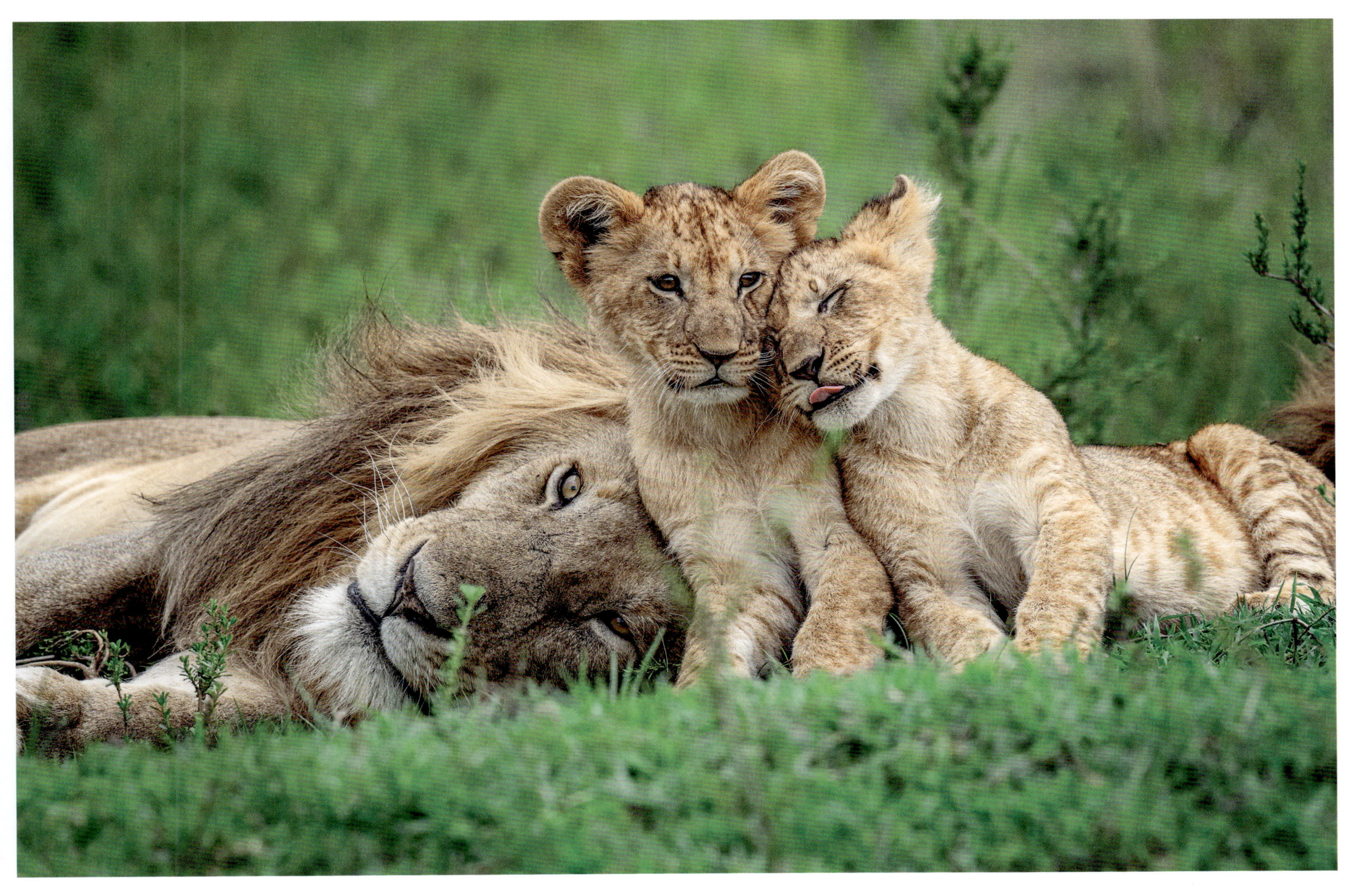

Jonathan and Angela Scott
African Lions
Maasai Mara National Reserve, Kenya

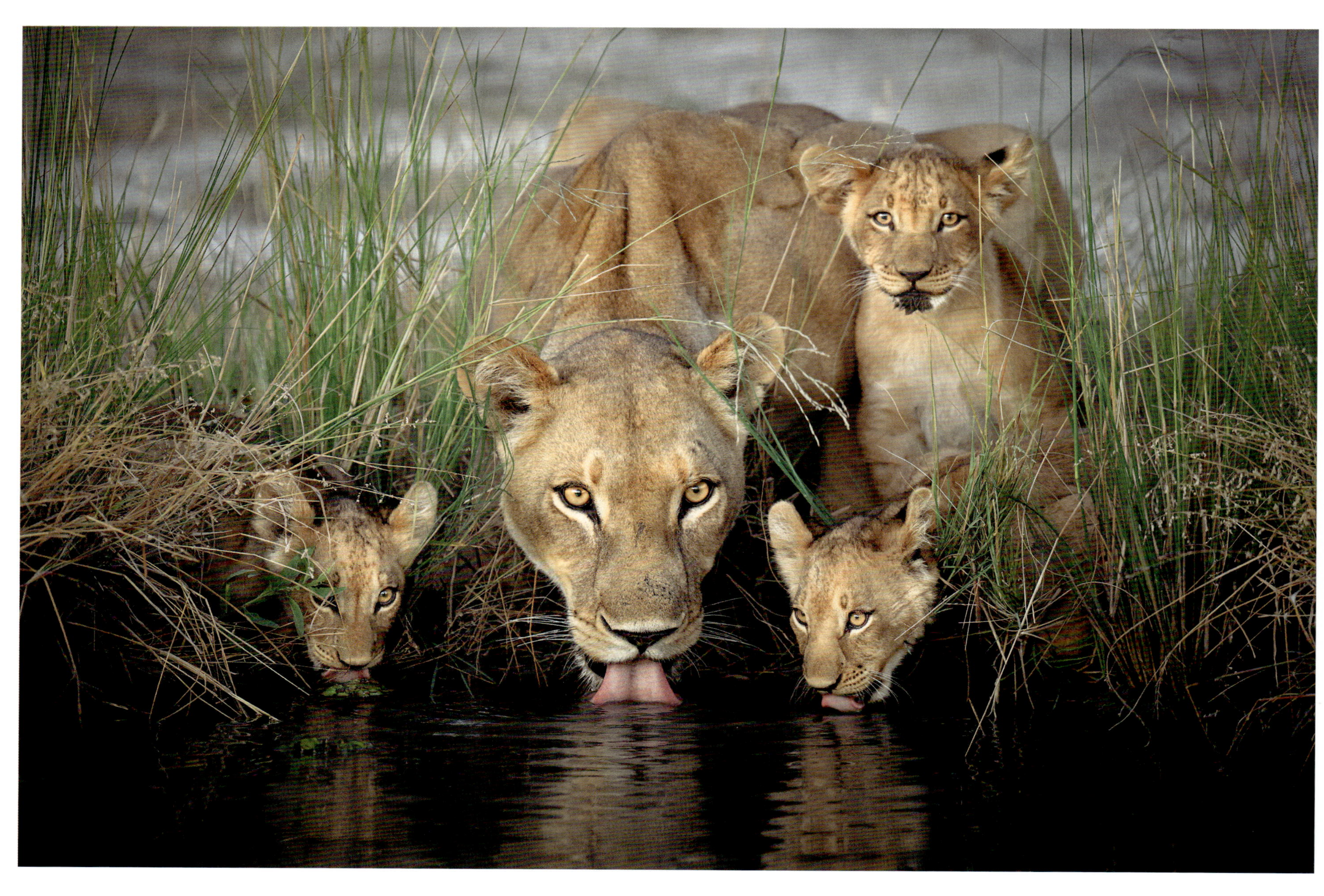

Marsel van Oosten
African Lions
Okavango Delta, Botswana

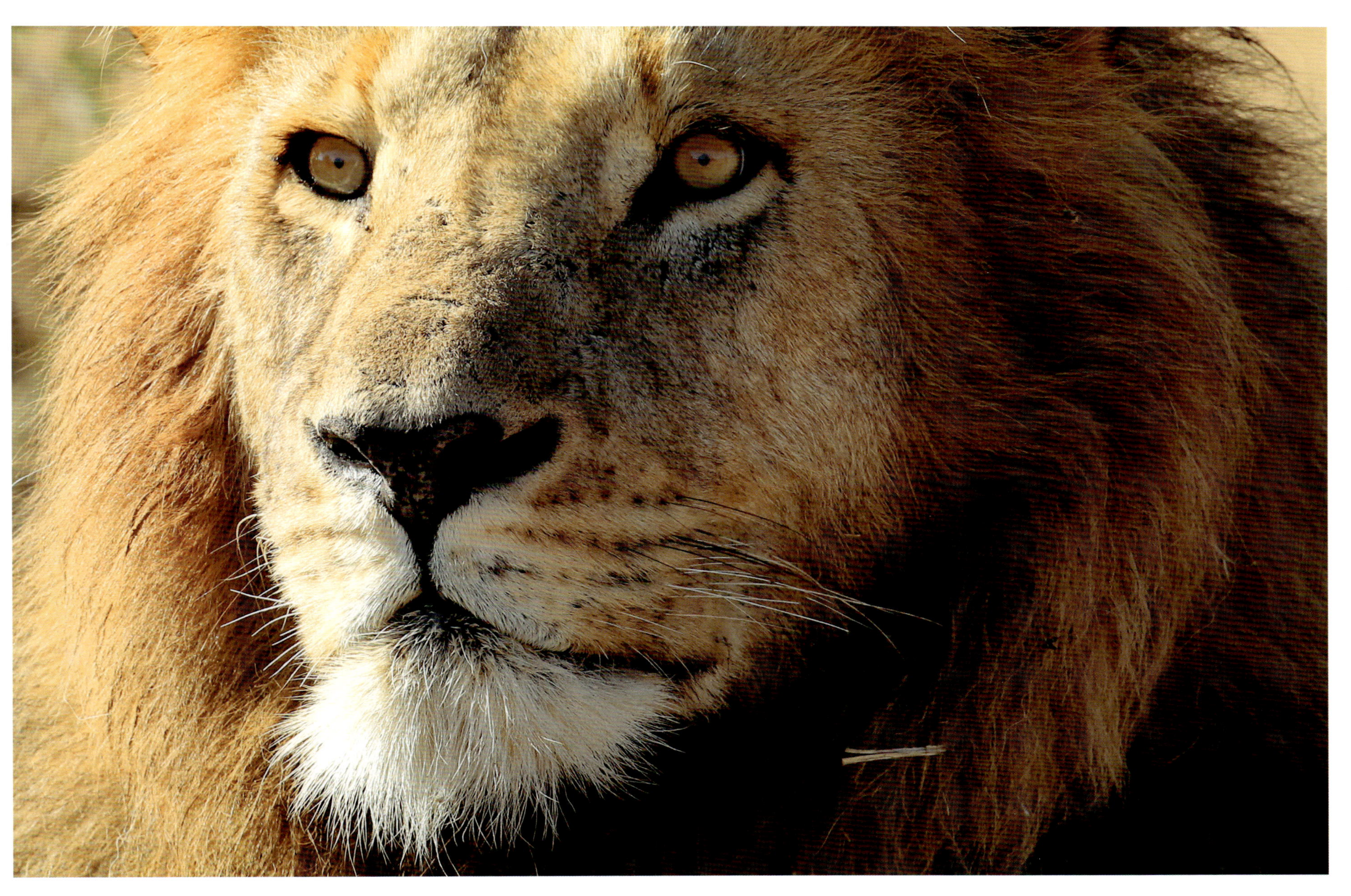

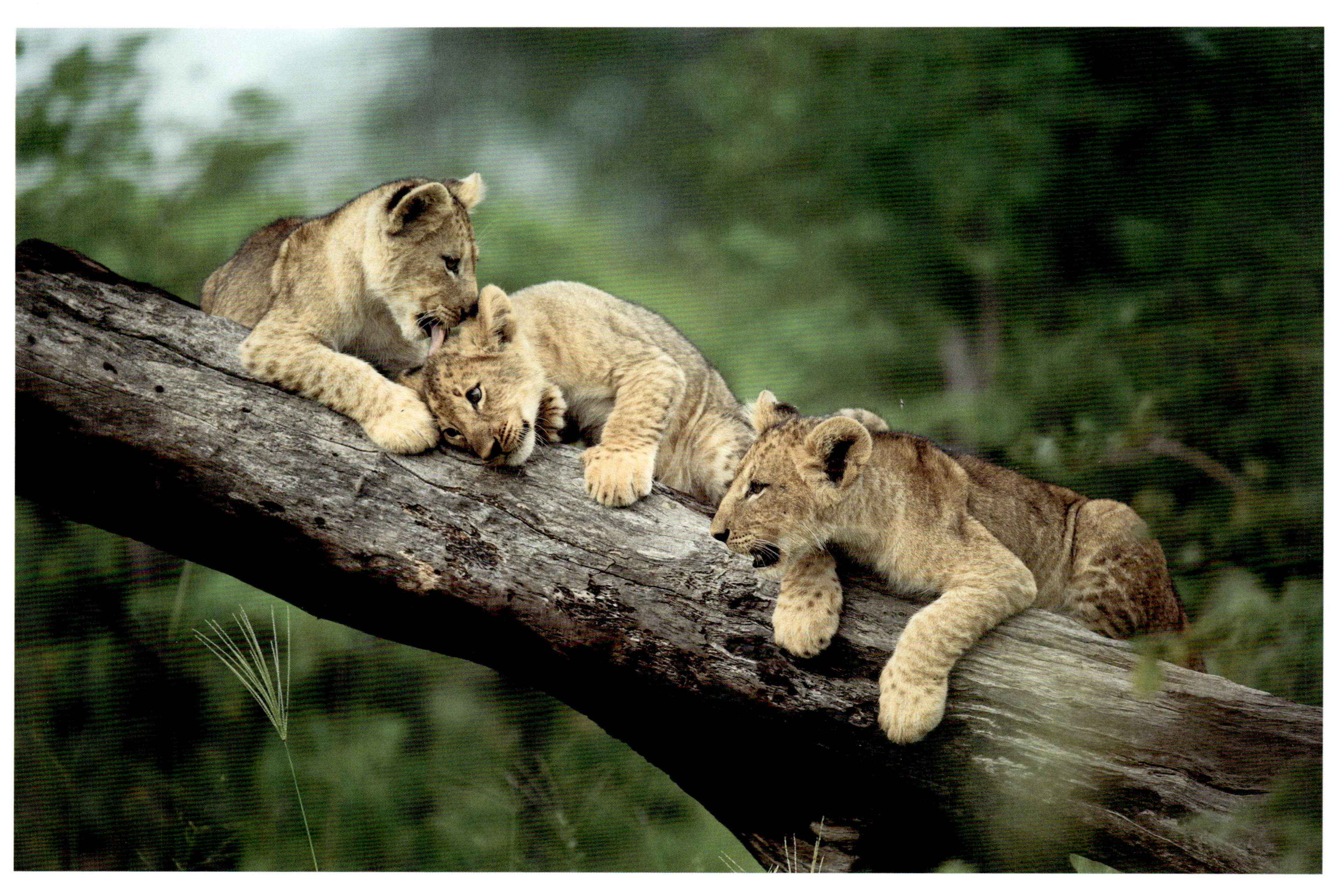

Carole Deschuymere
African Lions
Okavango Delta, Botswana

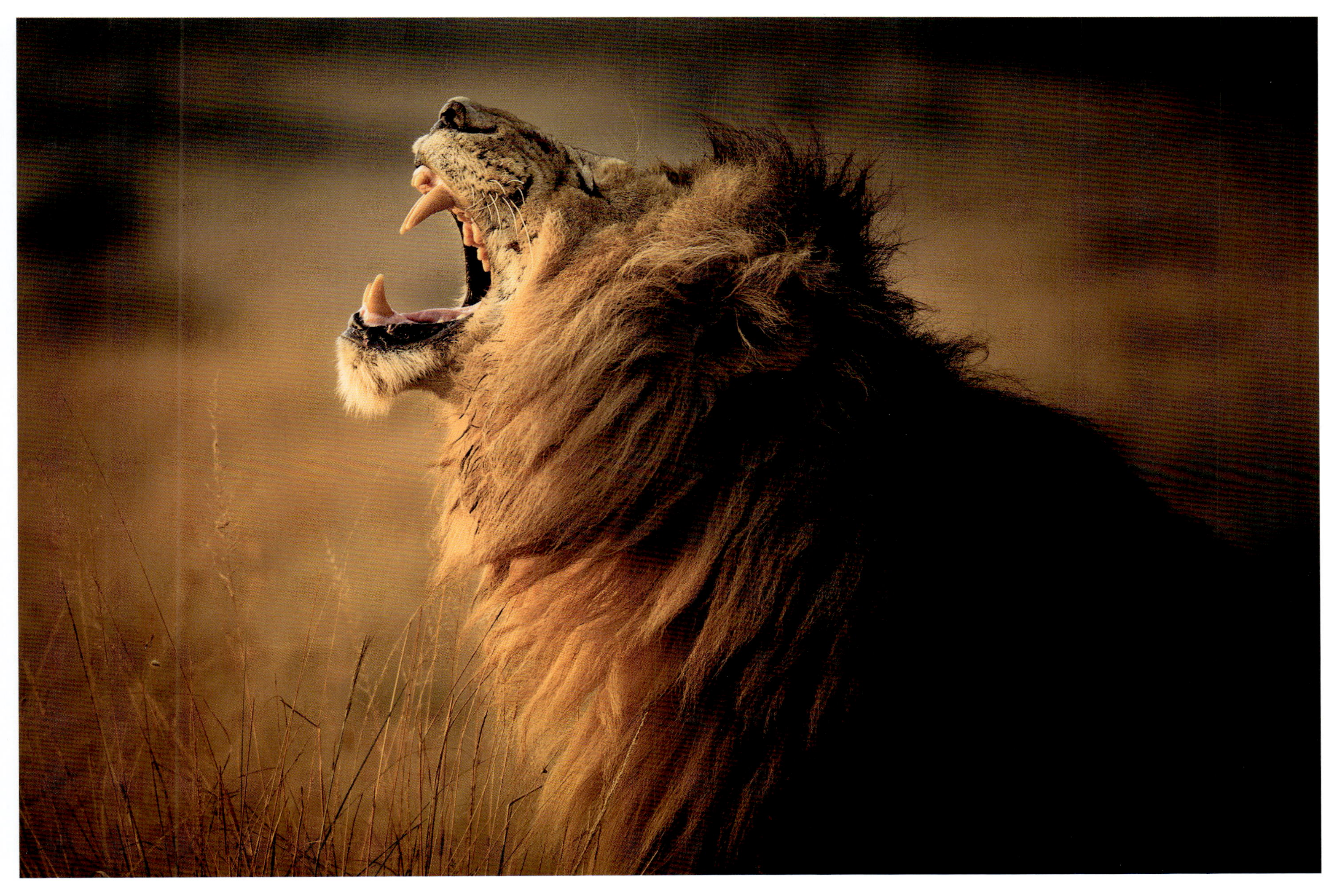

Clement Kiragu
African Lion
Maasai Mara National Reserve, Kenya

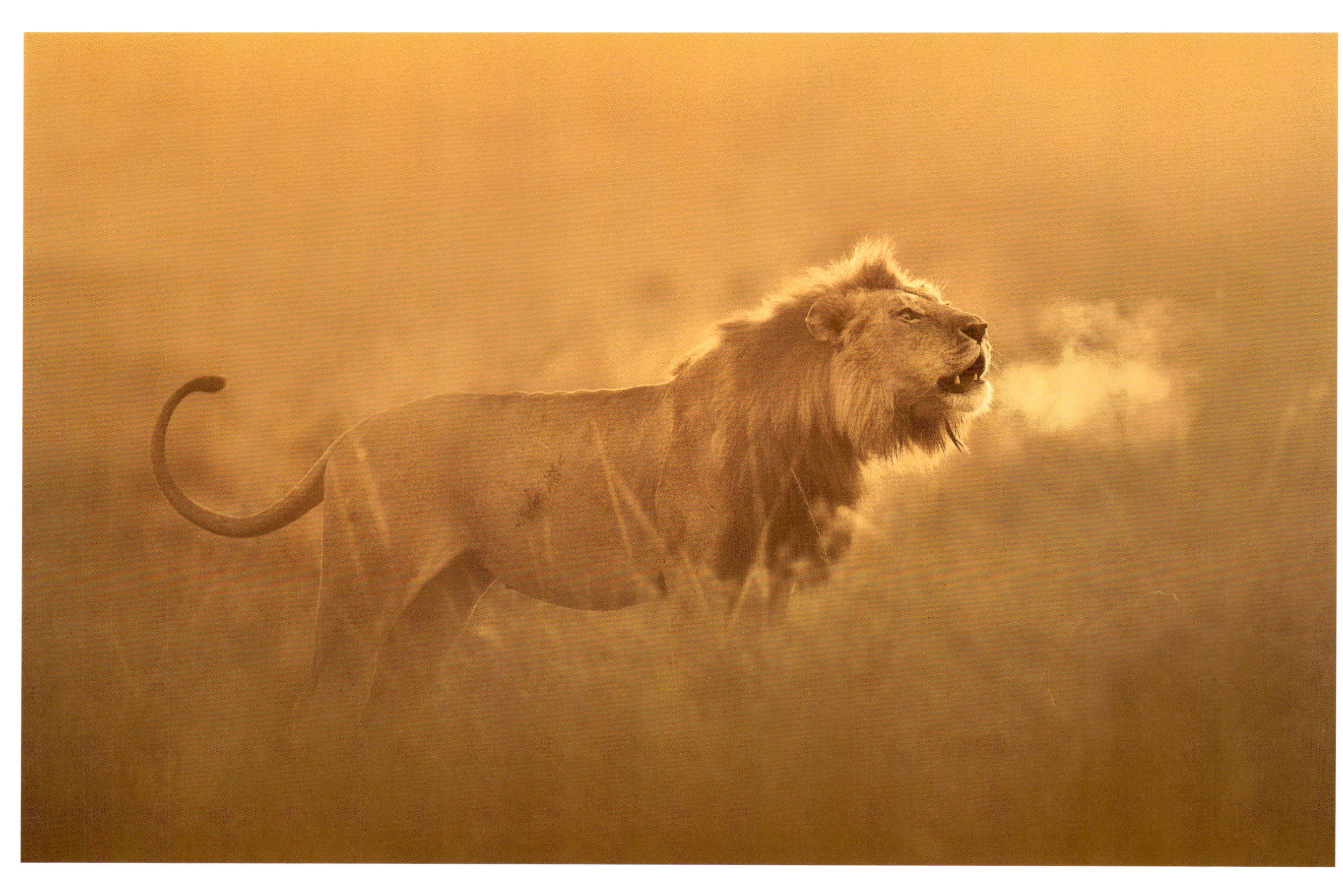

Marina Cano
African Lion
Maasai Mara National Reserve, Kenya

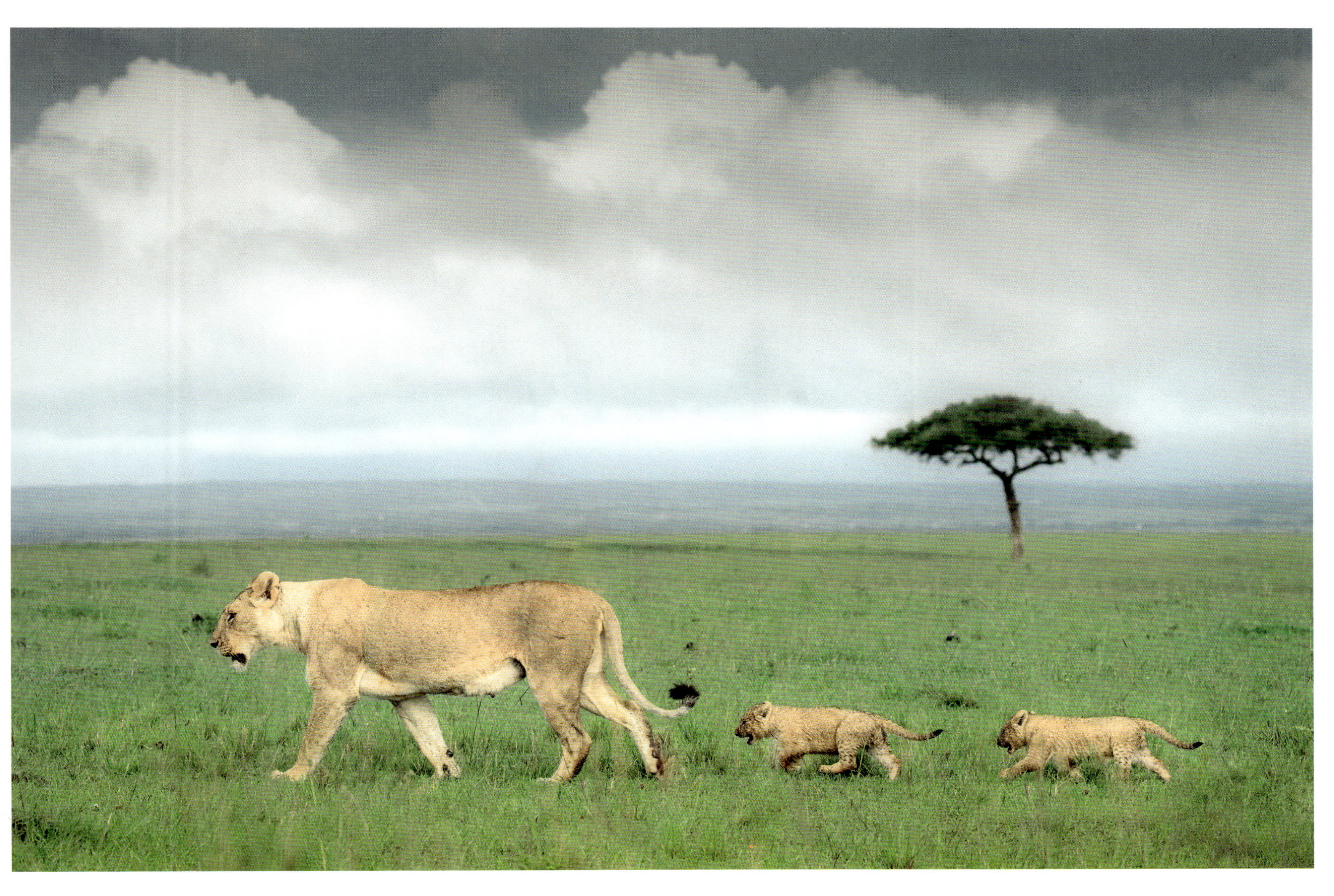

Marco Gaiotti
African Lions
Maasai Mara National Reserve, Kenya

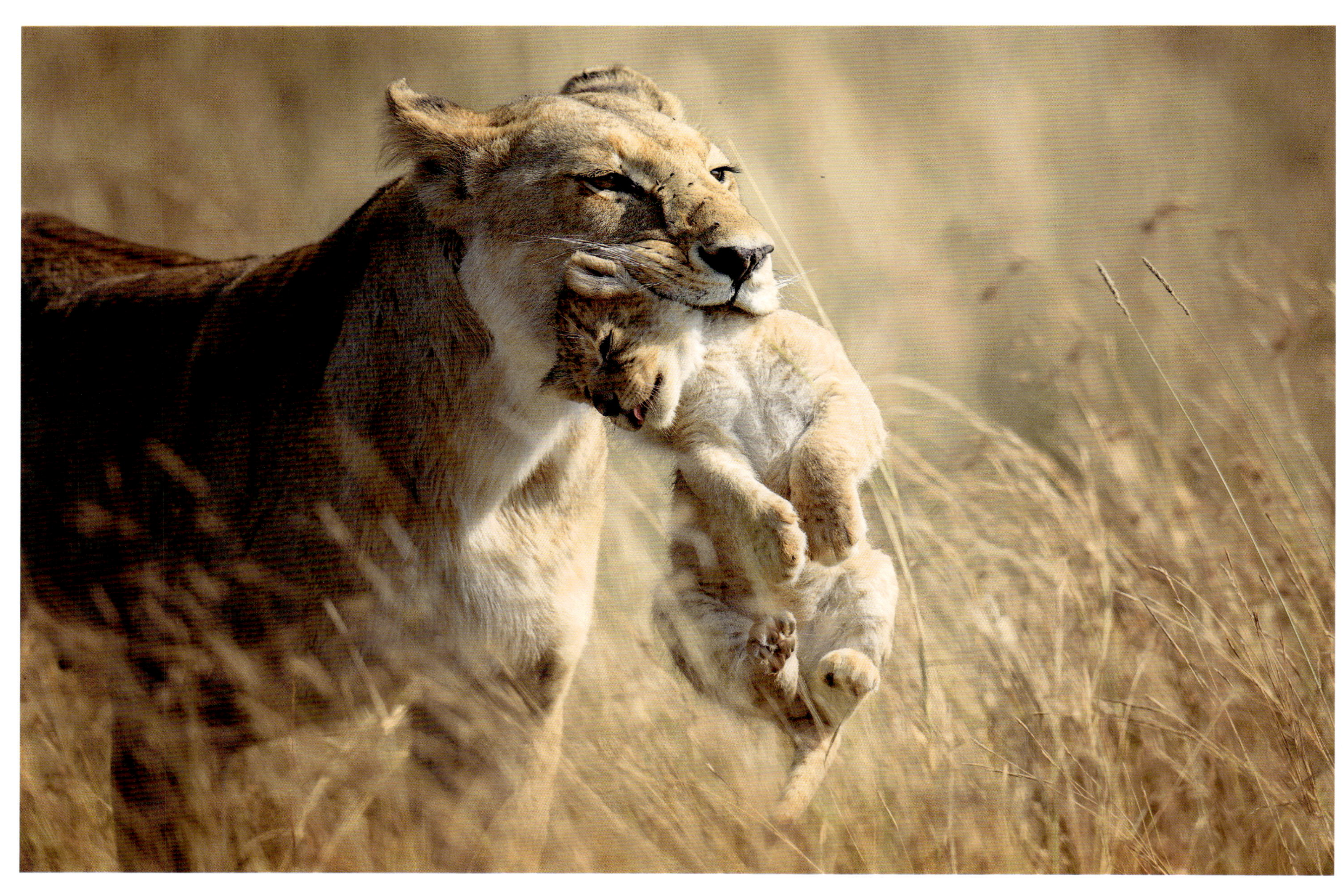

Vicki Jauron
African Lions
Maasai Mara National Reserve, Kenya

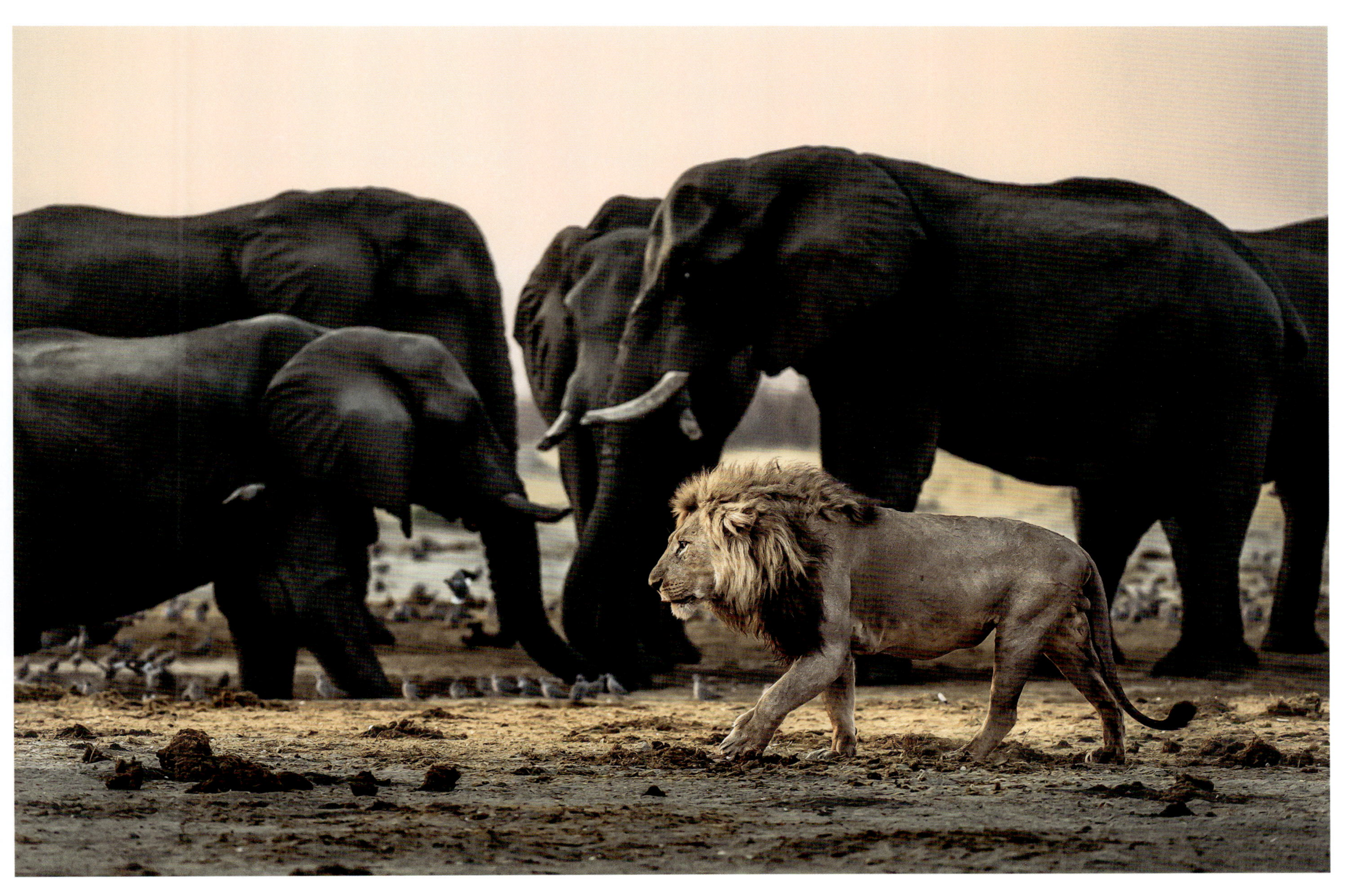

Hannes Lochner
African Lion
Chobe National Park, Botswana

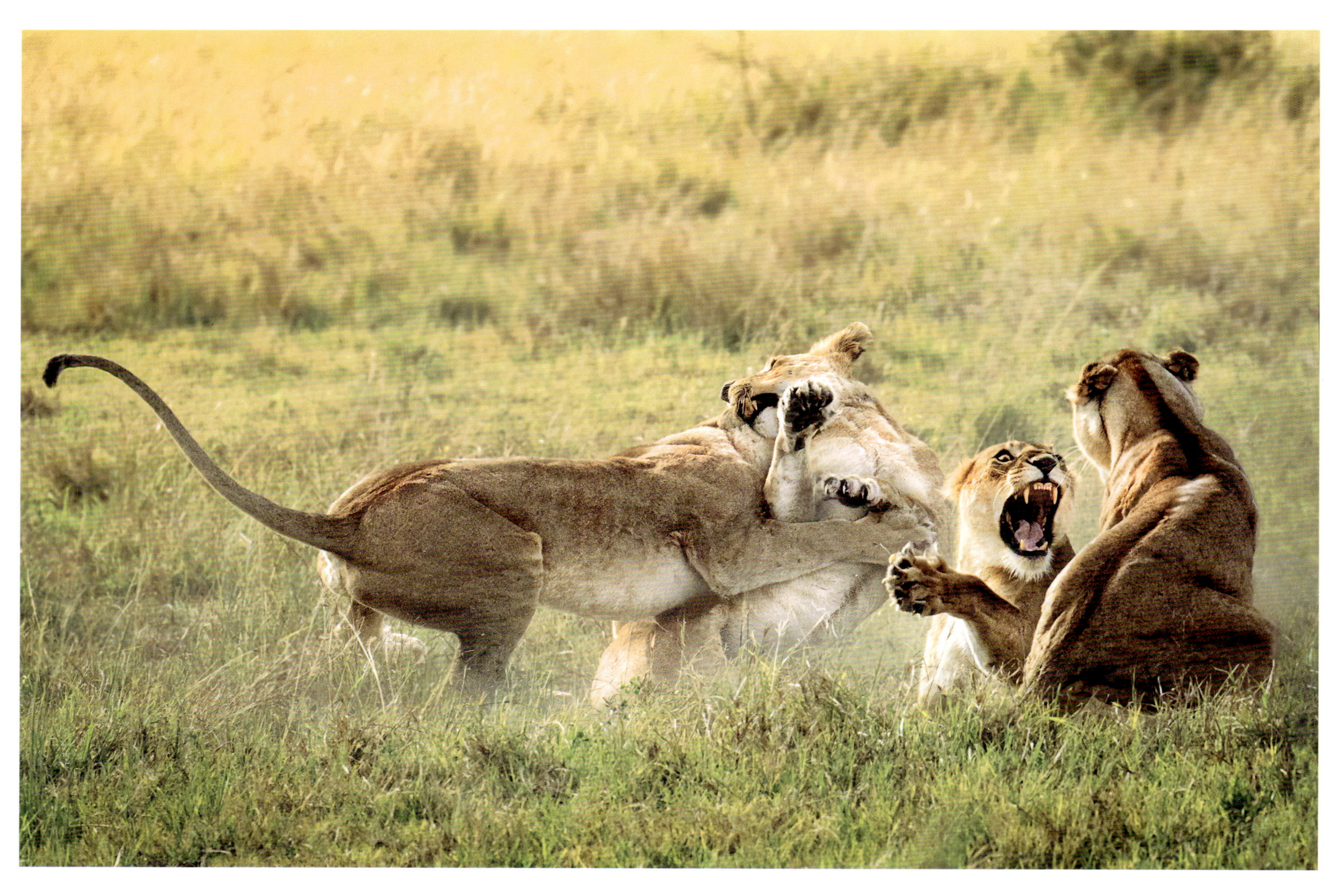

Alessandro Beconi
African Lions
Maasai Mara National Reserve, Kenya

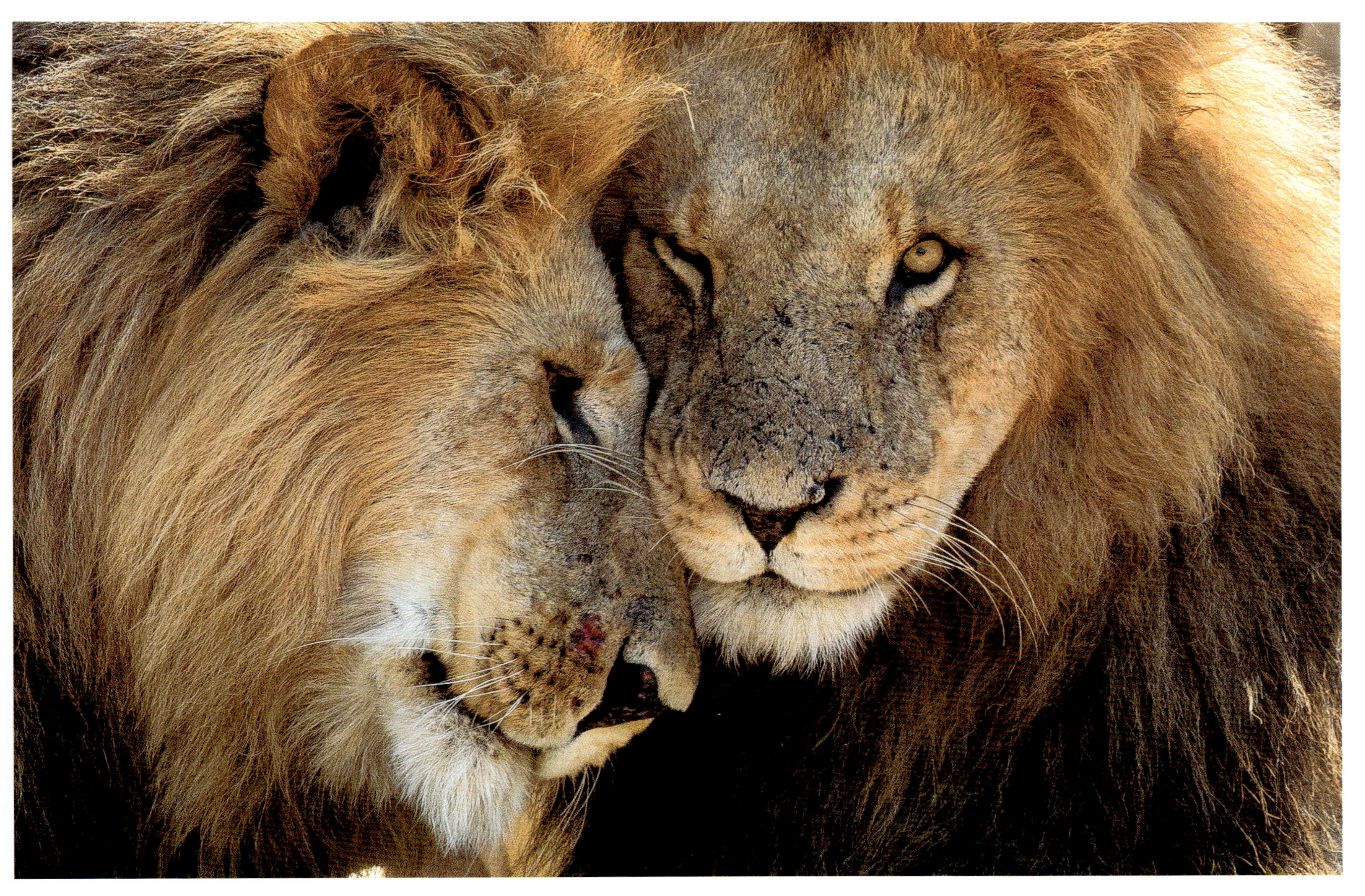

Graeme Green
African Lions
Mara Naboisho Conservancy, Kenya

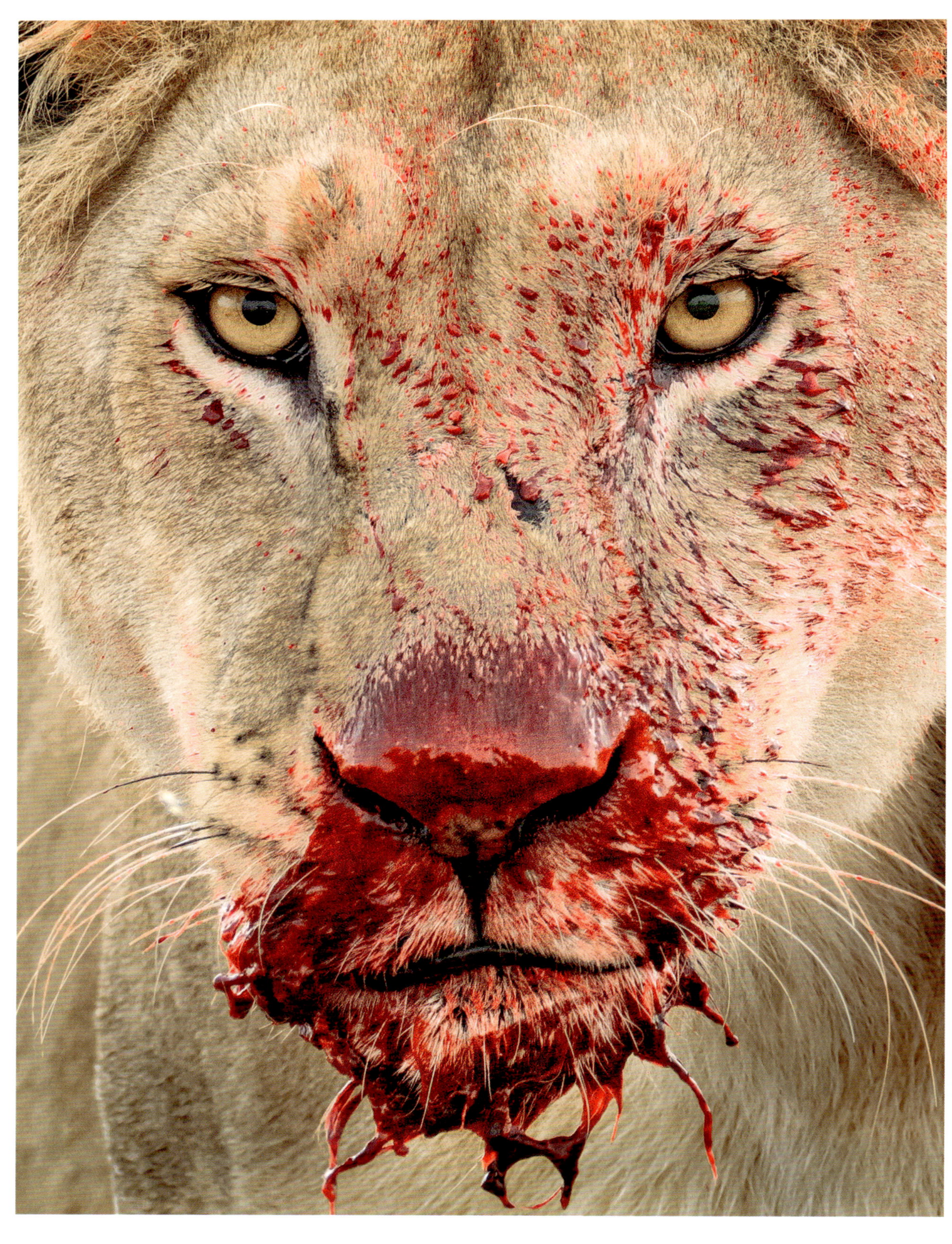

Lara Jackson
African Lion
Serengeti National Park, Tanzania

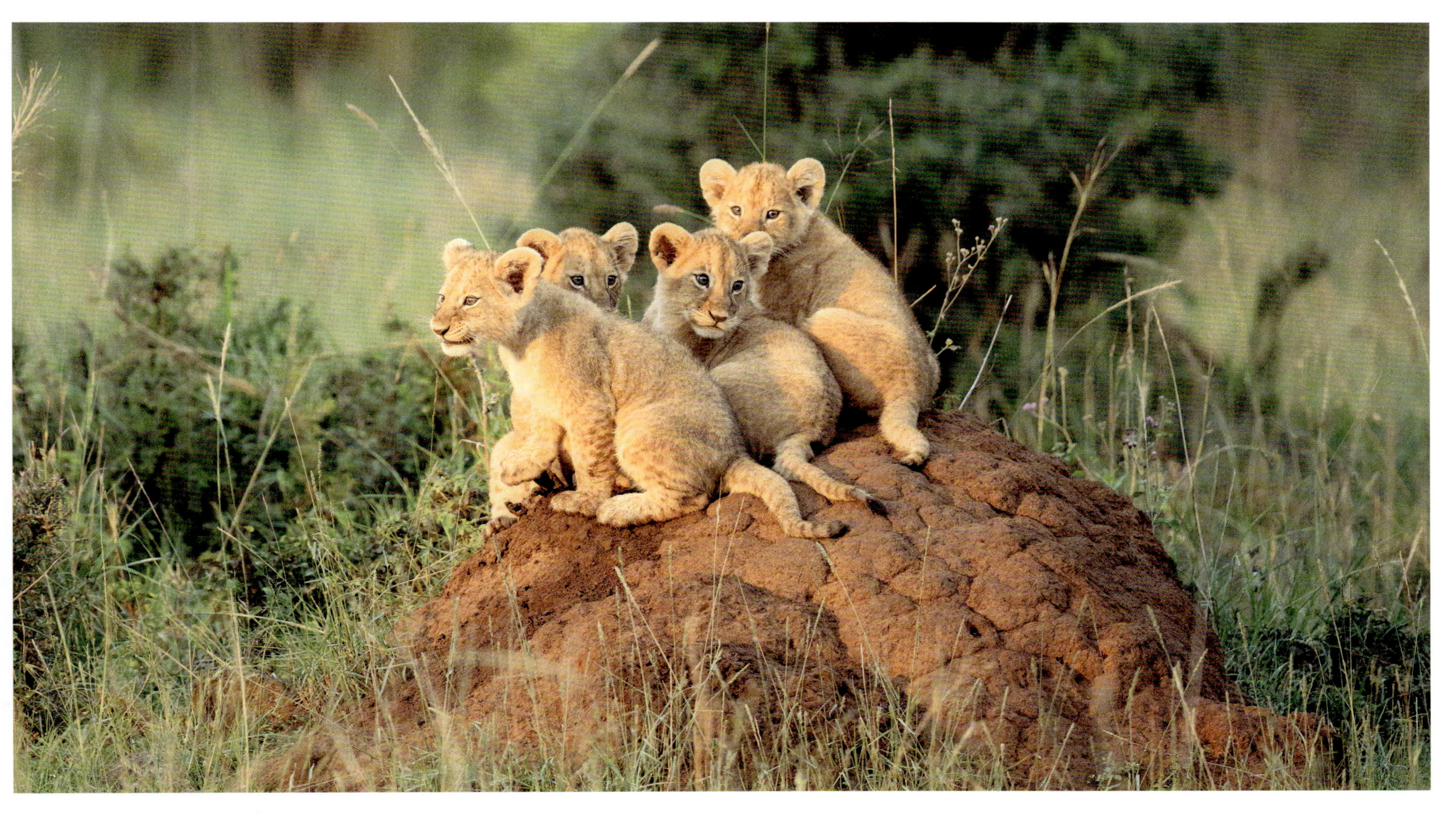

Lance van de Vyver
African Lions
Mara North Conservancy, Kenya

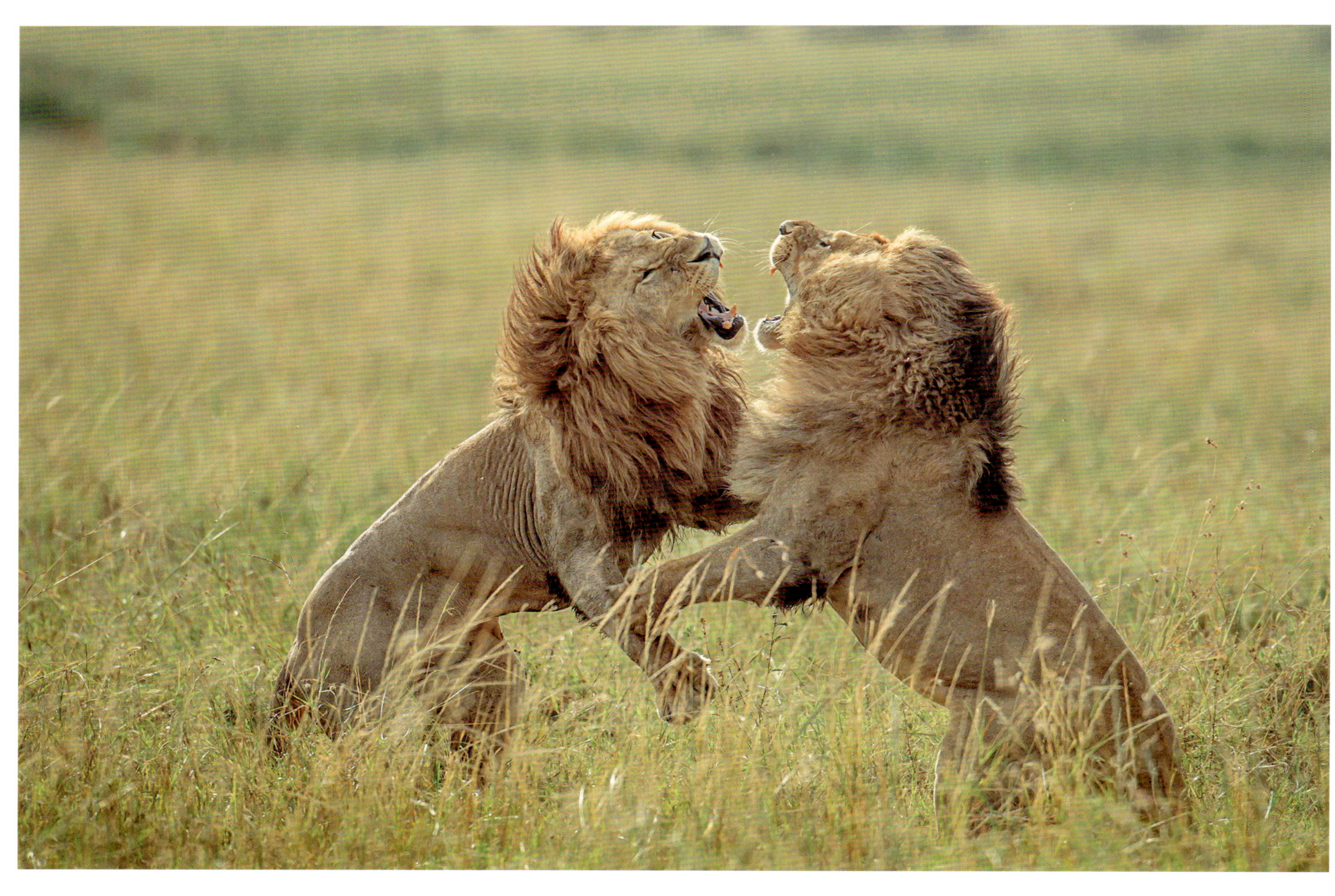

Paul Goldstein
African Lions
Maasai Mara National Reserve, Kenya

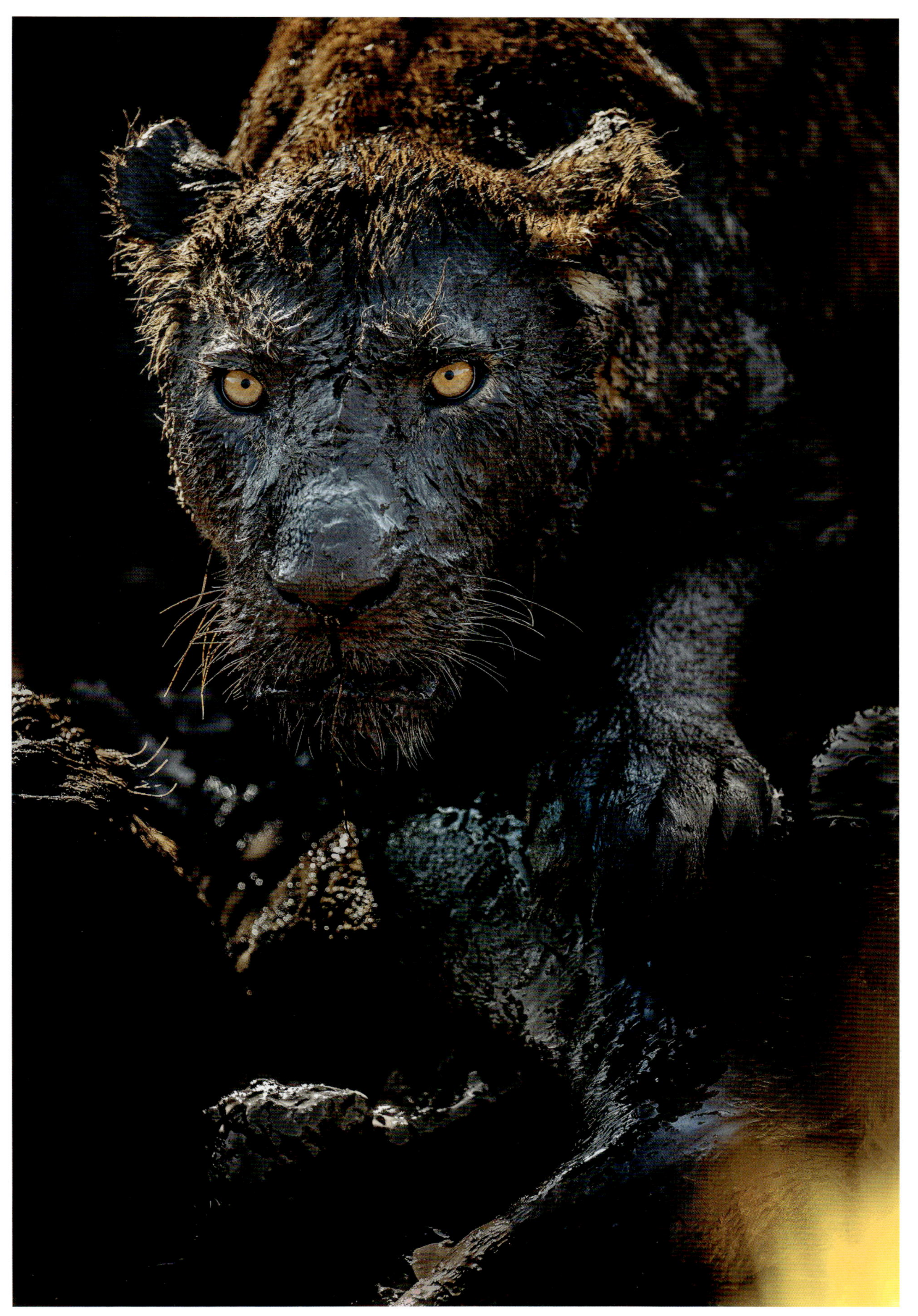

David Lloyd
African Lion
Maasai Mara National Reserve, Kenya

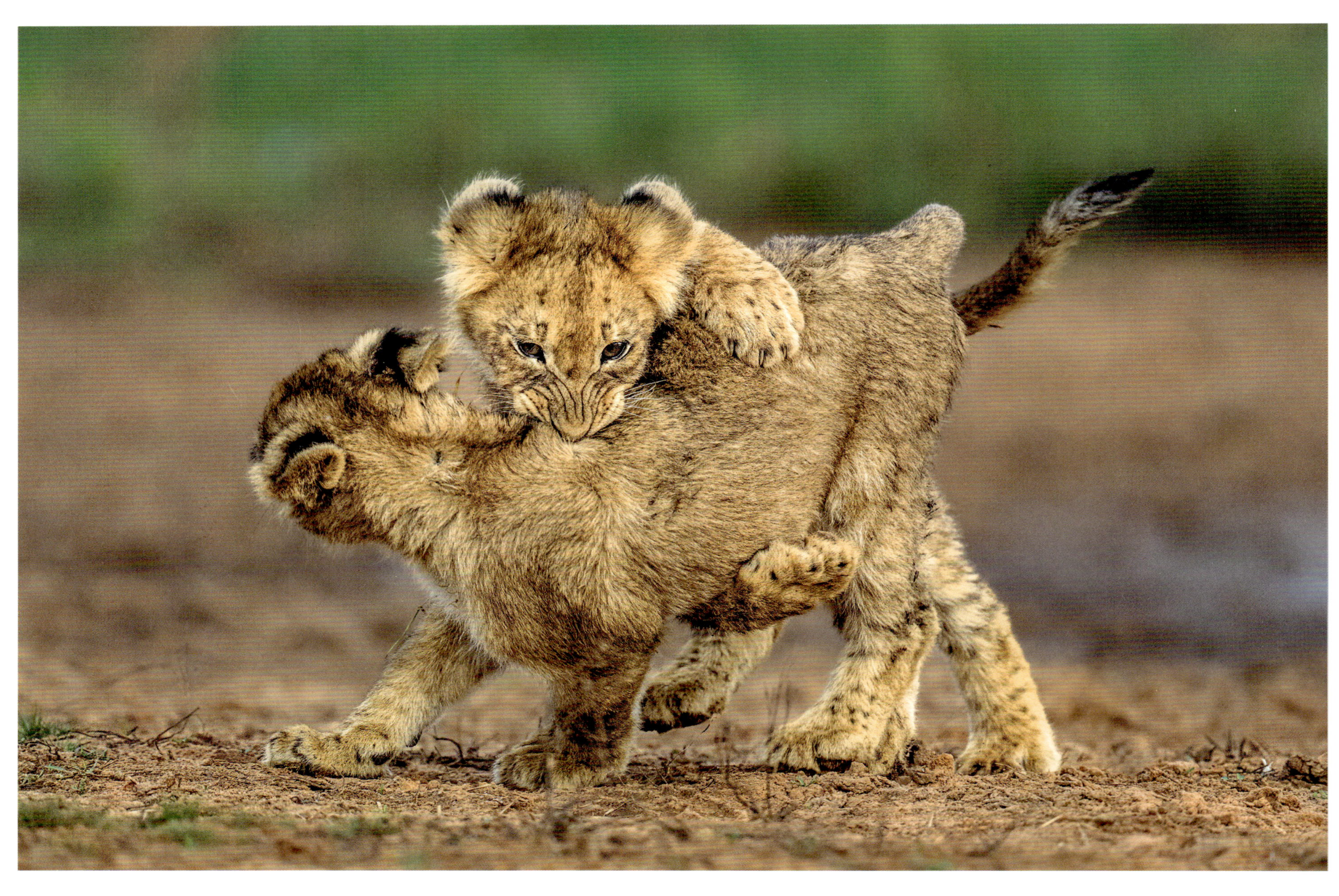

Marcus Westberg
African Lions
Tswalu Kalahari Reserve, South Africa

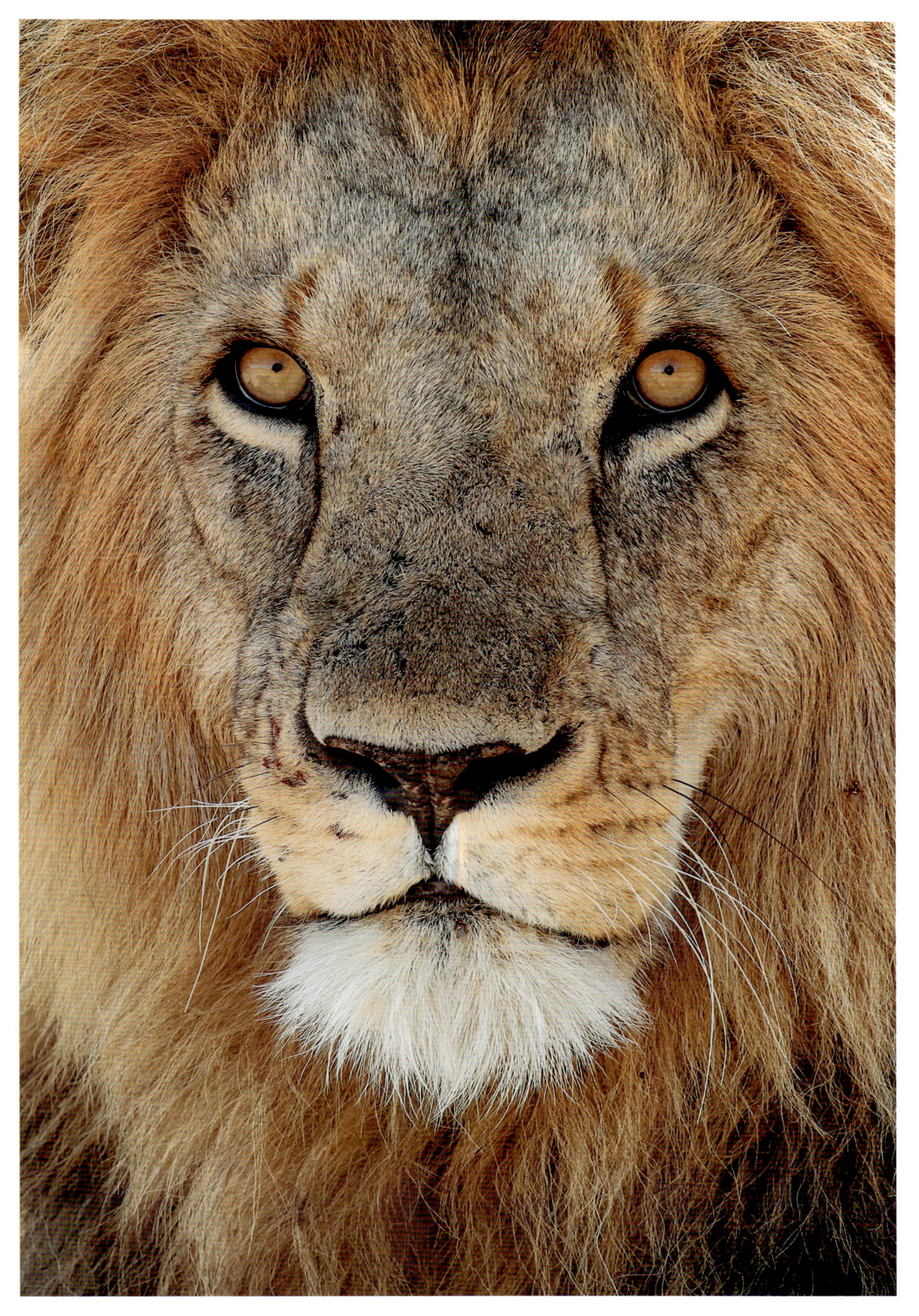

Graeme Green
African Lion
Mara Naboisho Conservancy, Kenya

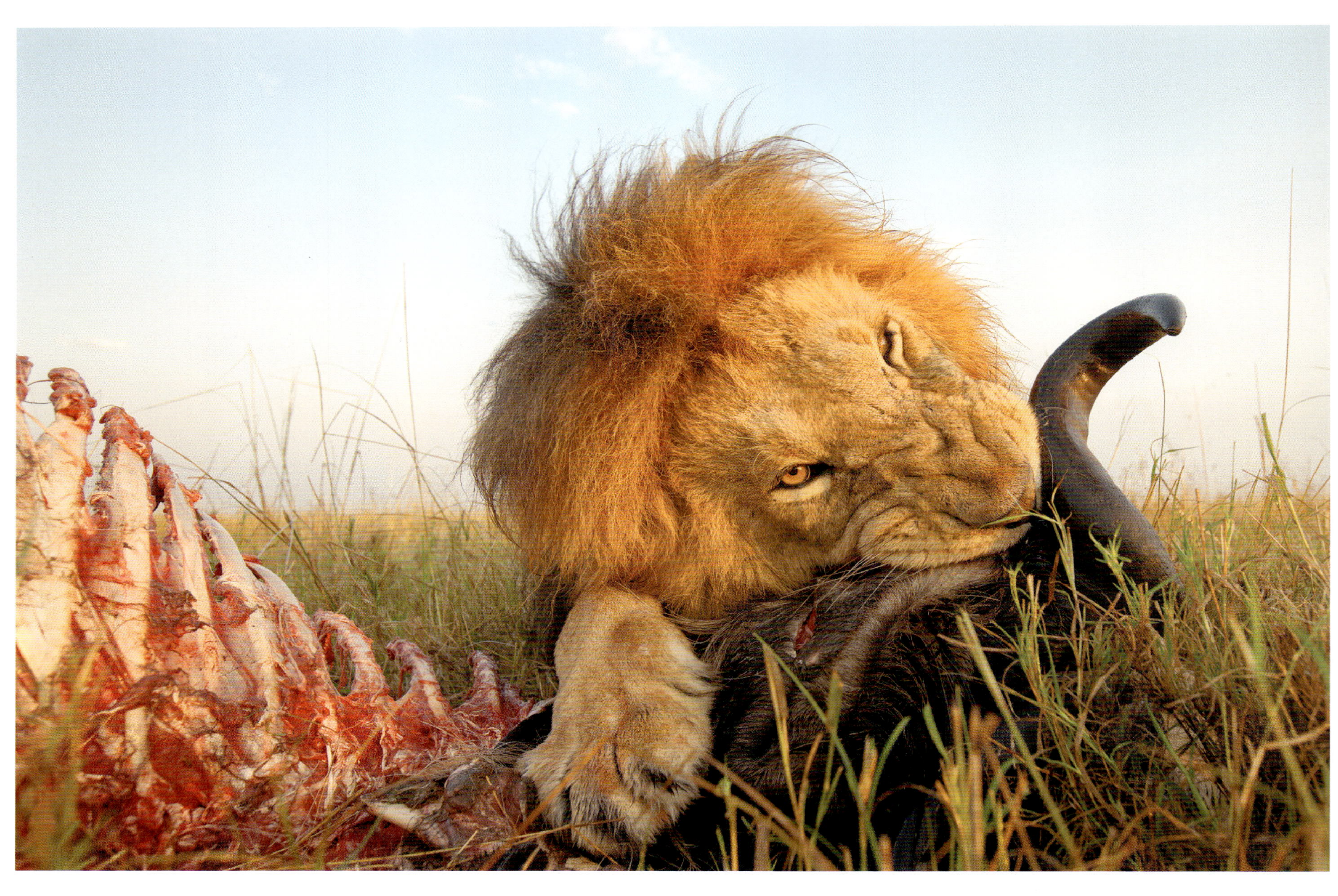

Will Burrard-Lucas
African Lion
Maasai Mara National Reserve, Kenya

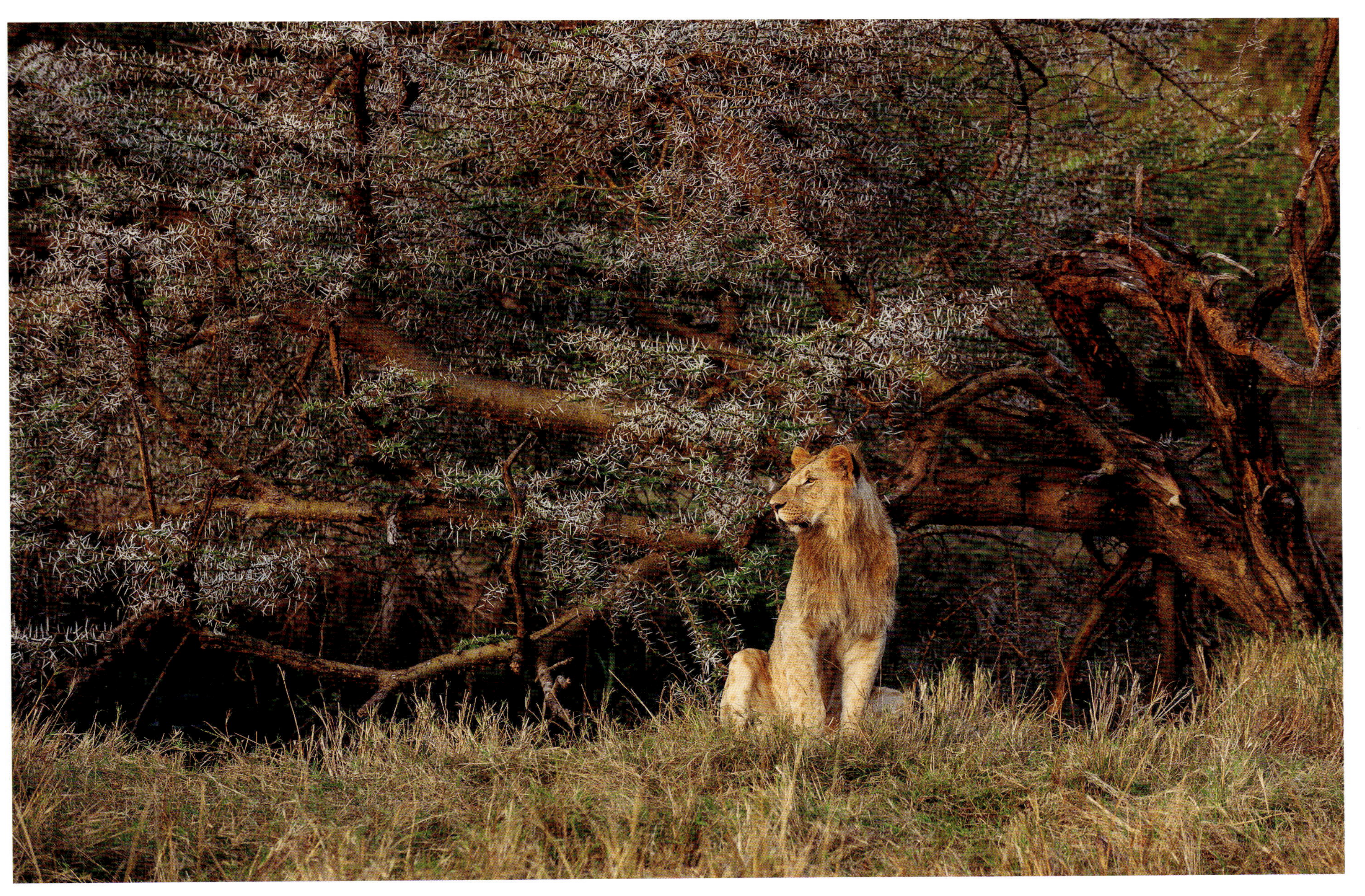

Sergio Pitamitz
African Lion
Maasai Mara National Reserve, Kenya

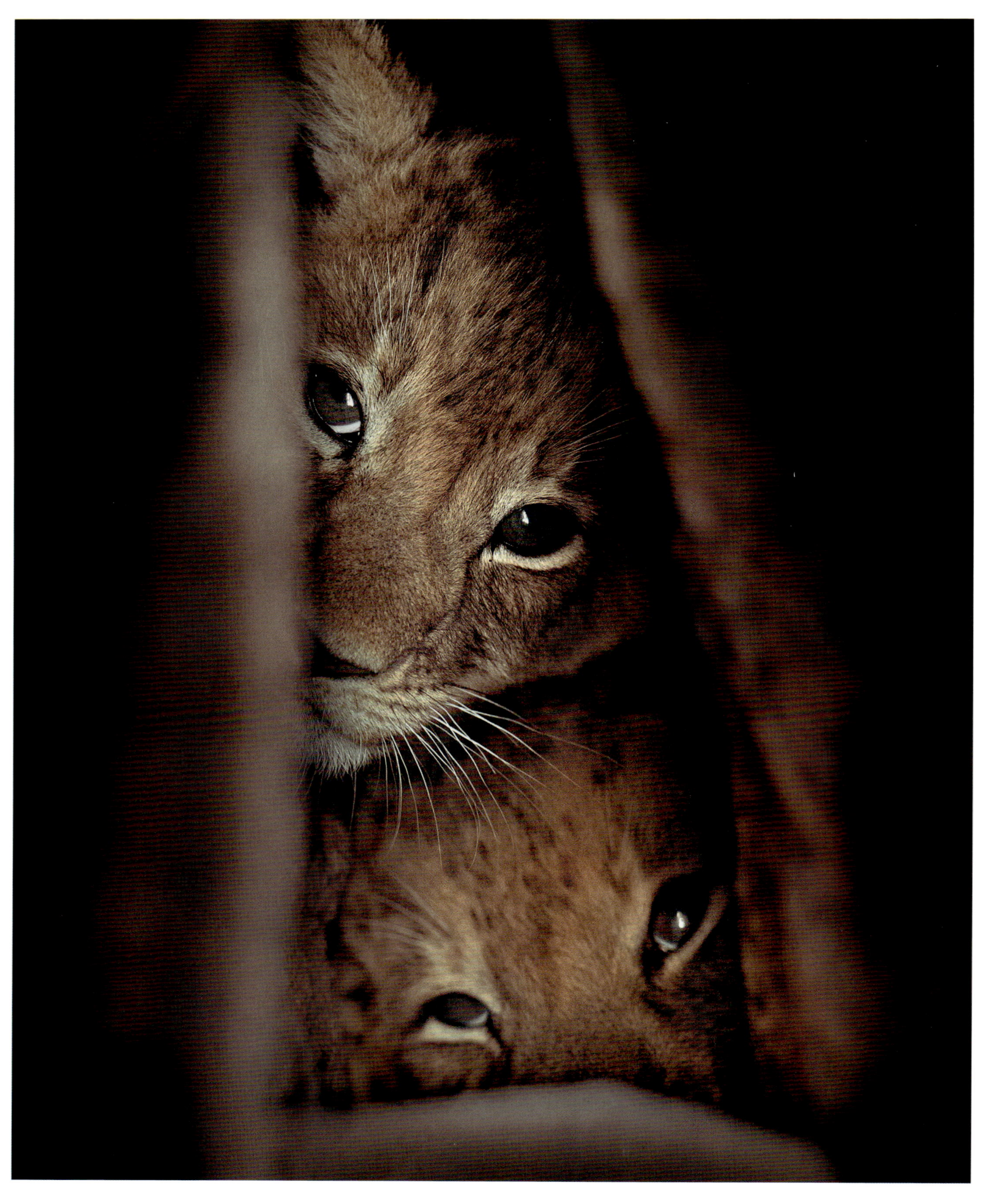

Priyanshi Bachhawat Nahata
African Lions
Maasai Mara National Reserve, Kenya

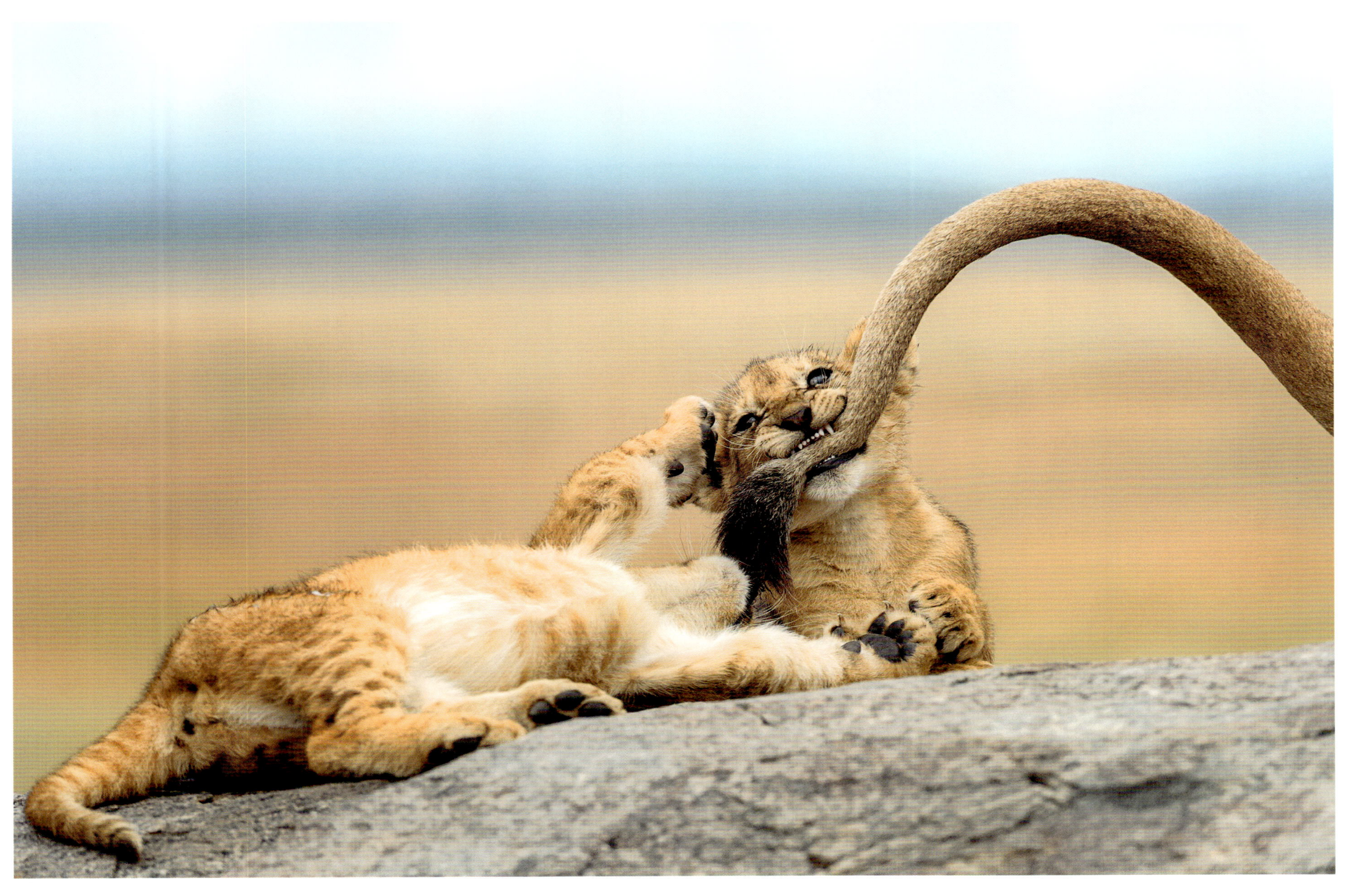

Yaron Schmid
African Lions
Serengeti National Park, Tanzania

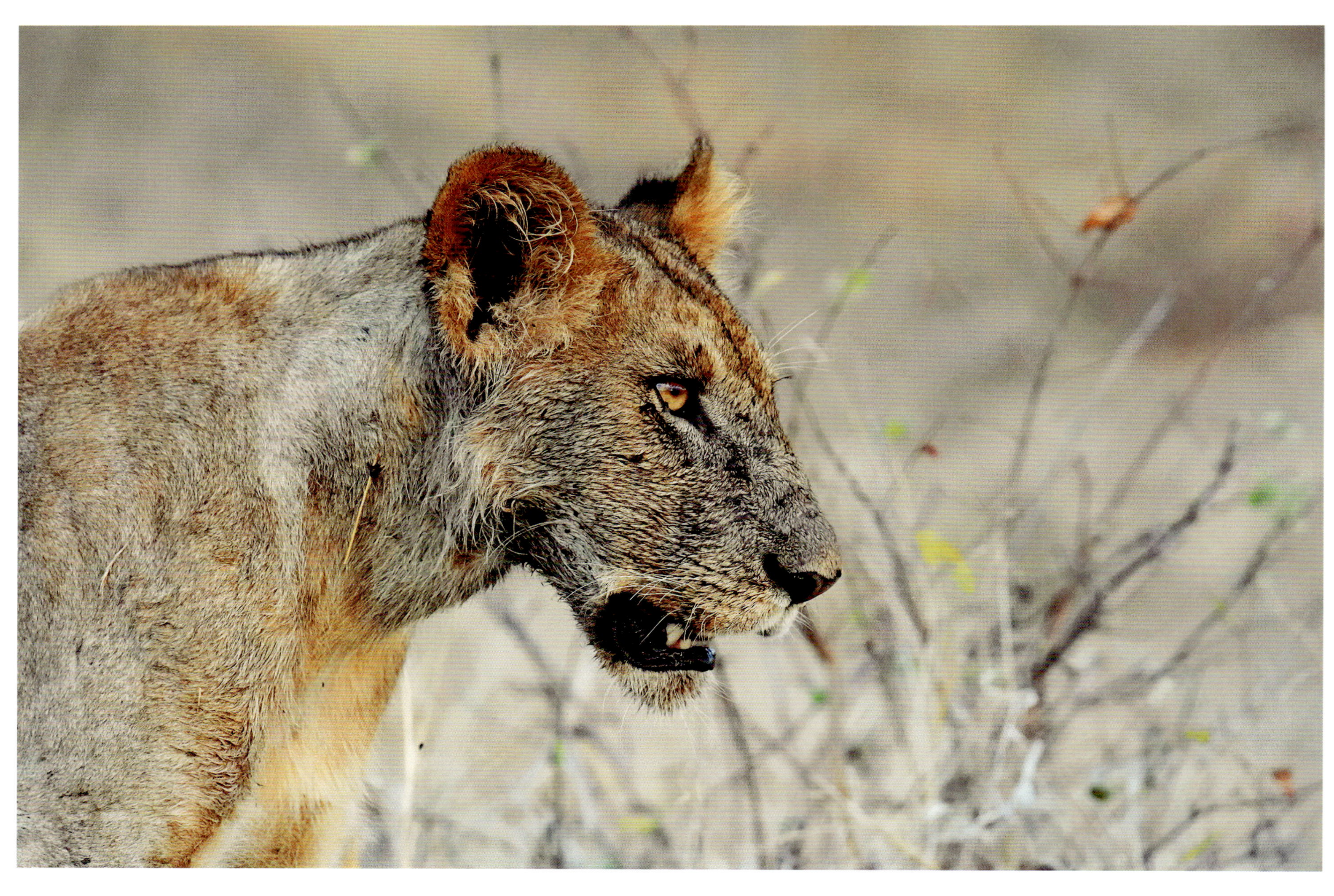

Graeme Green
African Lion
Ruaha National Park, Tanzania

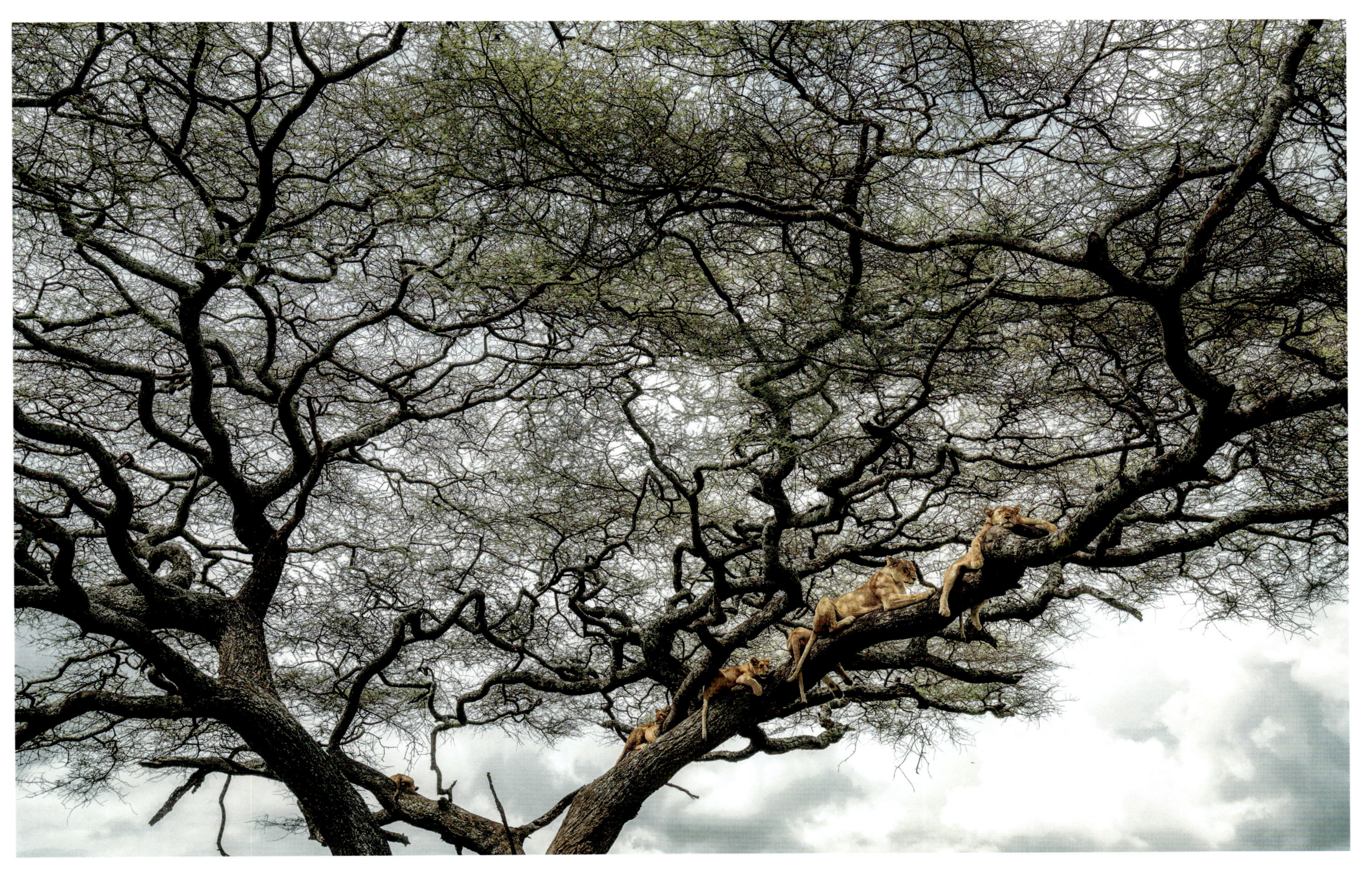

Chris Schmid
African Lions
Serengeti National Park, Tanzania

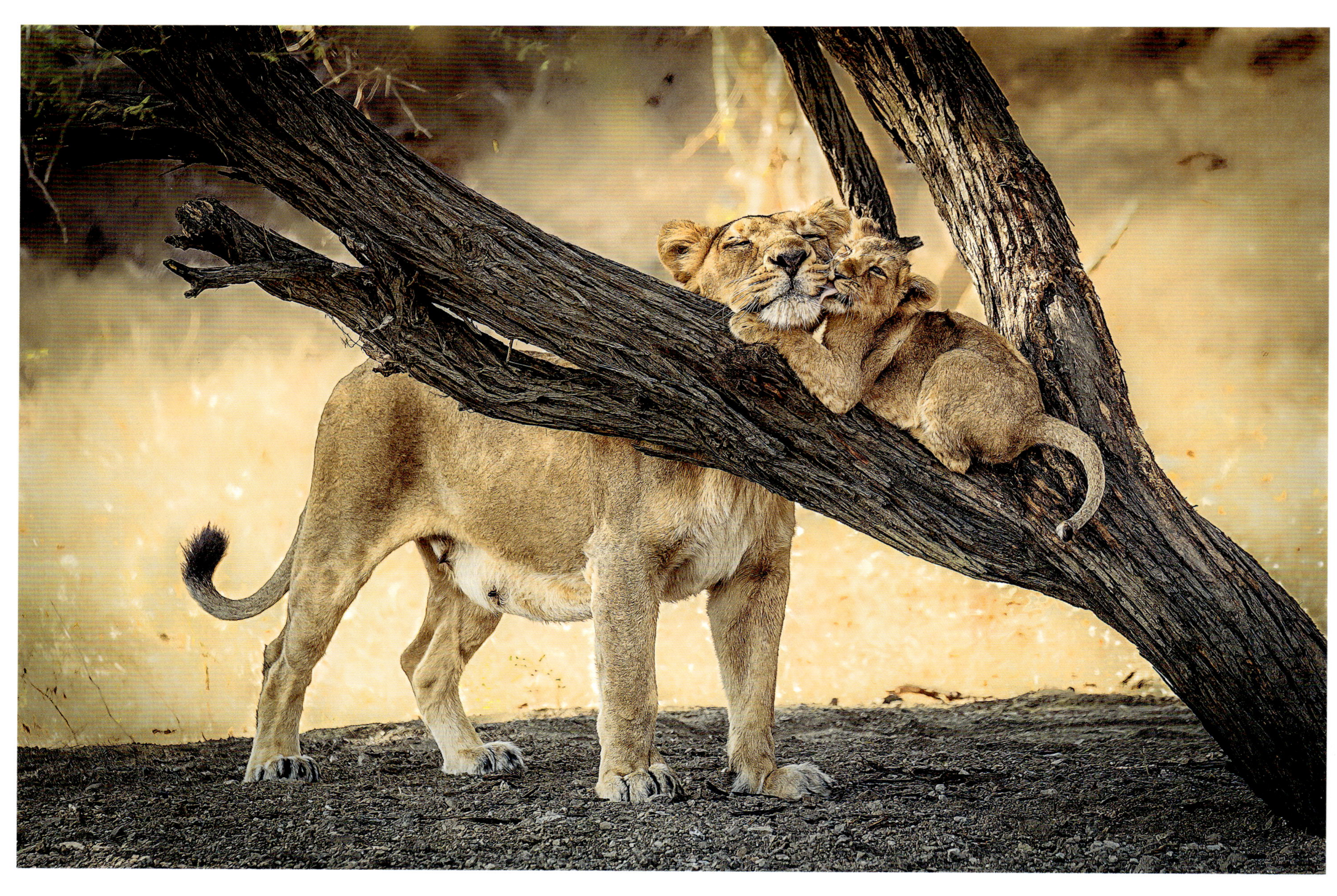

Pinkesh C. Tanna
Asiatic Lions
Gir National Park, India

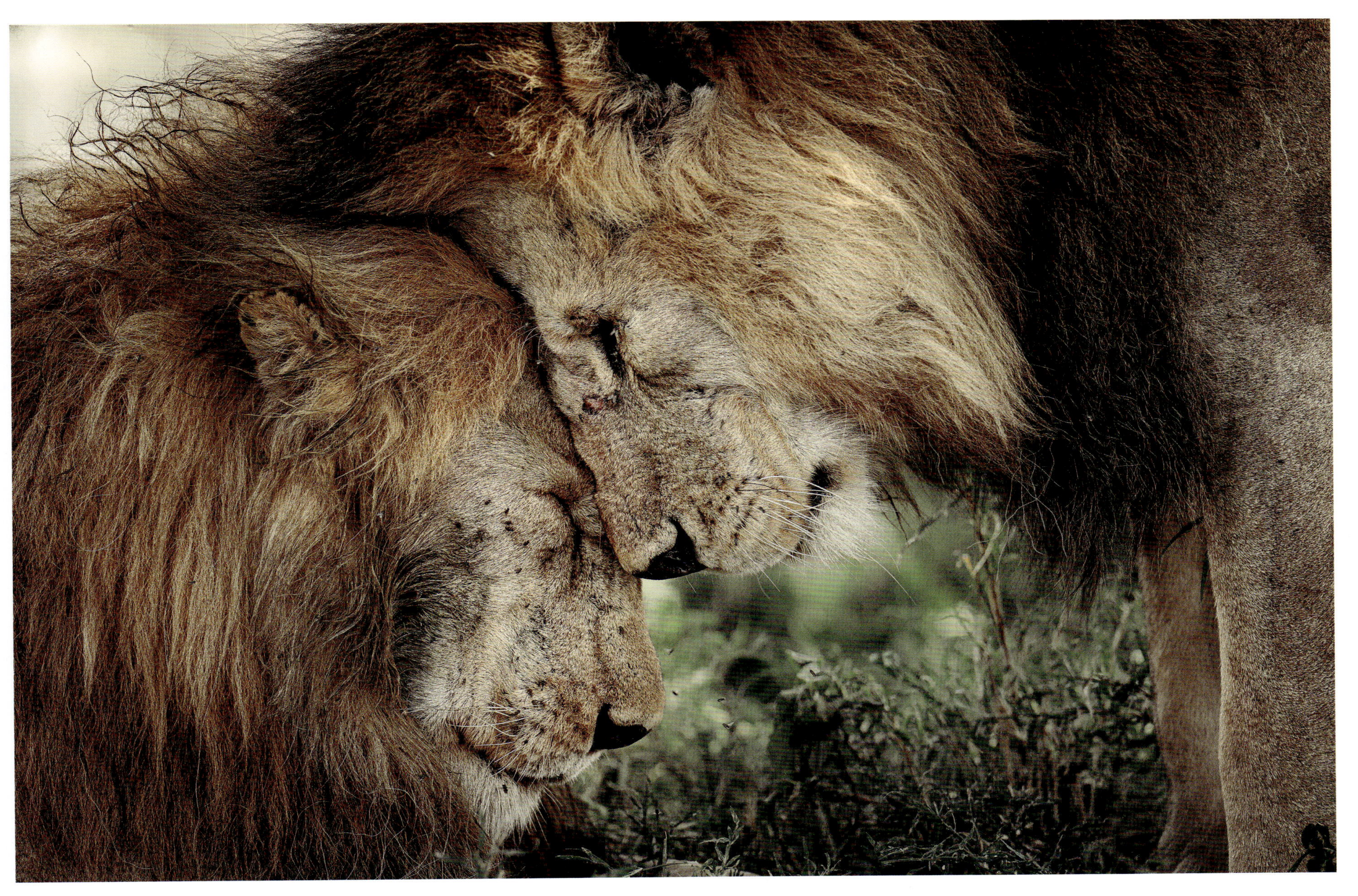

David Lloyd
African Lions
Serengeti National Park, Tanzania

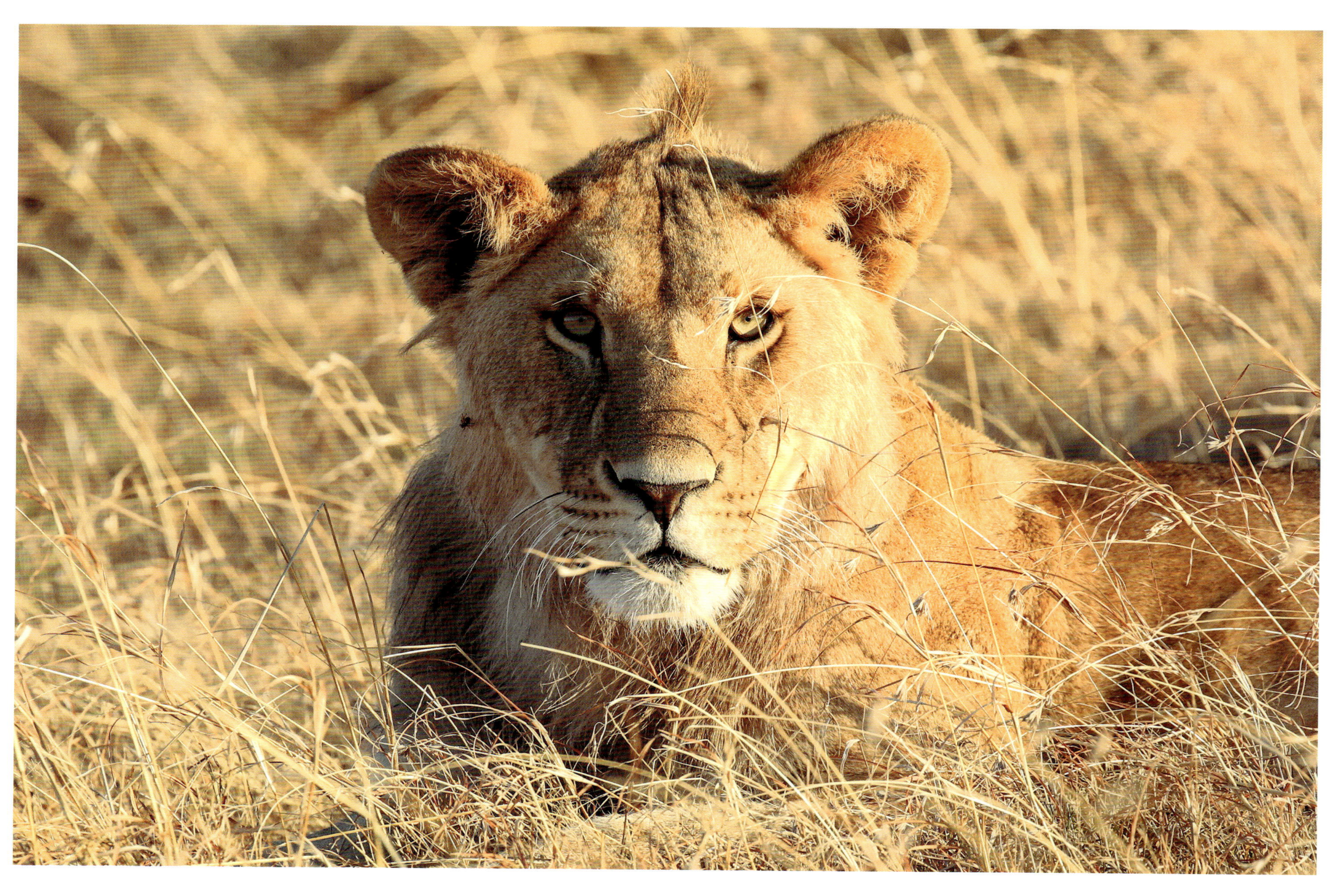

Graeme Green
African Lion
Mara Naboisho Conservancy, Kenya

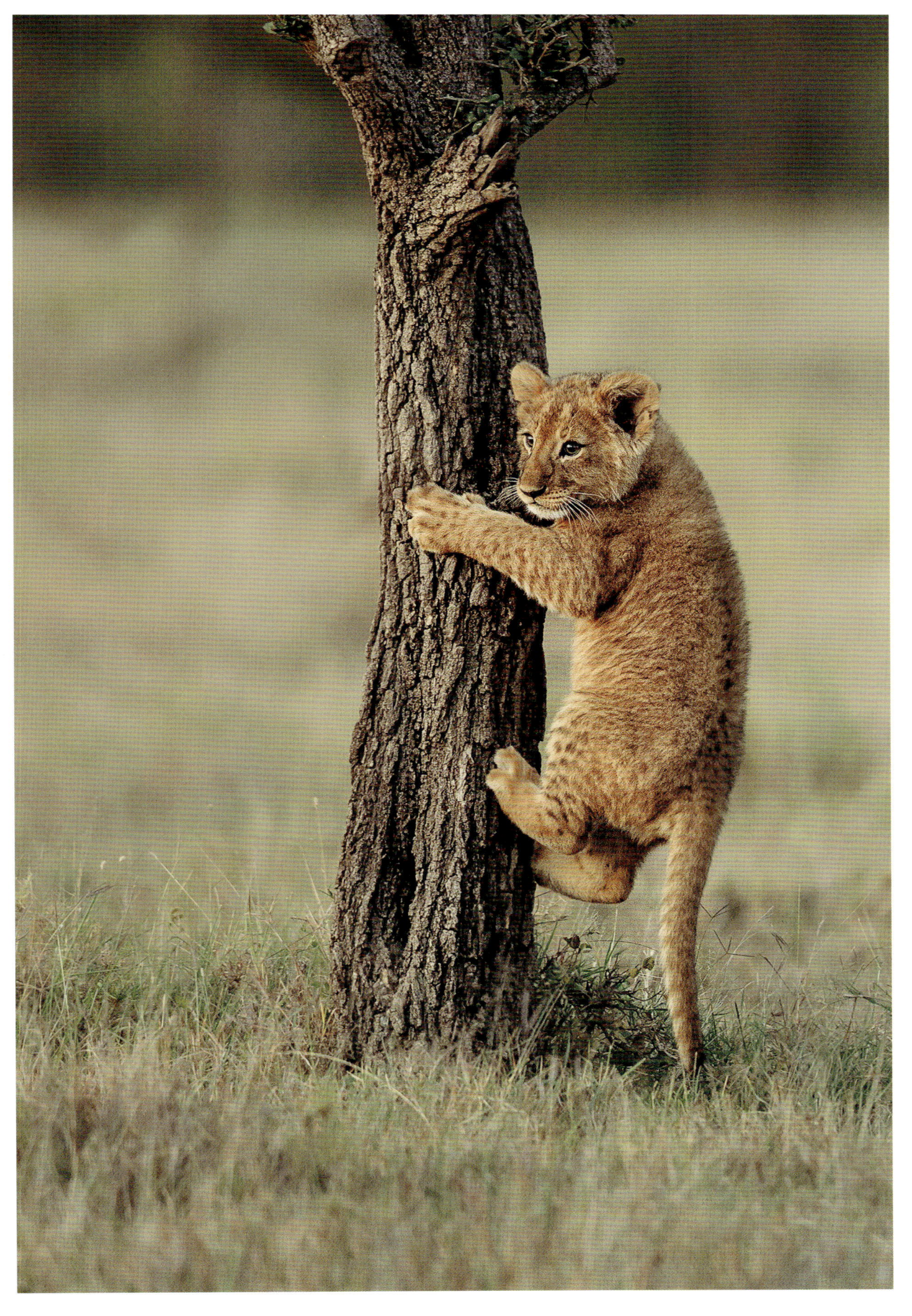

Sara Jenner
African Lion
Ol Kinyei Conservancy, Kenya

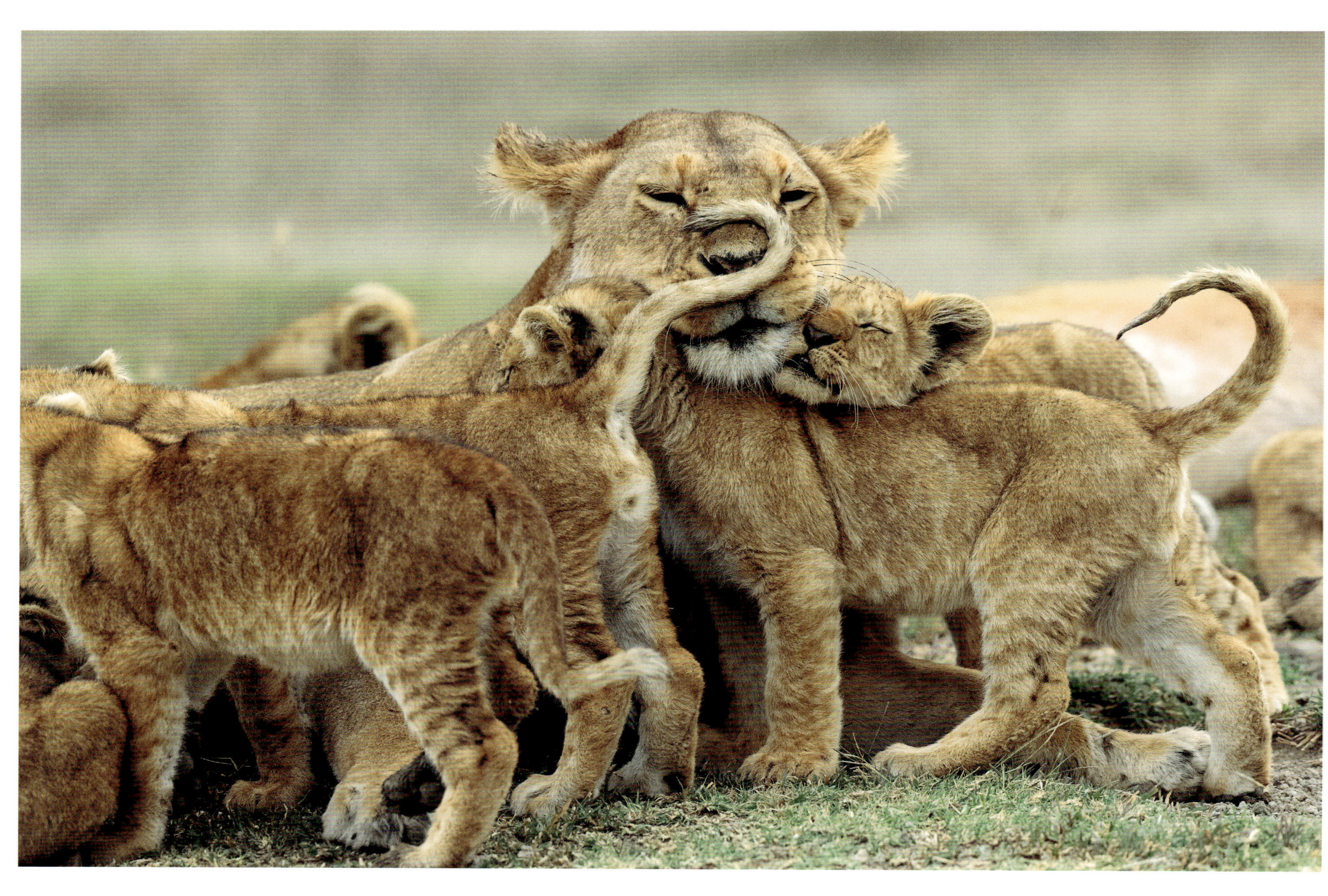

Ketan Khambhatta
African Lions
Serengeti National Park, Tanzania

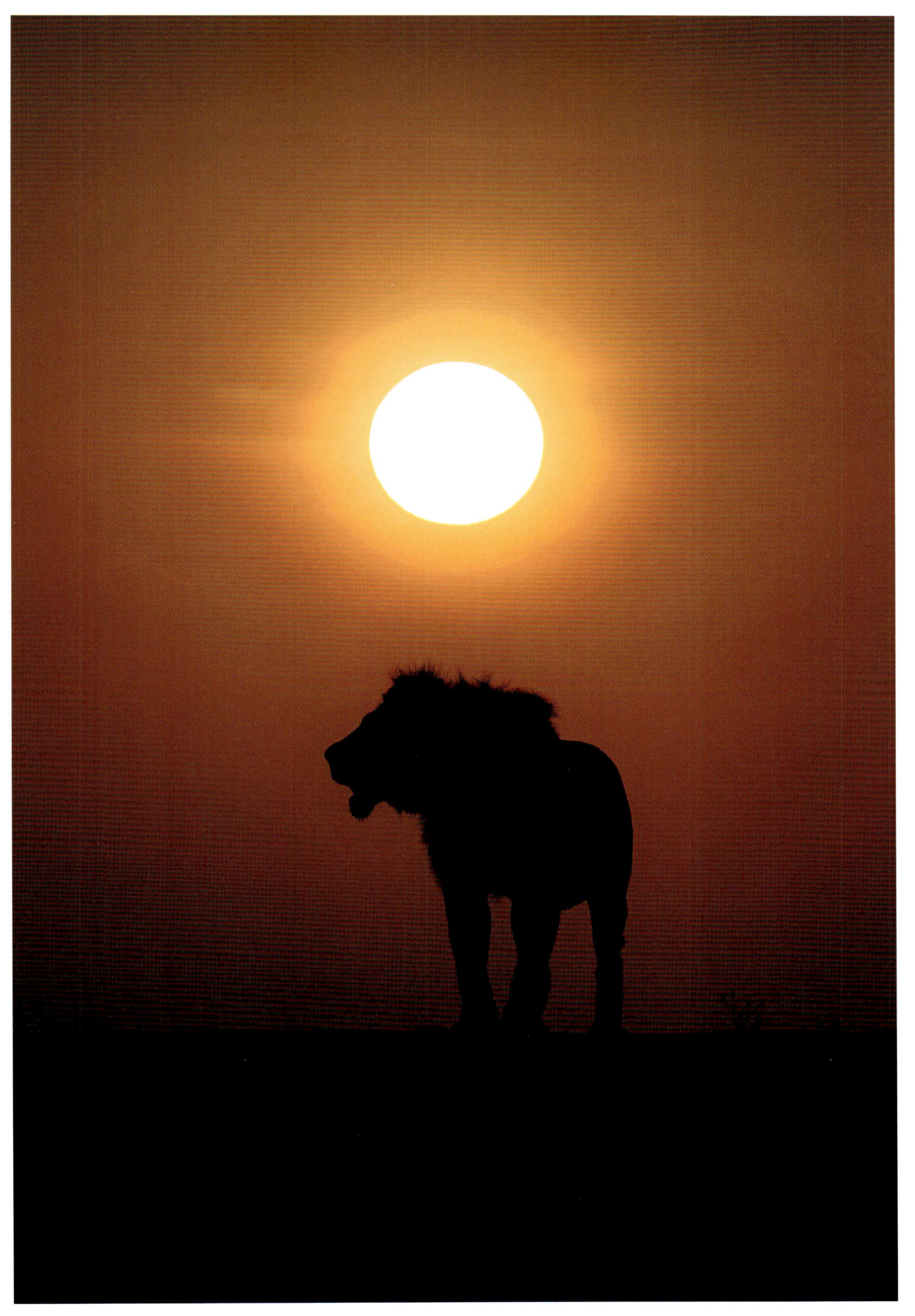

Gurcharan Roopra
African Lion
Nairobi National Park, Kenya

GORILLAS

Gorillas

Dr. Tara Stoinski

President, CEO, and Chief Scientific Officer, Dian Fossey Gorilla Fund

GORILLAS HAVE LONG FASCINATED US because we see ourselves in them. When you spend time with them, you can't help but see so much of our behavior reflected back. Like us, they have friends and enemies. They form relationships that last for decades and risk their lives defending their families. They laugh, fight, and hug their babies. They enjoy good meals and naps in the sun. They care for their most vulnerable and grieve their dead. When a silverback called Titus died in 2009 in Rwanda's Volcanoes National Park, his family stayed beside his body, grieving, trying to rouse him for three full days. I mourned along with them, as I do every time we lose a gorilla.

The world's largest primates, gorillas share 98 percent of our DNA. Every day we see evidence of just how similar they are to humans. Empathy was once thought to be a uniquely human trait. But it's something we now know we share with our closest relatives and many other animal species. In 2017, a young gorilla named Fasha was healing from a snare wound when her family encountered a river they needed to cross in search of dinner. Fasha seemed afraid to cross the river, unable to maneuver across the slippery rocks. When her family saw her struggling, they stopped on the far bank and waited patiently. Her sister, Icyororo, reached out to encourage Fasha as she tentatively picked her way across. When she finally made it to the other side, her sister threw her arms around Fasha, embracing her tightly, before the entire group moved off into the trees to eat and rest together.

Gorillas are also smart. They're able to navigate their often inhospitable home with its cold, rainy, steep terrain. They've even learned to protect themselves from snares. Fortunately, mountain gorillas are not hunted today as they were when Dian Fossey first started her work. But poachers still enter the forest to set up snares, hoping to catch an antelope to eat. After long years of experience, mountain gorillas have become snare aware; they've figured out how to spot these snares and even go one step further, a story best illustrated by the famous silverback Cantsbee.

Cantsbee got his name from Dian Fossey herself; Dian had misidentified his mother as a male, so when she showed up one day and discovered that what she thought was the male had given birth, she exclaimed, "It can't be." Cantsbee grew into a powerful silverback who led the largest group of gorillas every recorded and sired more than thirty offspring. A caring father, he was often seen babysitting, surrounded by youngsters, while the babies' mothers were off feeding or catching a needed rest.

One day, when our trackers found his group, Cantsbee was showing uncharacteristic aggression toward the juveniles playing near him, emitting what sounded like a pig grunt, a mildly aggressive gorilla vocalization, whenever the youngsters approached him. The young gorillas gave Cantsbee his space. When our team approached to get a closer look, they received the same pig grunt. After the group moved away, we saw Cantsbee had been sitting next to a snare. His warning sounds had kept his family members out of harm's way. We couldn't help but feel he was protecting us, too.

Moments like these remind me of the importance of what those of us working in conservation do. I was thirty-two when I saw my first gorilla in the wild. The first word that came to mind back then, when I saw a giant silverback emerge from the trees in front of me, was *amazing*. Even now, twenty years later, I am still absolutely amazed. I've been honored to spend so much time with the mountain gorillas of Rwanda, privileged to do my small part to protect them.

Despite our common humanity and our close genetic ties, gorillas are one of the planet's at-risk species. Dian Fossey predicted gorillas would be extinct by the year 2000. But thanks to her dedication, people became aware of their plight. Conservationists and government leaders stepped in to find ways to protect them, and today the population of mountain gorillas Fossey set out to study in Rwanda more than fifty years ago has grown to an estimated 600 individuals, up from a low of 250 in the 1980s. Decades of conservation action and leadership by the countries where mountain gorillas live (Rwanda, Uganda, and the Democratic Republic of the Congo) and conservation organizations have resulted in an all-too-rare success story. Mountain gorillas are the only great ape whose population is increasing. With just over a thousand individuals remaining, we need to remember that it is a fragile success.

Mountain gorillas still face numerous threats. Their small population size and limited habitat (their two ranges total less than 300 square miles, around one tenth the size of Yellowstone National Park), combined with the risks posed by disease, climate change, and human encroachment, make their future anything but secure. Unfortunately, the news for gorillas as a whole is more dire. In the DRC, the mountain gorillas' close cousins, Grauer's gorillas (also known as eastern lowland gorillas), have declined in numbers by more than 60 percent in the last two decades alone. The DRC is the only place where Grauer's gorillas are found. The majority live outside of national parks, with no formal protection. Their decline is a result of direct poaching, a tragic side effect of the race for rare minerals that are found in the gorillas' forest home.

The hope for me is that if we can change the trajectory in the same way we did with mountain gorillas, there is still time to save them. And, luckily, there's still lots of intact forest left. Local communities are working to secure ownership over their lands and provide protection to these globally important forests and biodiversity. The international community needs to support the Congolese people's efforts, which may be our best hope at preventing further forest loss and ensuring a future for Grauer's gorillas.

Grauer's gorillas are just one example of what is happening during the Anthropocene, the period when human activity has been the dominant influence on climate and the environment. Around the world, wildlife and the ecosystems that they need to survive must be valued. Nature has to become a priority and we must act as if our lives depend on it, because they do. It has to become a priority that governments realize that ultimately our health as a species depends on the health of these ecosystems.

Look at the last two years: pandemics happen because of spillover events when humans and animals come together. Keeping ecosystems intact and protecting species is essential for our survival. Governments, corporations, and global citizens will hopefully realize that and make the investments necessary to protect these areas.

Mountain gorillas are a great case study showing that a difference can be made. The reasons so many animals are threatened are some of the biggest challenges we face on the planet, whether it's poverty, hunger, lack of education, or lack of resources. Protecting wildlife is a long-term, concerted effort. If we want gorillas, elephants, or orangutans to survive, it'll take a global effort—it can't just be the responsibility of the countries where they live. Local communities have to be part of the equation, too.

Gorillas share our humanity. We need them as much as they need us. Gorillas are the gardeners of Africa's immense rain forests, which are essential for the thousands of other species that live there, from chimpanzees to forest elephants. Their daily activities—foraging, nest building, roaming—keep the forests healthy by spreading seeds, clearing vegetation, and producing fertilizer. We need these forest ecosystems to remain intact because our own survival depends on them. They are the lungs of the planet. The Congo Basin houses the second largest tropical rain forest on the planet, and rain forests are one of our best natural defenses against climate change. If we can save these gorillas and their incredibly biodiverse forest home, we may save ourselves, too.

I'll never stop being amazed by these beautiful, intelligent animals, and I'll never stop fighting to protect them.

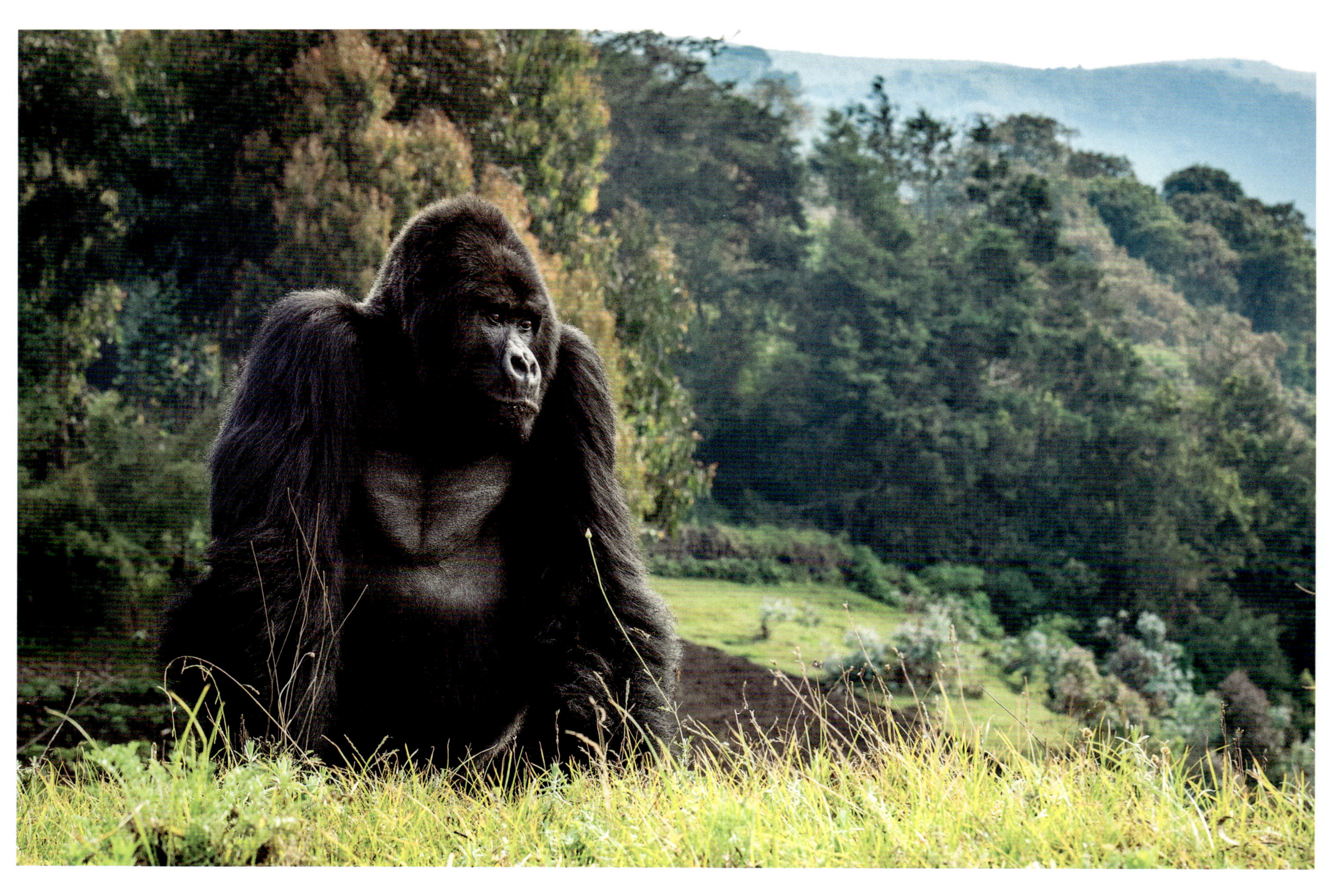

Daryl and Sharna Balfour
Mountain Gorilla
Volcanoes National Park, Rwanda

142

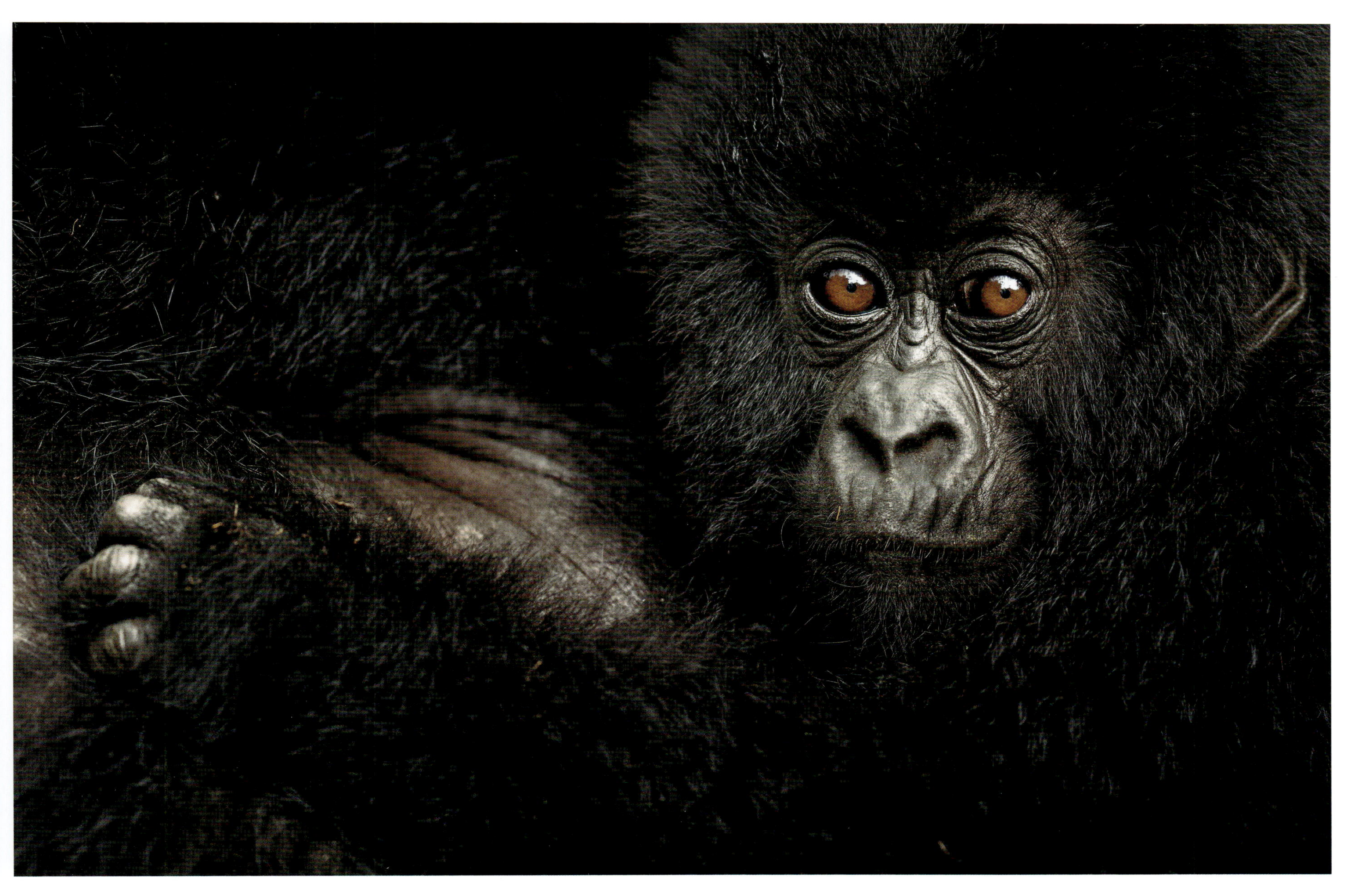

Nelis Wolmarans
Mountain Gorilla
Volcanoes National Park, Rwanda

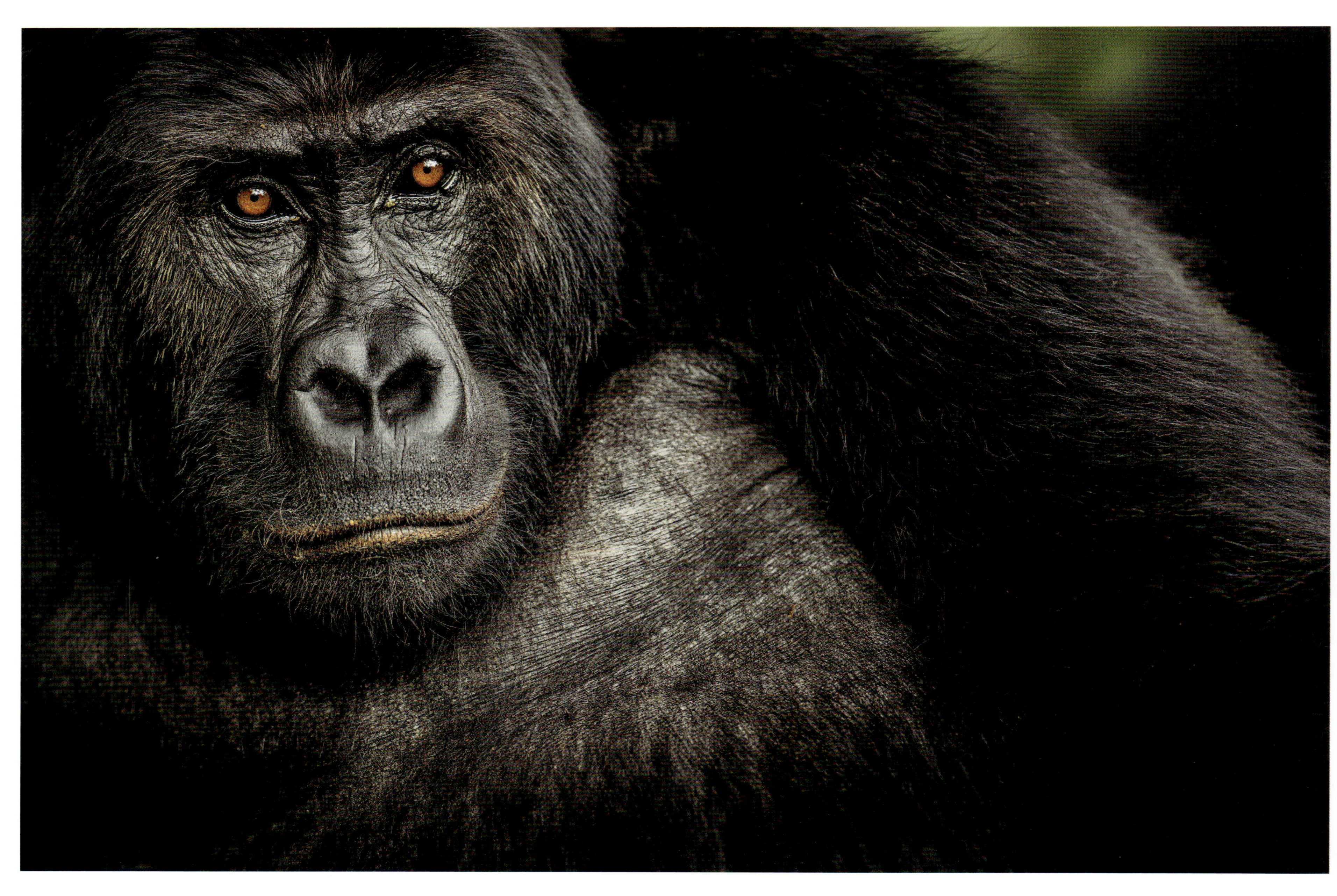

Marcus Westberg
Grauer's Gorilla
Kahuzi-Biega National Park,
Democratic Republic of the Congo

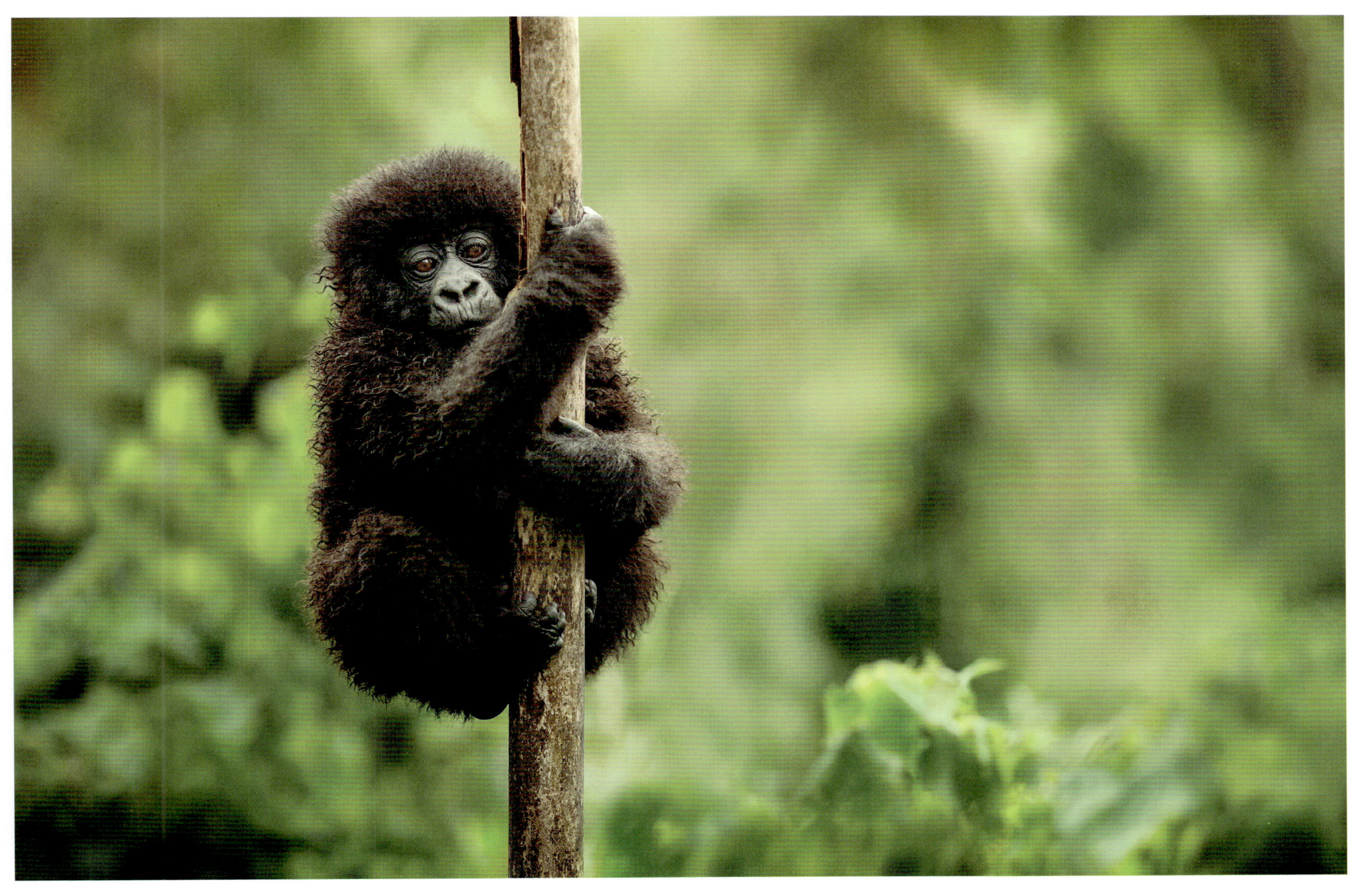

Vladimir Cech, Jr.
Mountain Gorilla
Volcanoes National Park, Rwanda

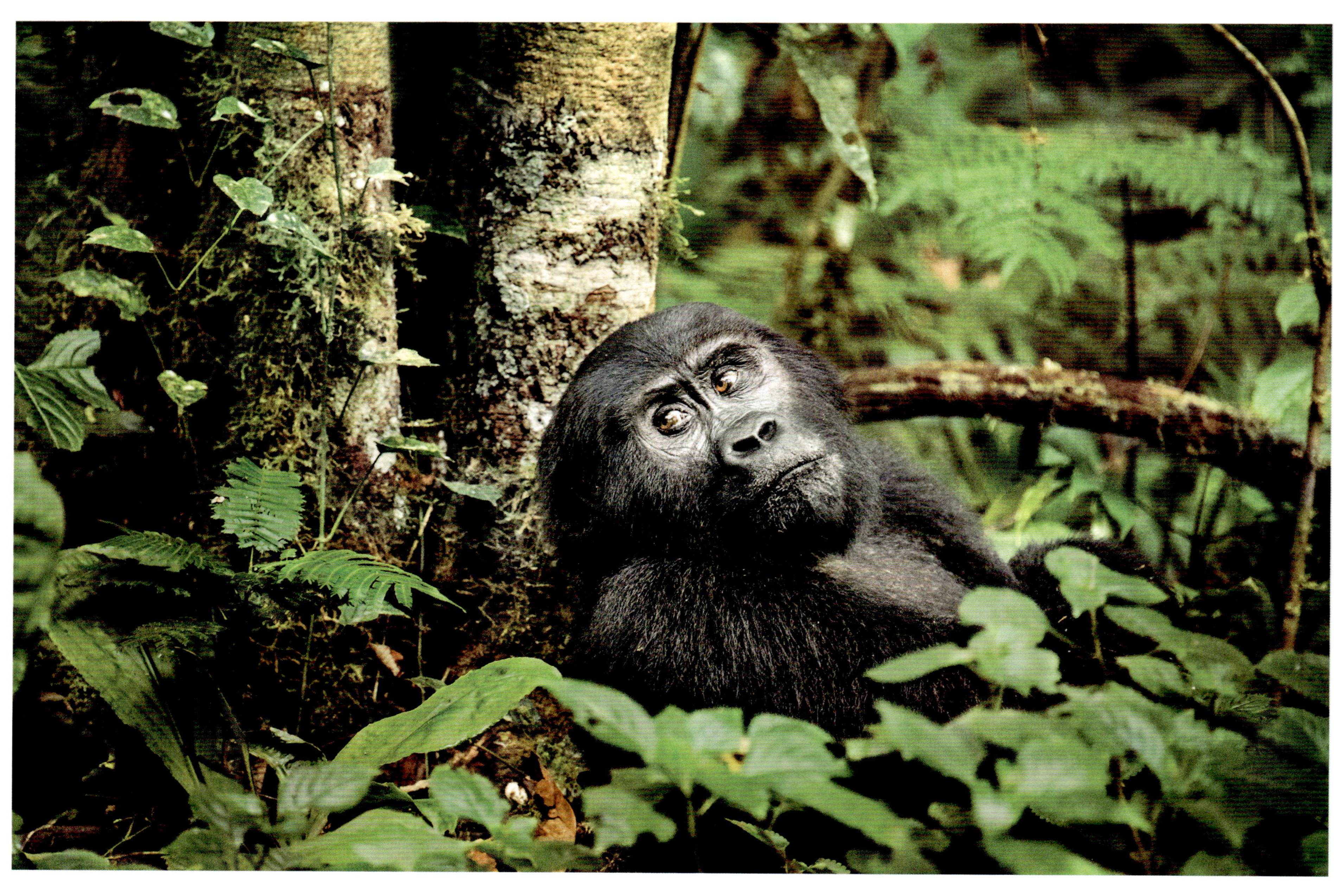

Steve McCurry
Mountain Gorilla
Bwindi Impenetrable Forest, Uganda

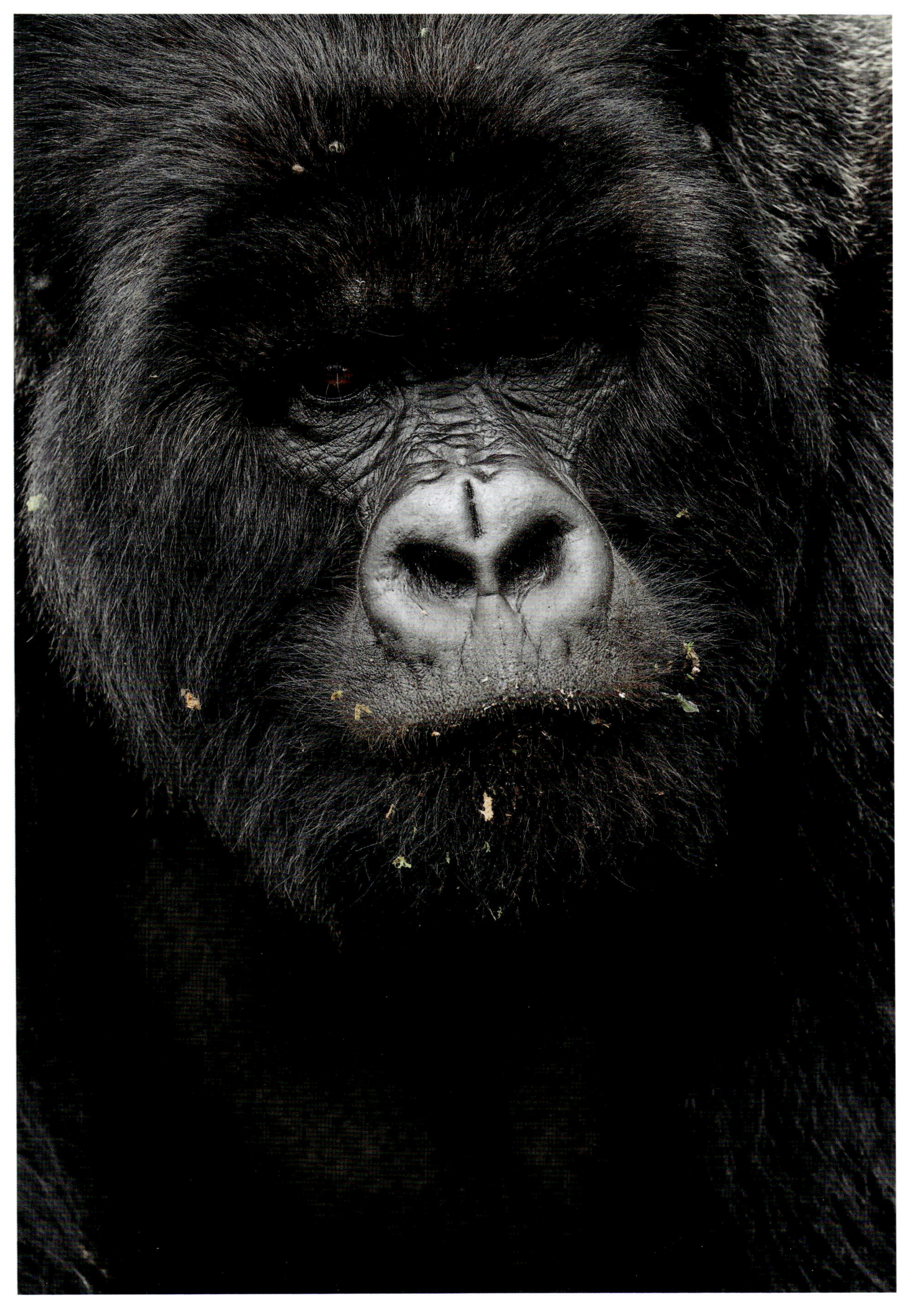

Graeme Green
Mountain Gorilla
Volcanoes National Park, Rwanda

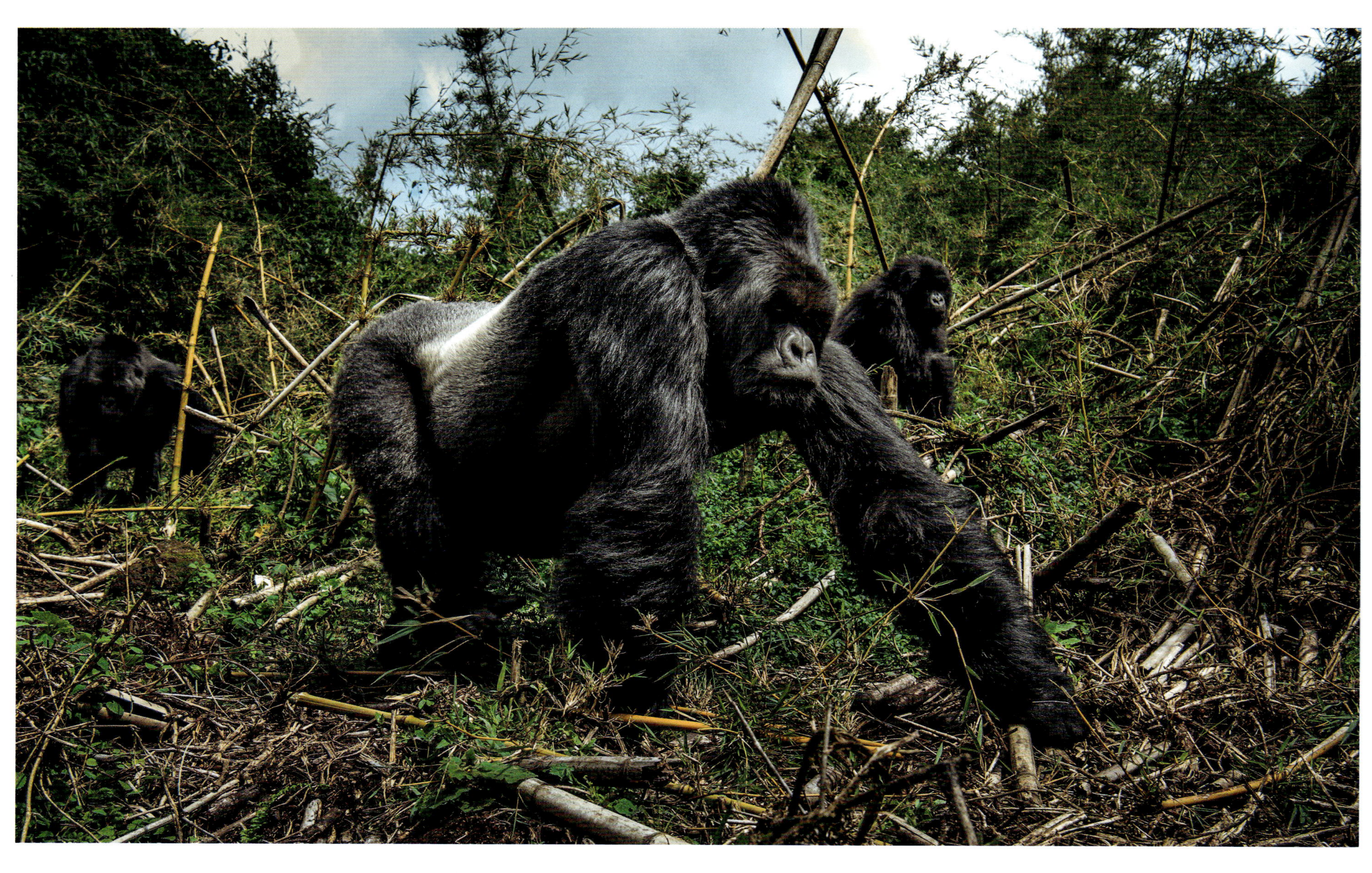

Ami Vitale
Mountain Gorillas
Volcanoes National Park, Rwanda

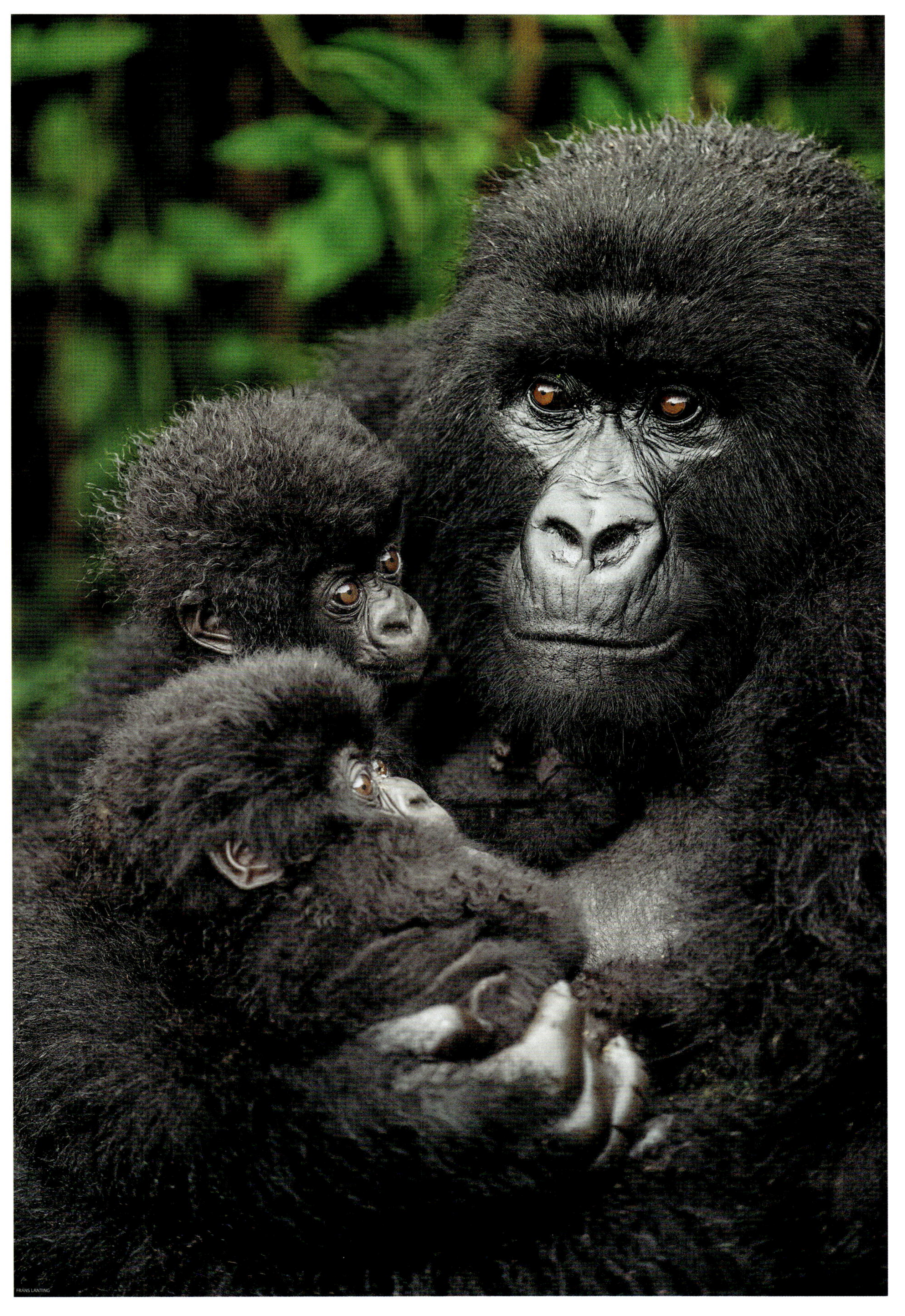

Frans Lanting
Mountain Gorillas
Volcanoes National Park, Rwanda

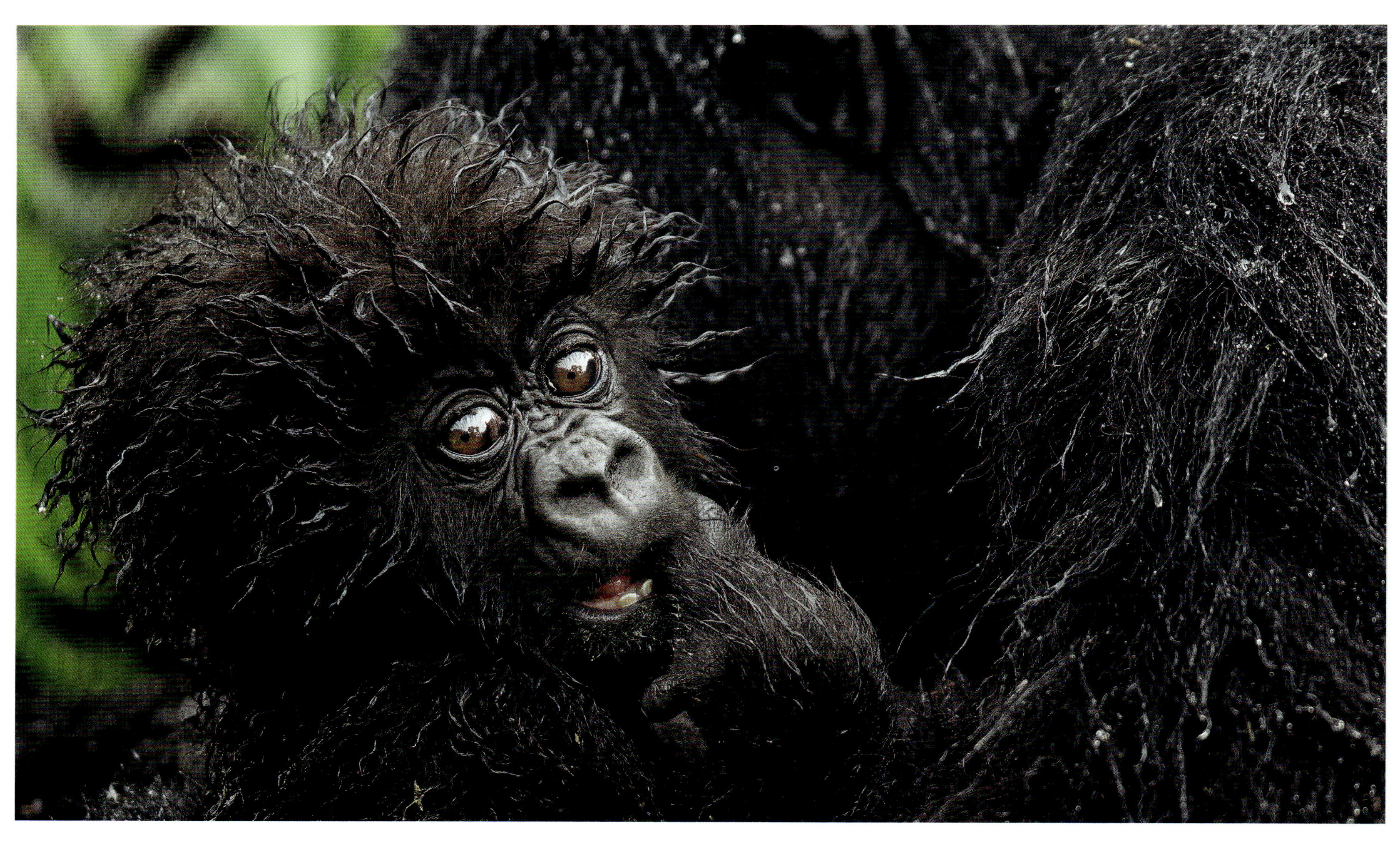

Brian W. Matthews
Mountain Gorilla
Volcanoes National Park, Rwanda

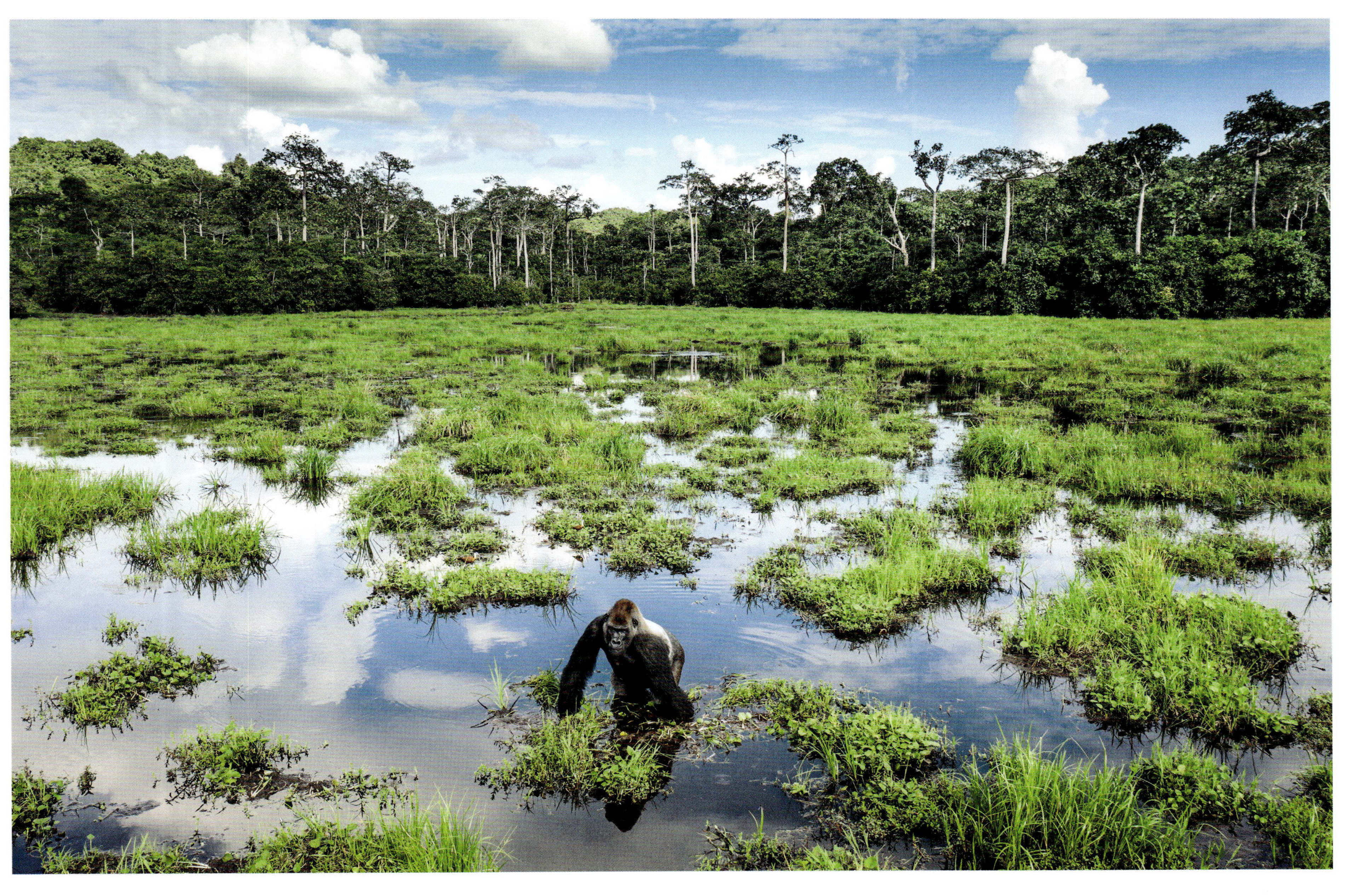

Scott Ramsay
Western Lowland Gorilla
Nouabalé-Ndoki National Park,
Republic of the Congo

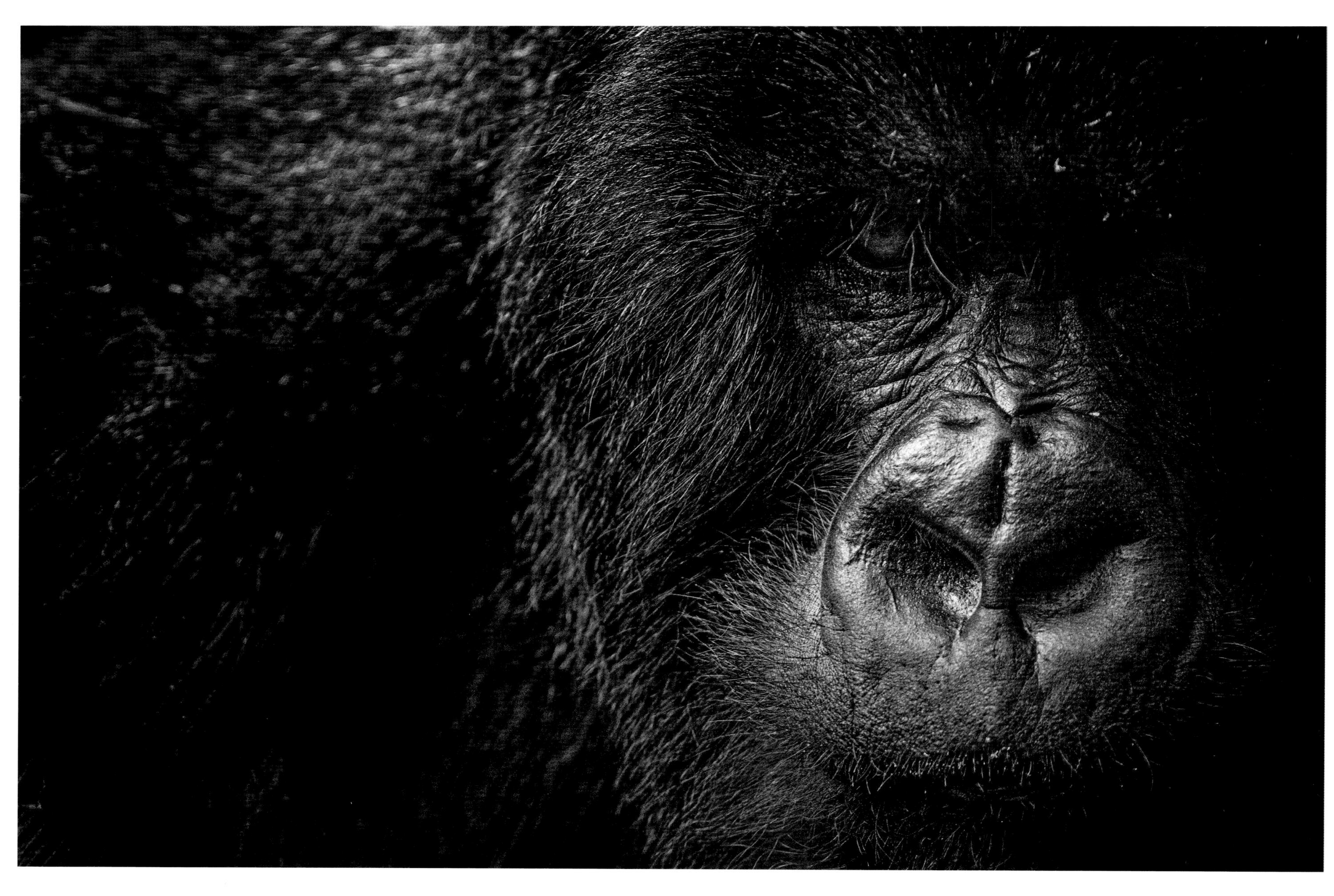

Gaël R. Vande weghe
Mountain Gorilla
Volcanoes National Park, Rwanda

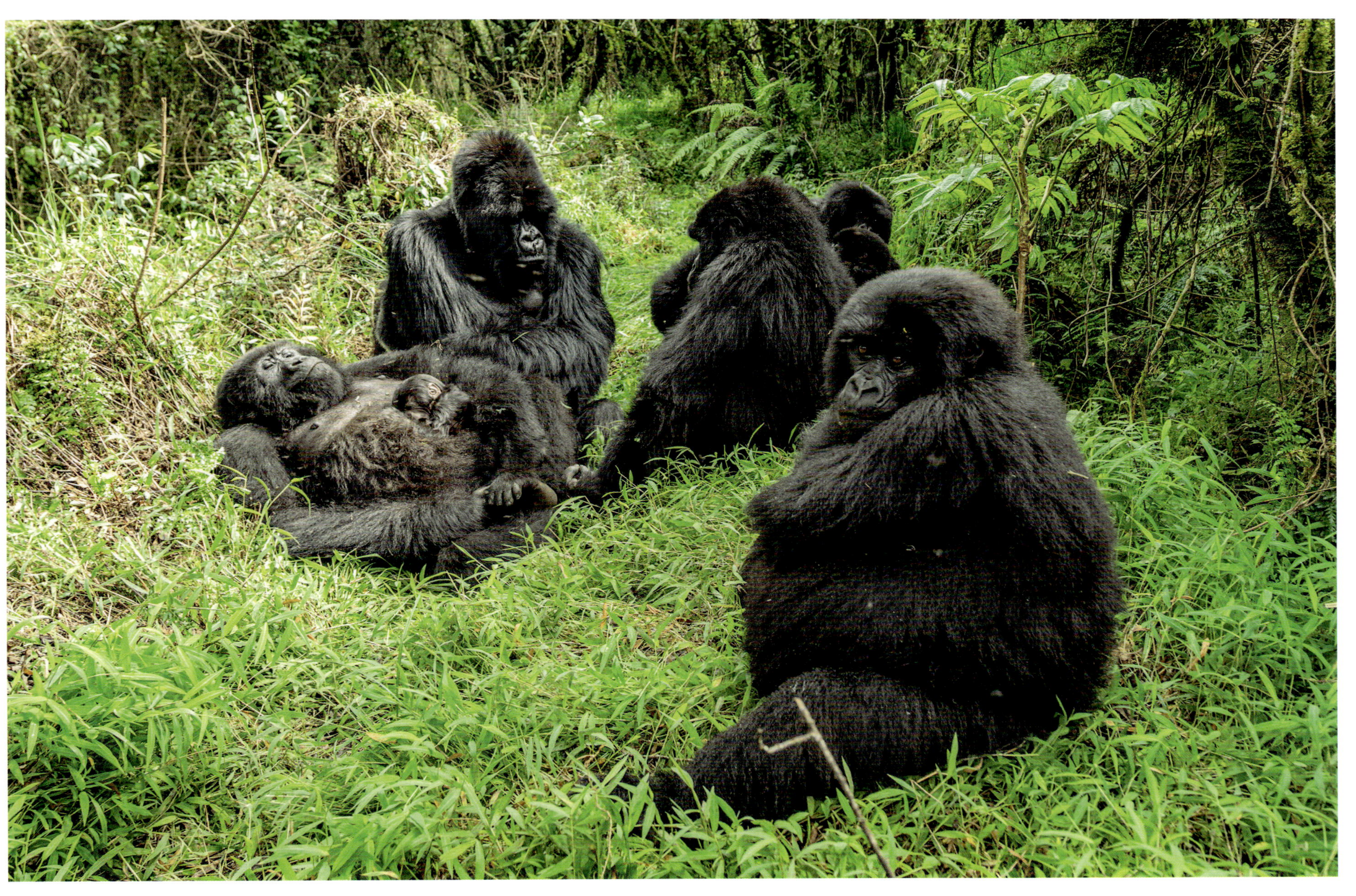

Usha Harish
Mountain Gorillas
Mgahinga Gorilla National Park, Uganda

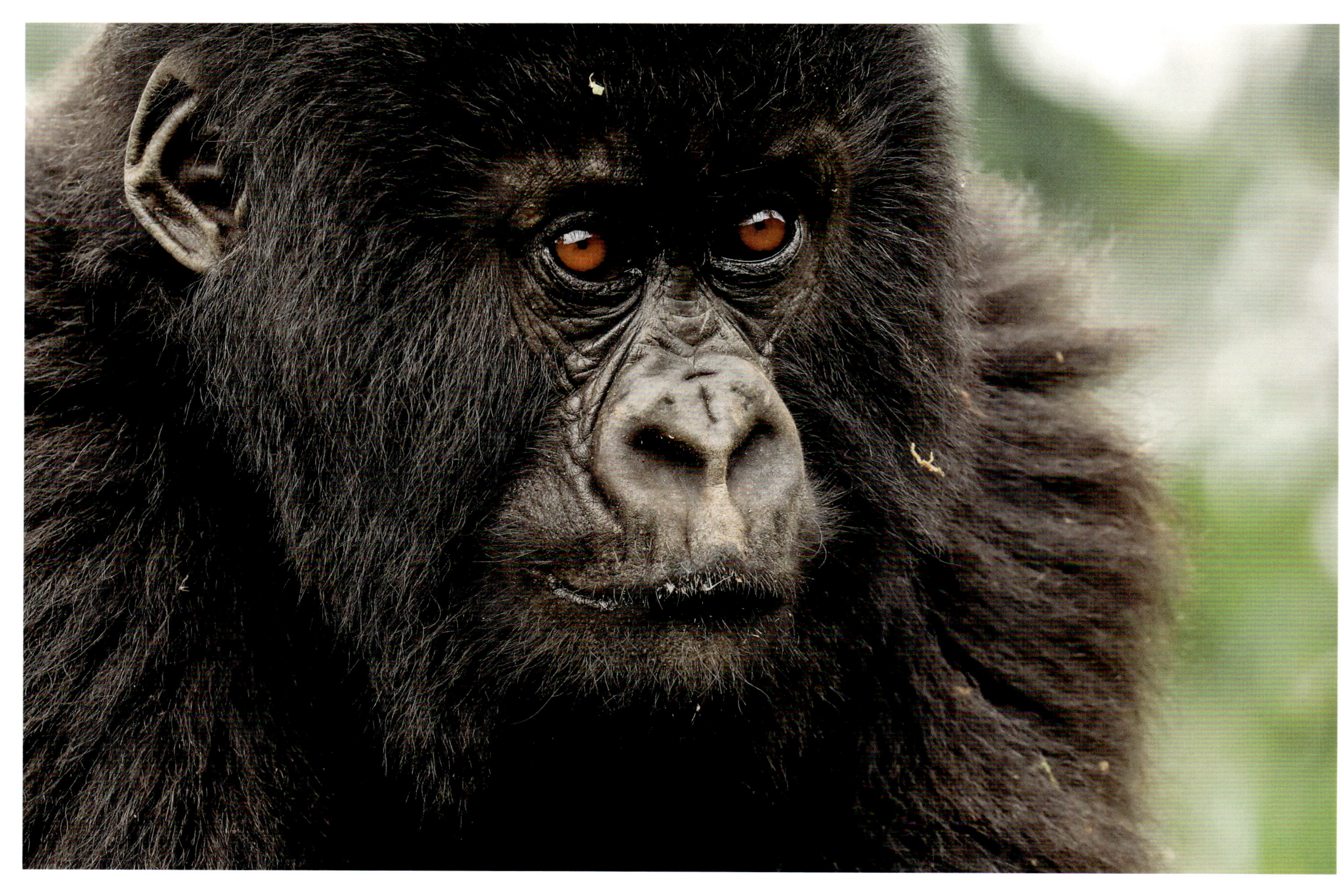

Graeme Green
Mountain Gorilla
Volcanoes National Park, Rwanda

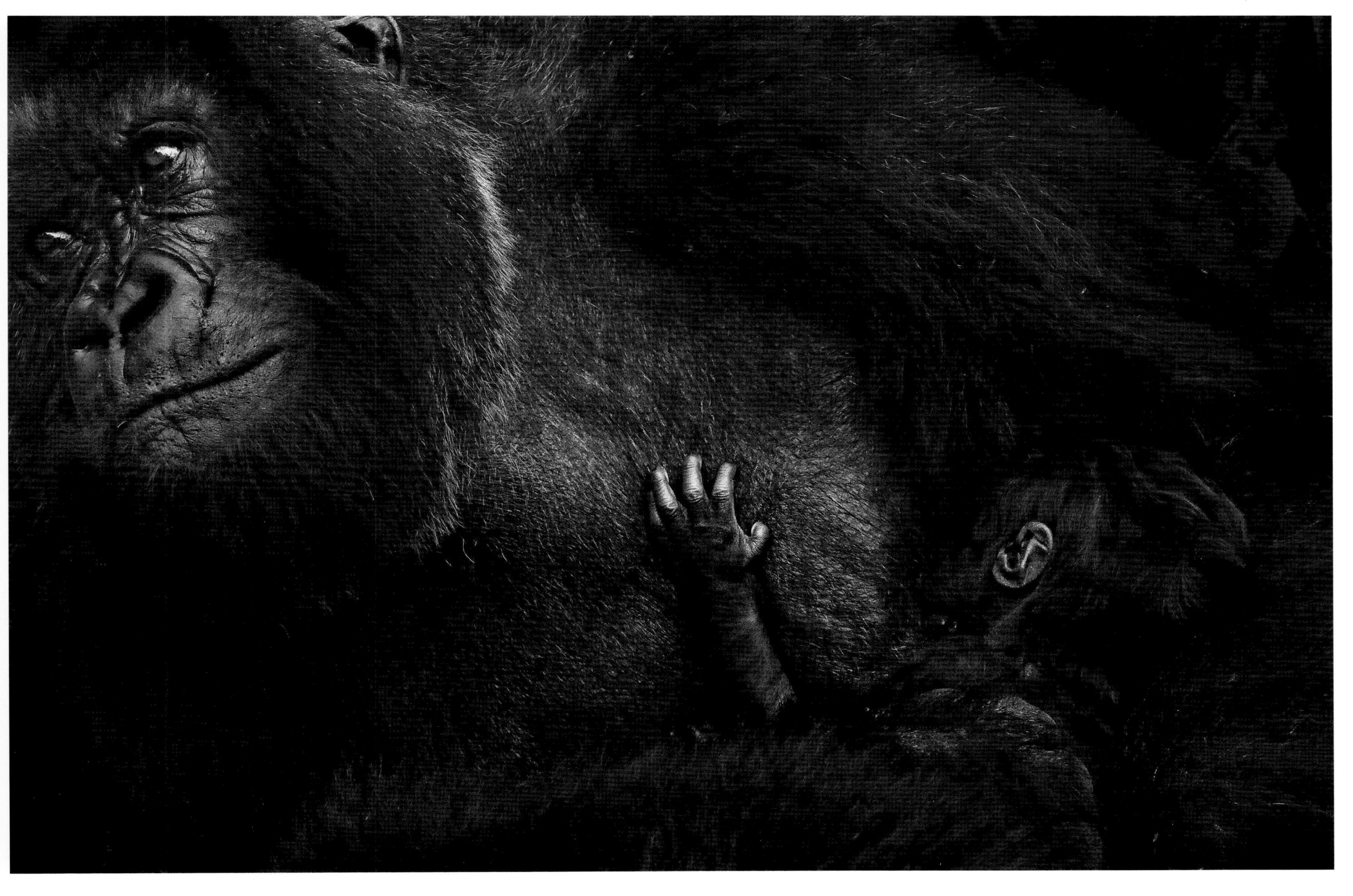

Piper Mackay
Mountain Gorillas
Volcanoes National Park, Rwanda

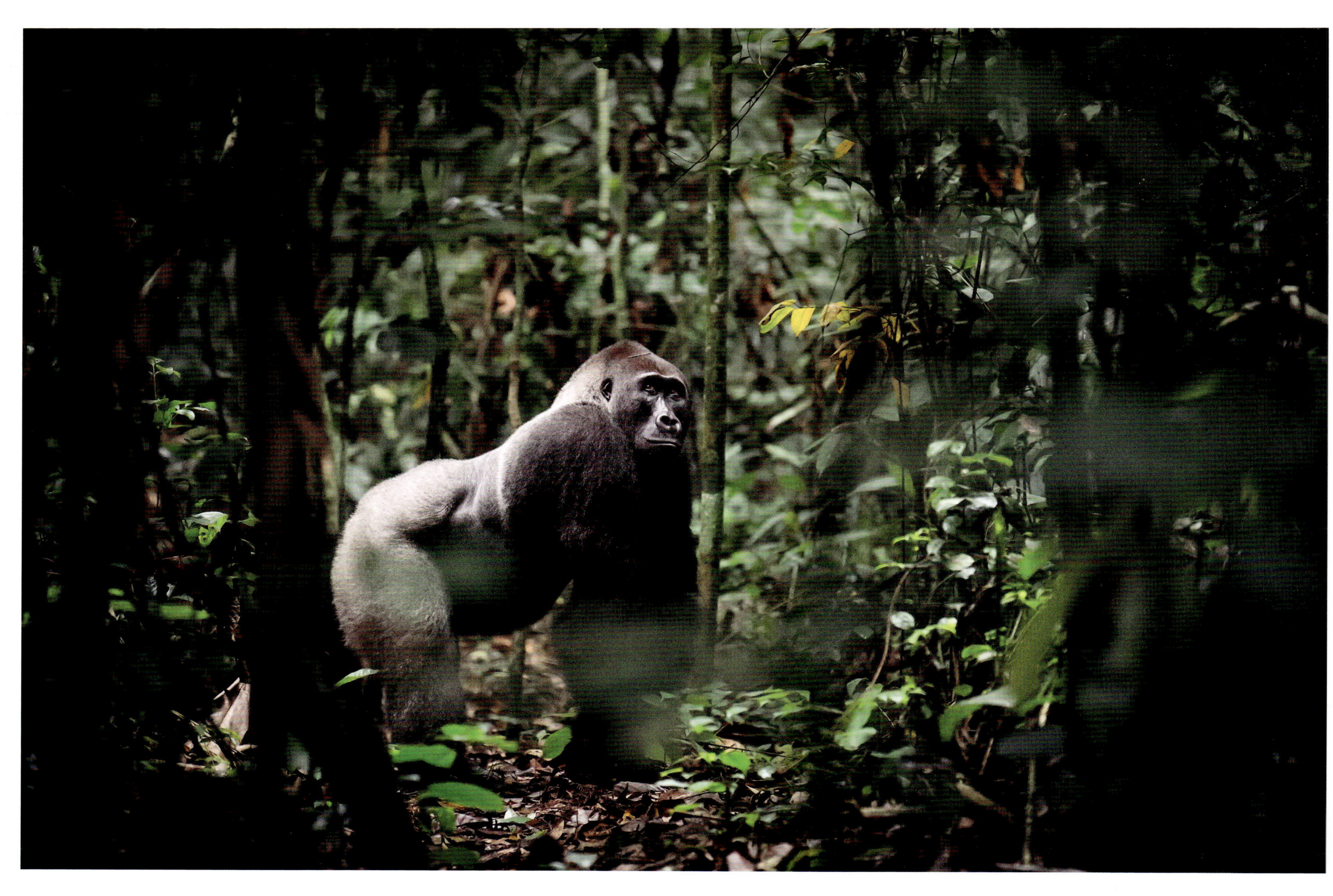

Will Burrard-Lucas
Western Lowland Gorilla
Odzala-Kokoua National Park,
Republic of the Congo

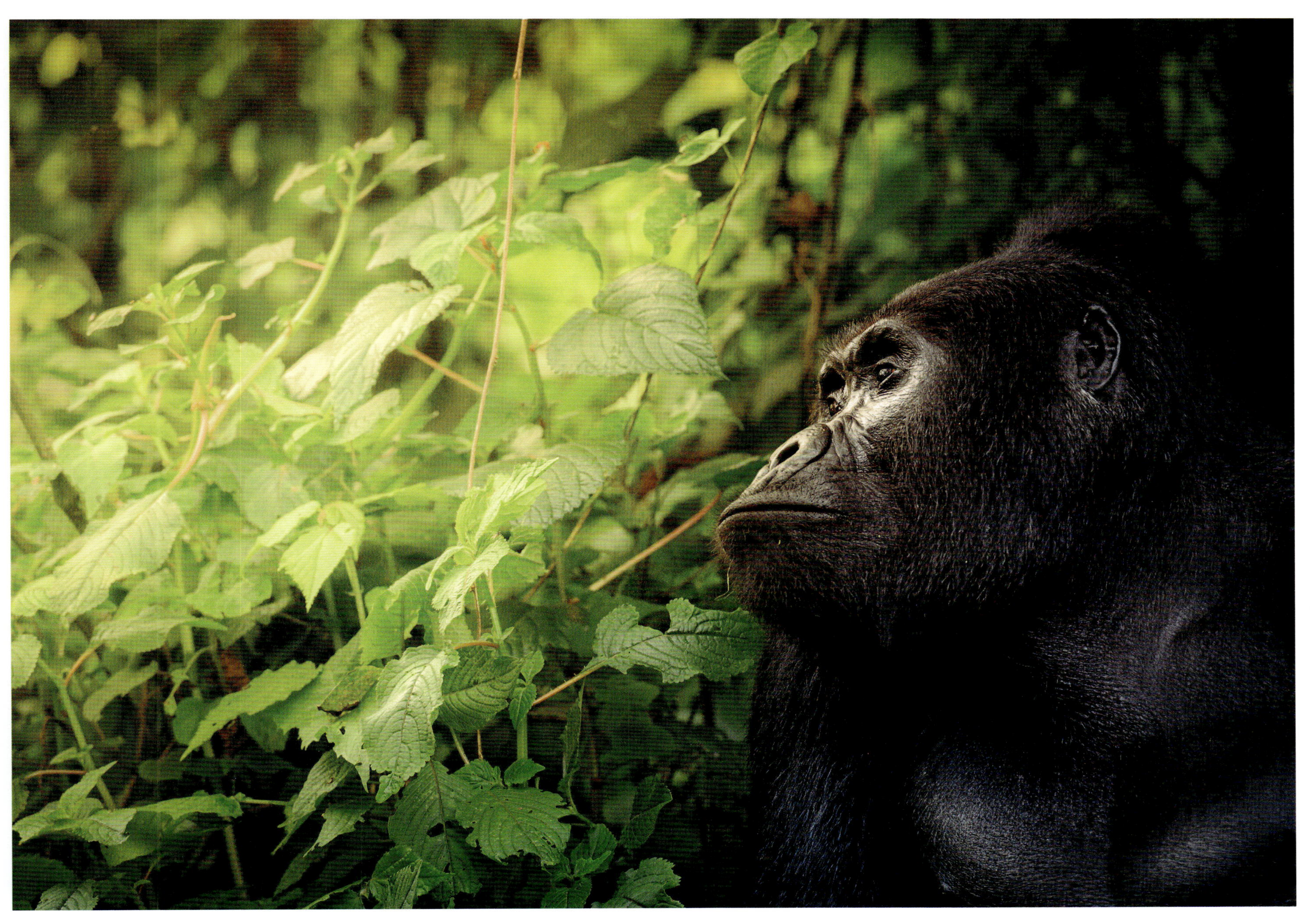

Majed Alzaabi
Mountain Gorilla
Bwindi Impenetrable Forest, Uganda

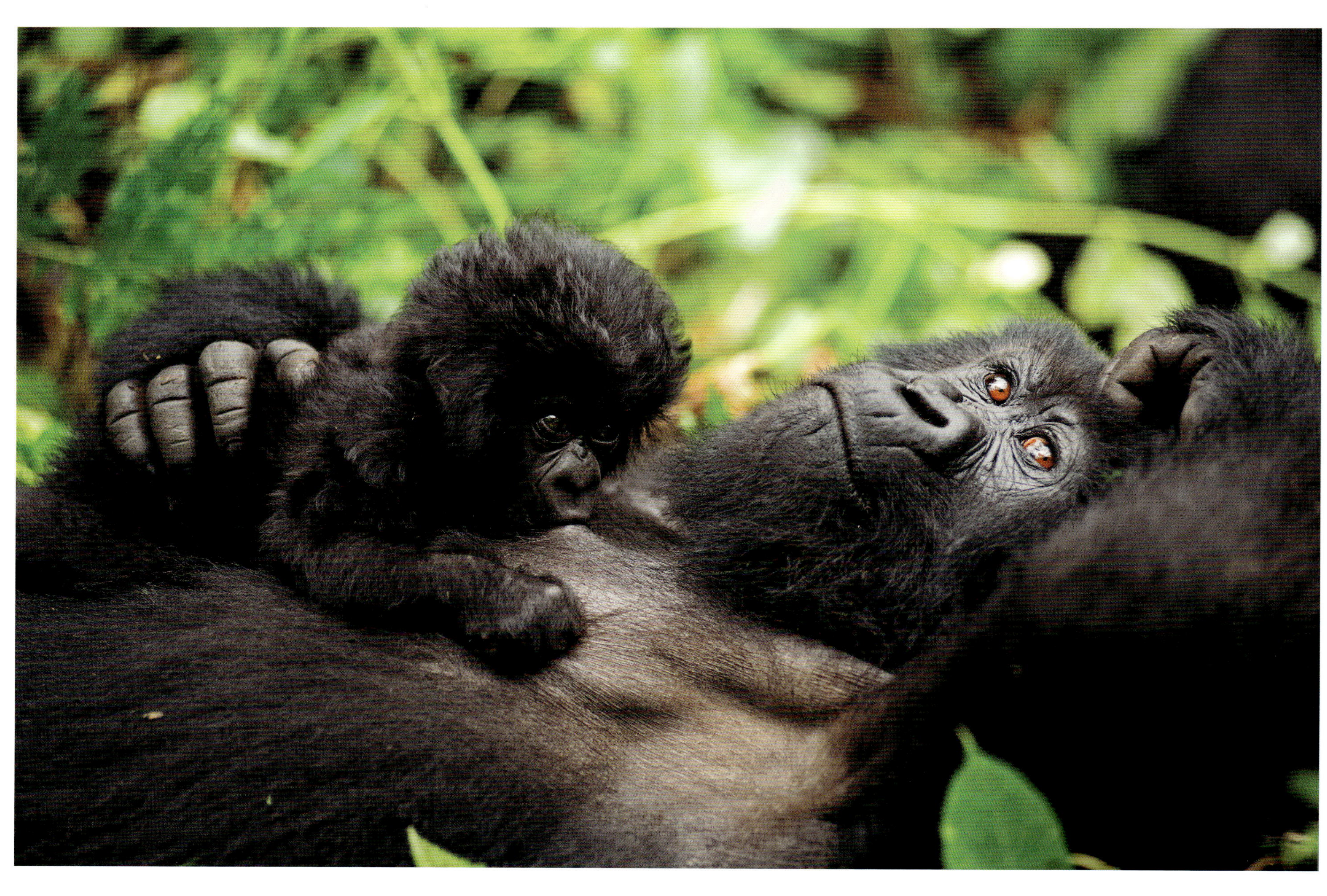

Amy Gulick
Mountain Gorillas
Volcanoes National Park, Rwanda

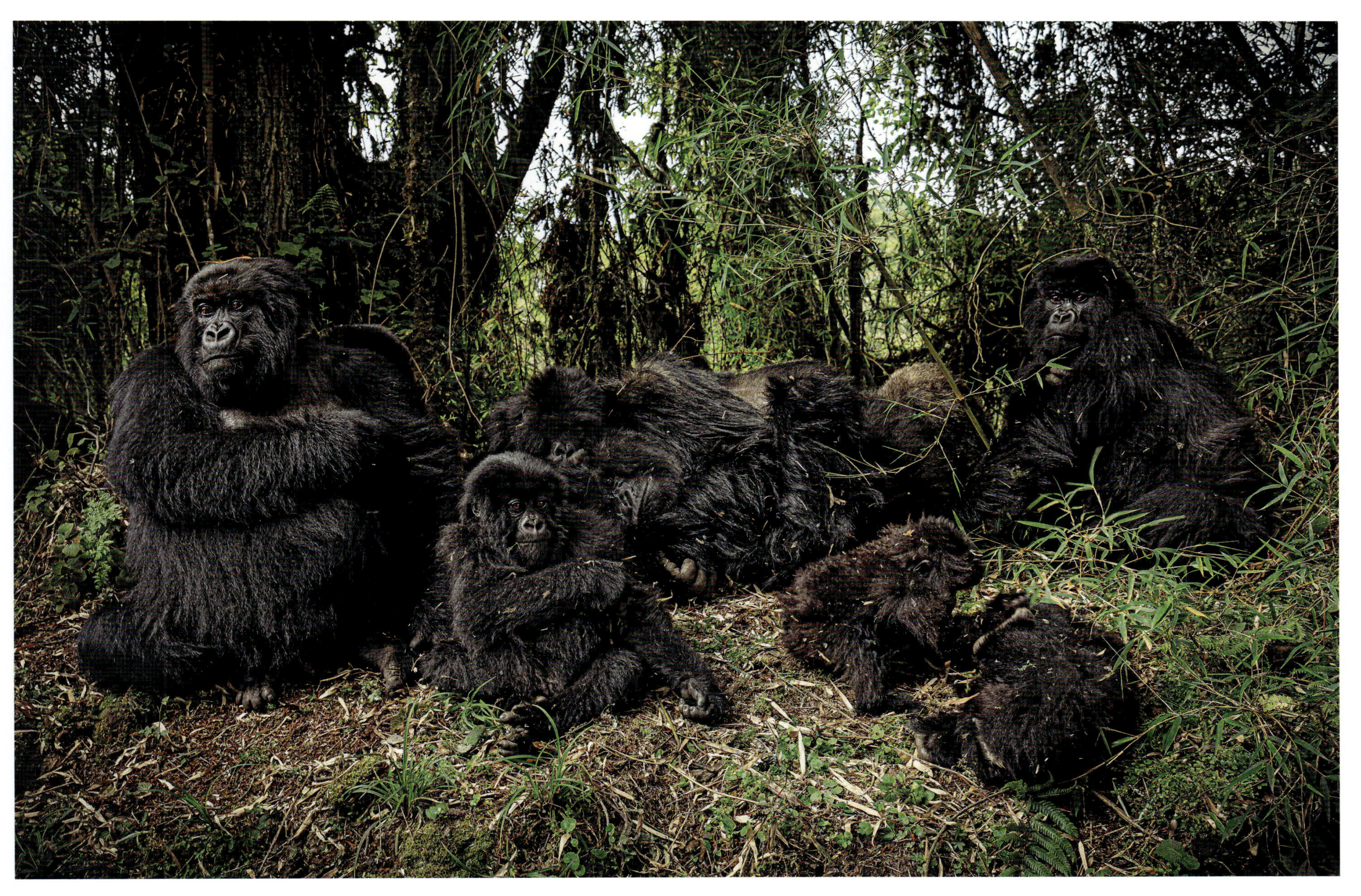

Ronan Donovan
Mountain Gorillas
Volcanoes National Park, Rwanda

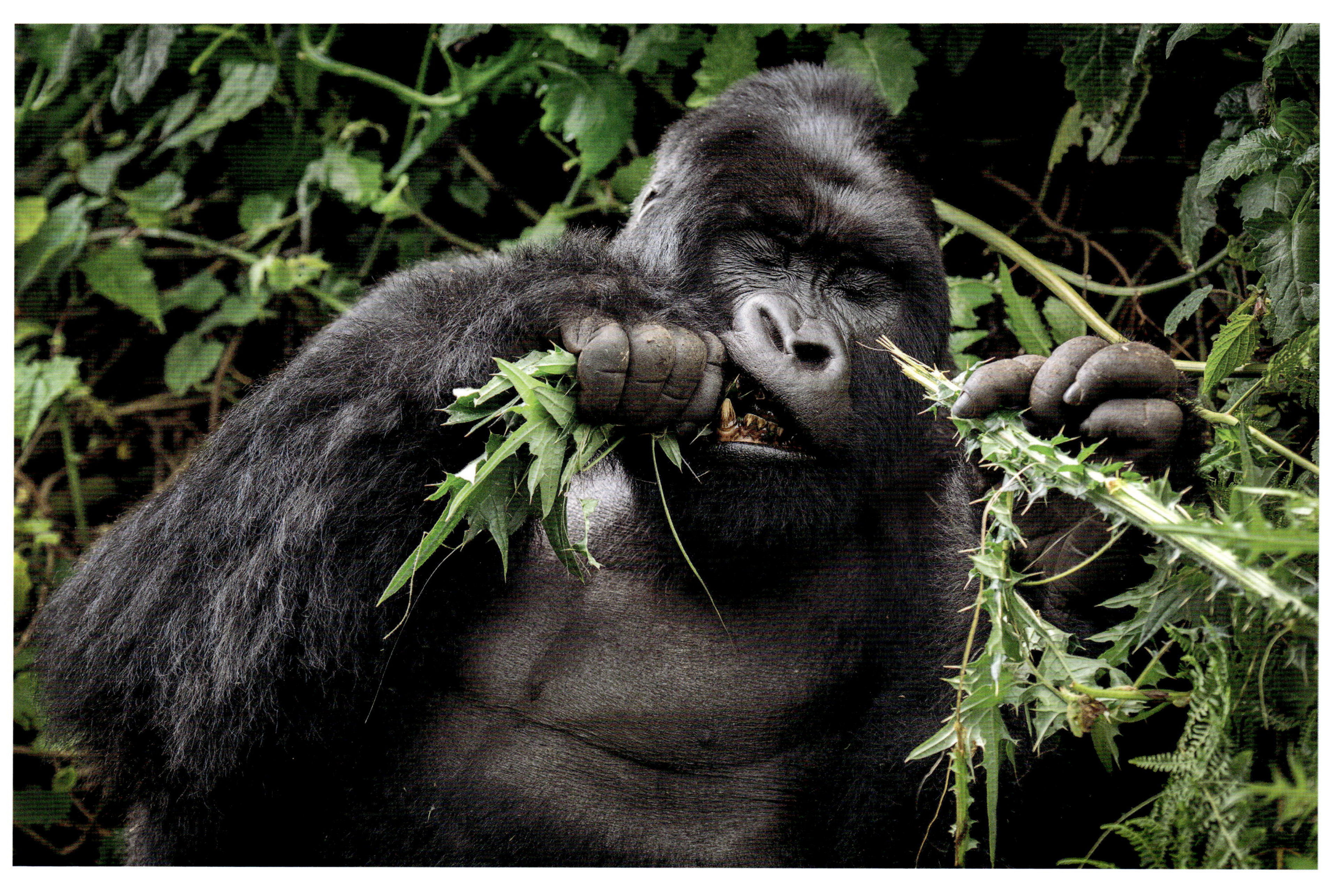

Mark Edward Harris
Mountain Gorilla
Volcanoes National Park, Rwanda

Vladimir Cech, Jr.
Mountain Gorilla
Volcanoes National Park, Rwanda

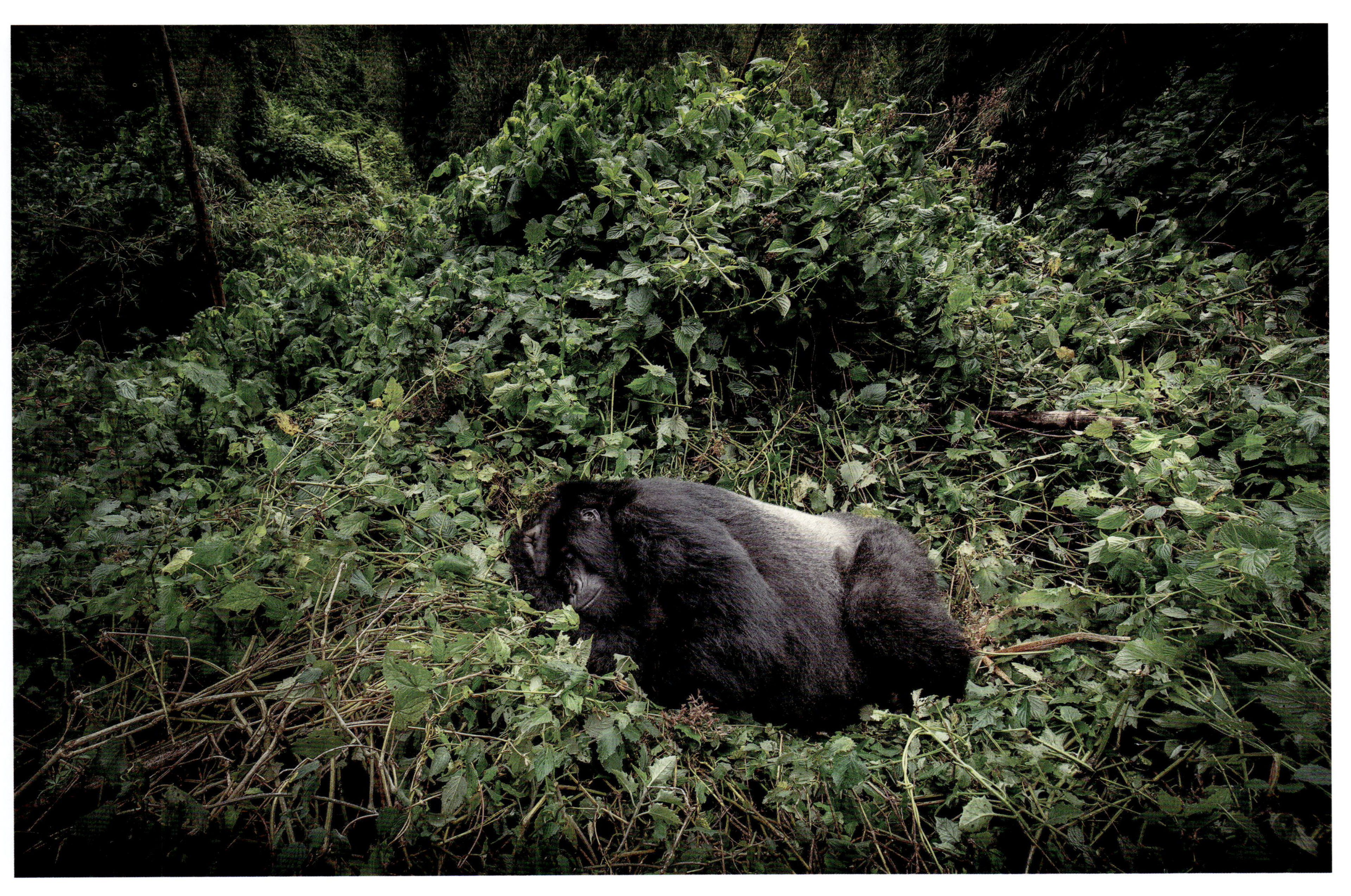

161

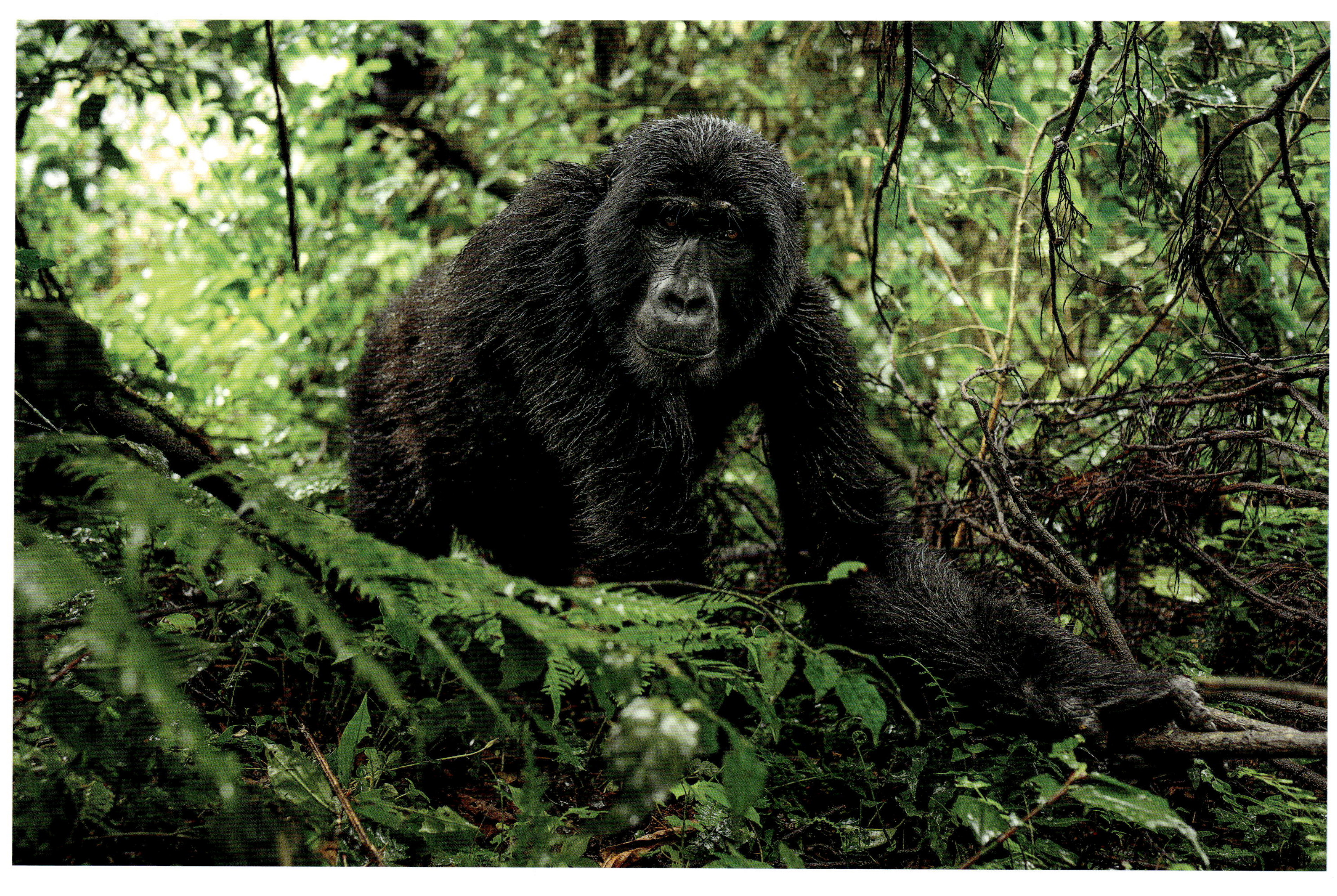

Richard Peters
Mountain Gorilla
Bwindi Impenetrable Forest, Uganda

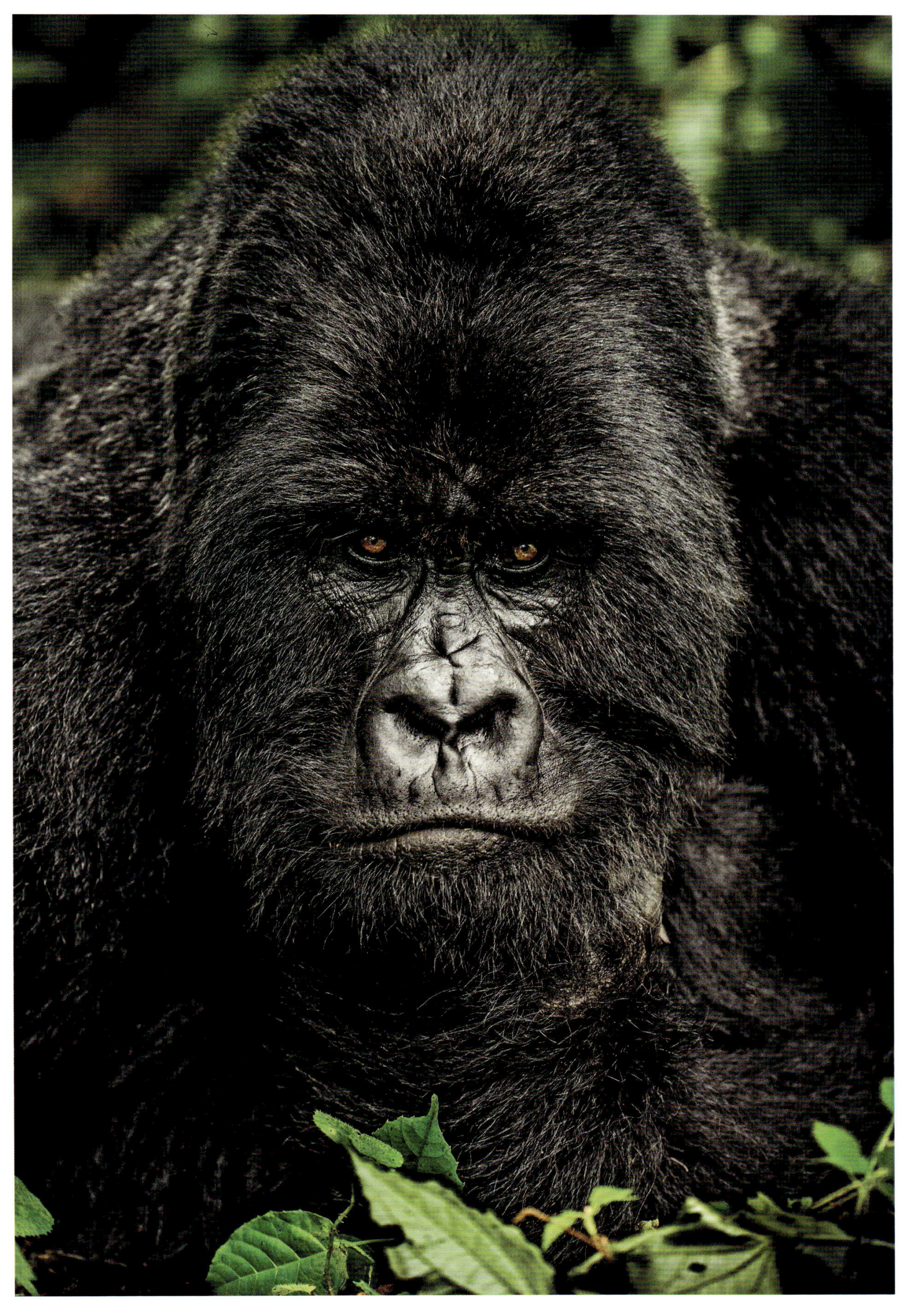

Nelis Wolmarans
Mountain Gorilla
Virunga National Park,
Democratic Republic of the Congo

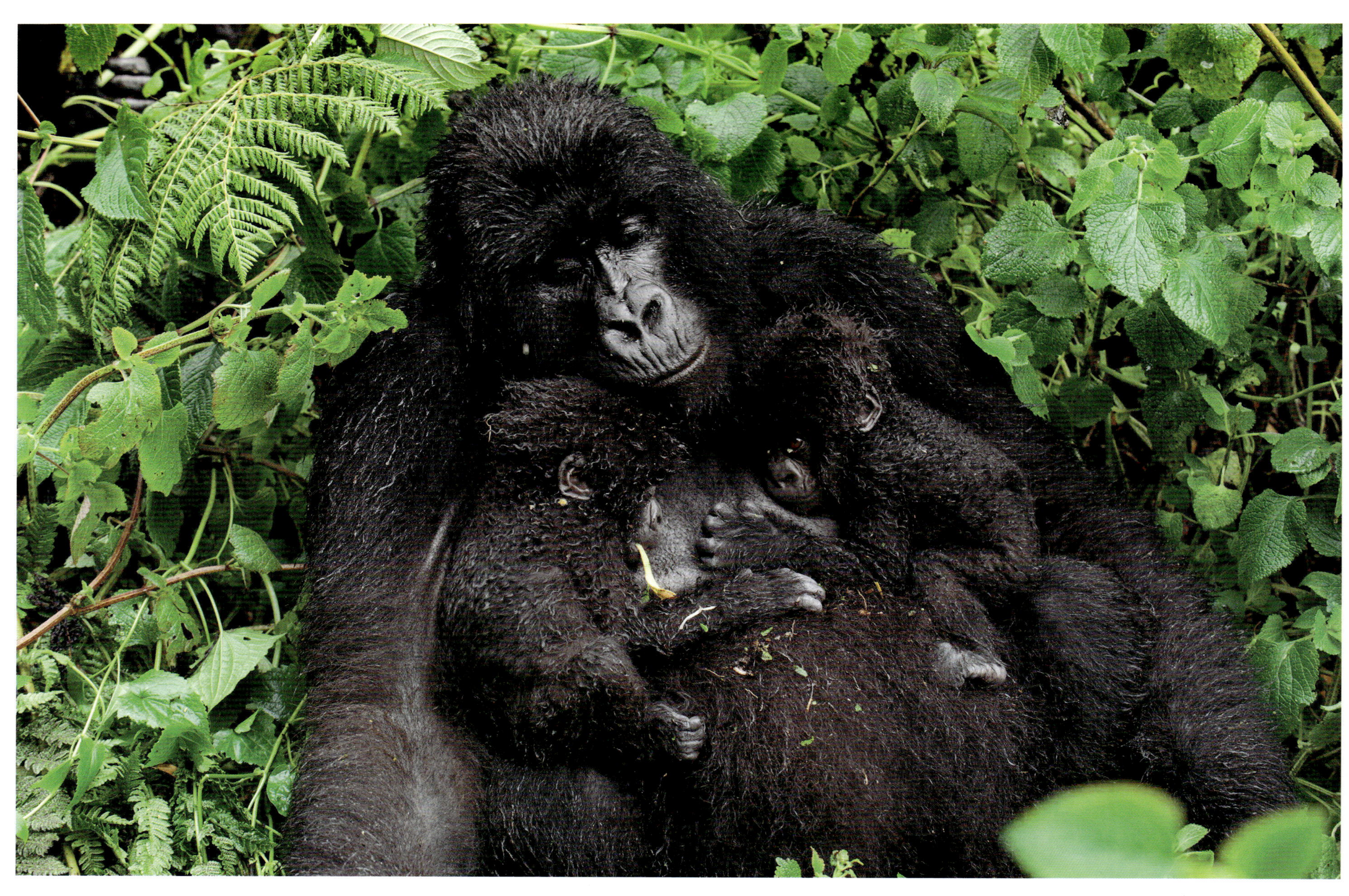

Suzi Eszterhas
Mountain Gorillas
Volcanoes National Park, Rwanda

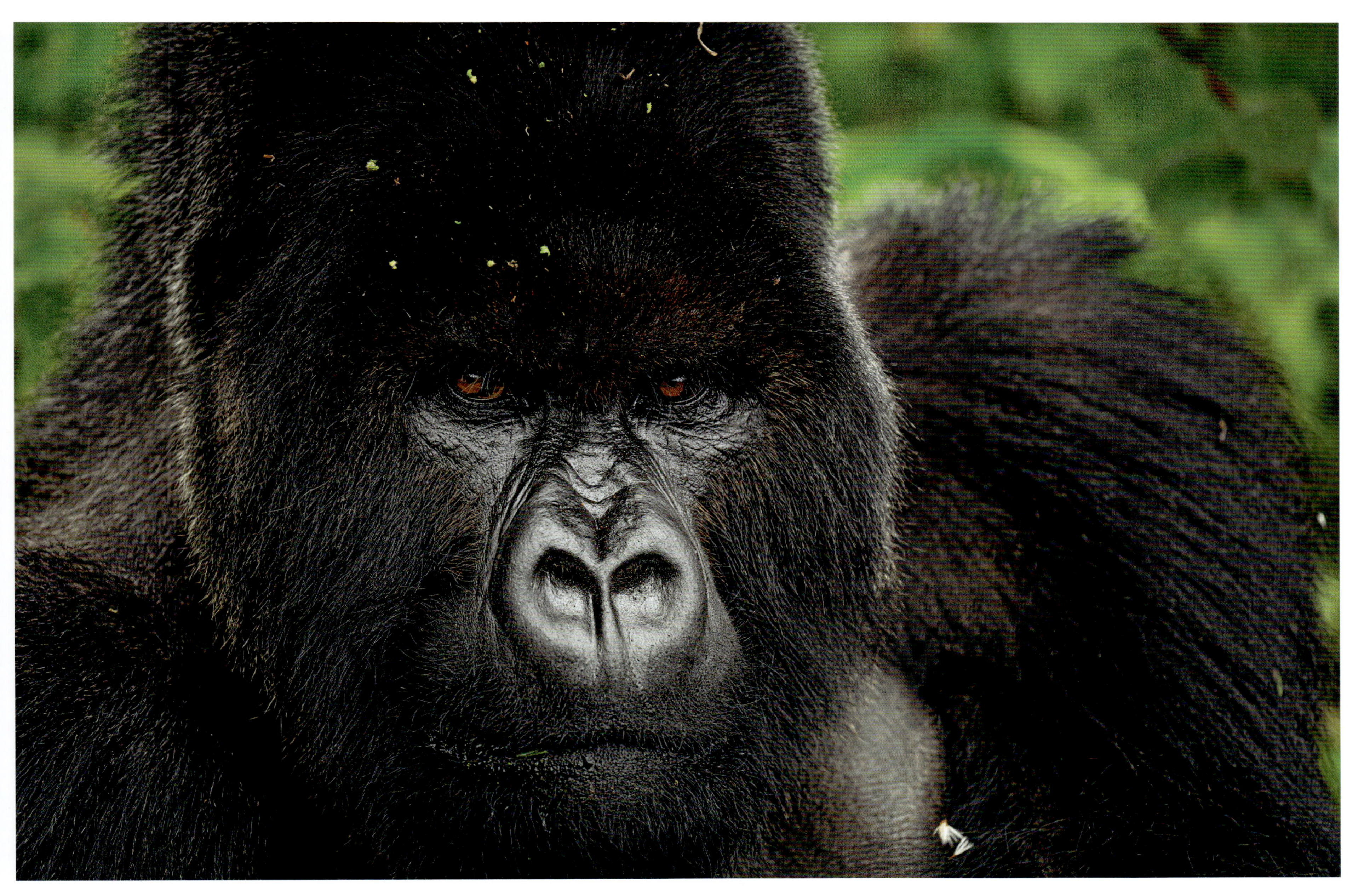

Ronan Donovan
Mountain Gorilla
Volcanoes National Park, Rwanda

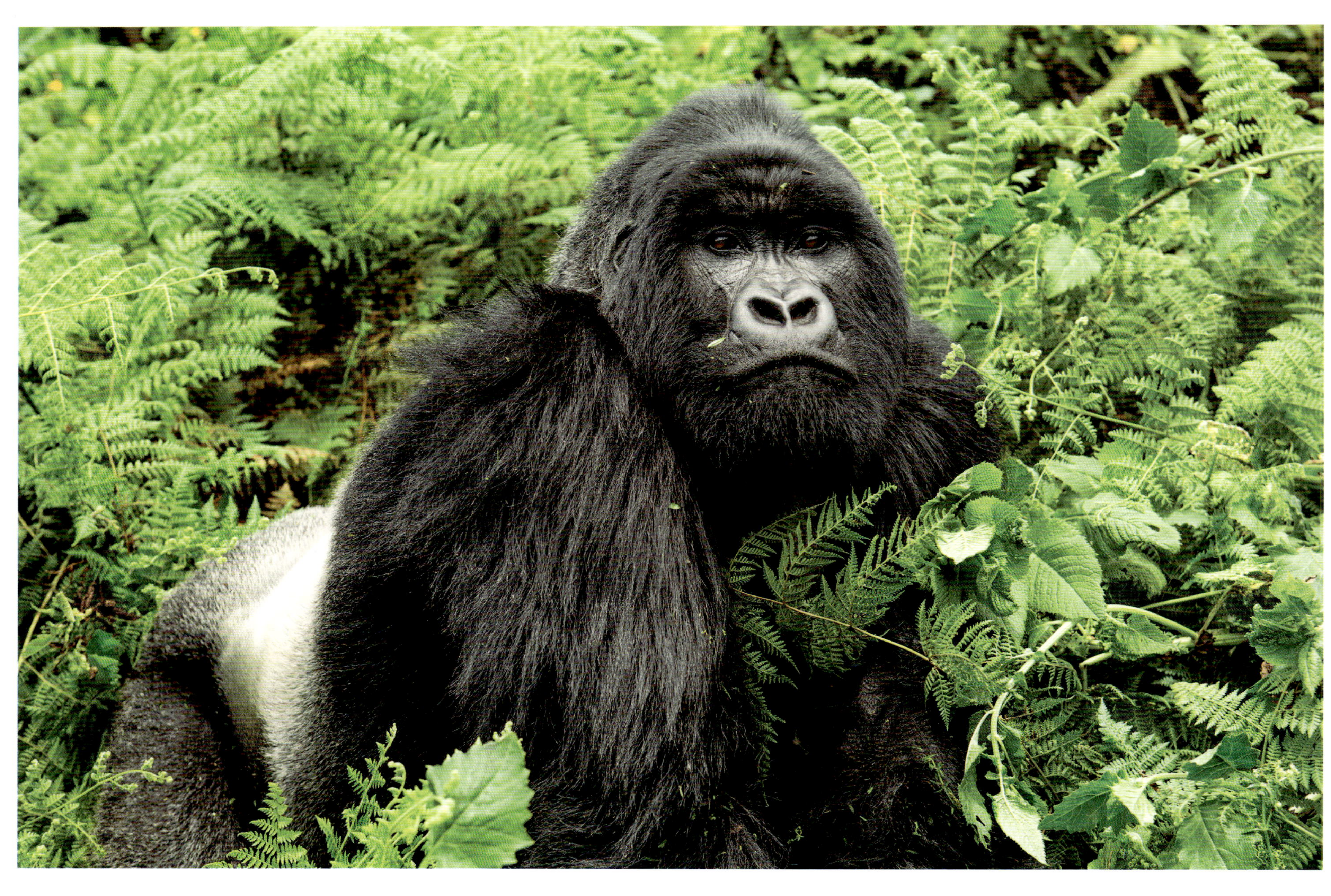

Sandesh Kadur
Mountain Gorilla
Volcanoes National Park, Rwanda

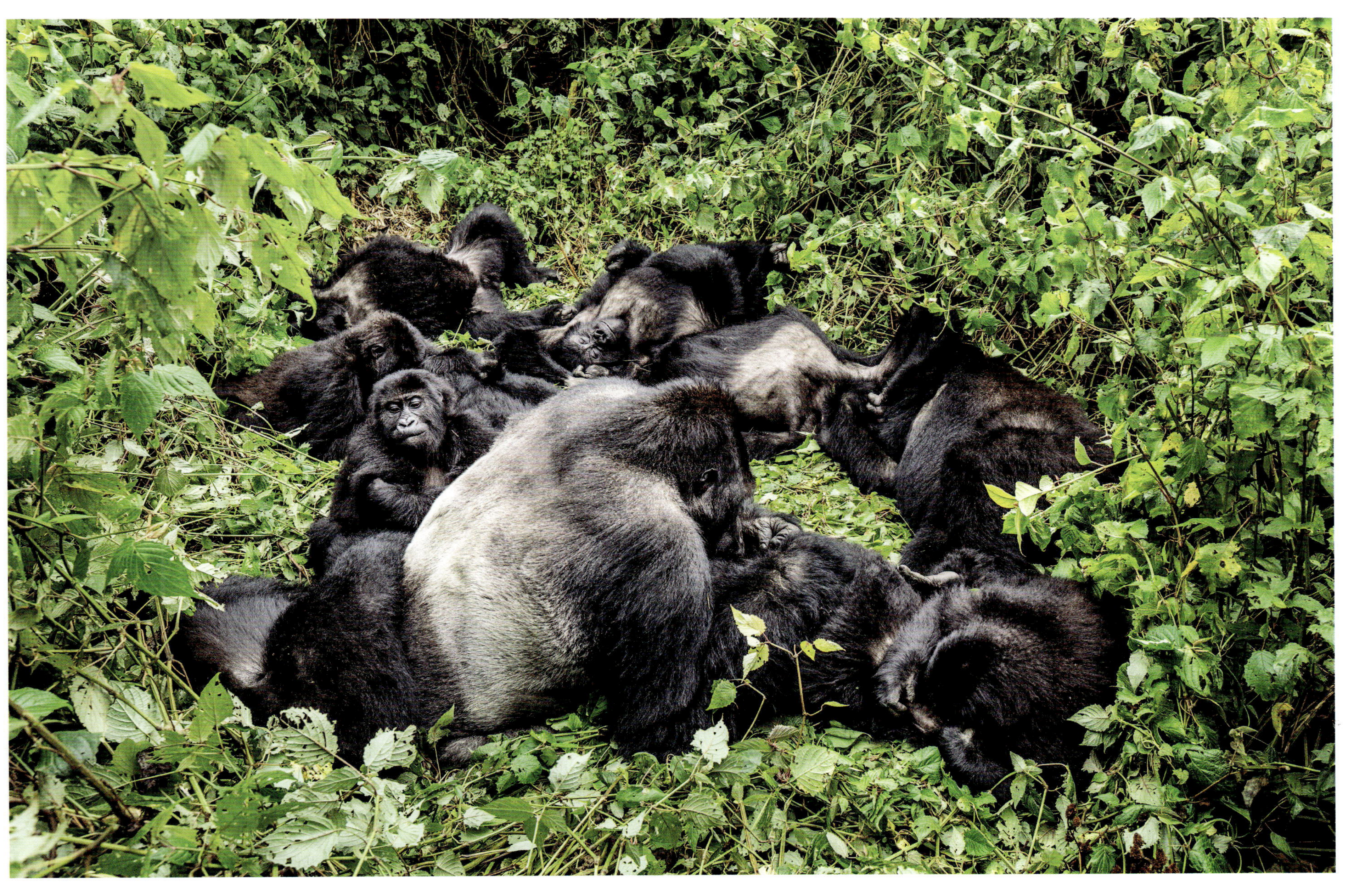

Marcus Westberg
Grauer's Gorillas
Kahuzi-Biega National Park,
Democratic Republic of the Congo

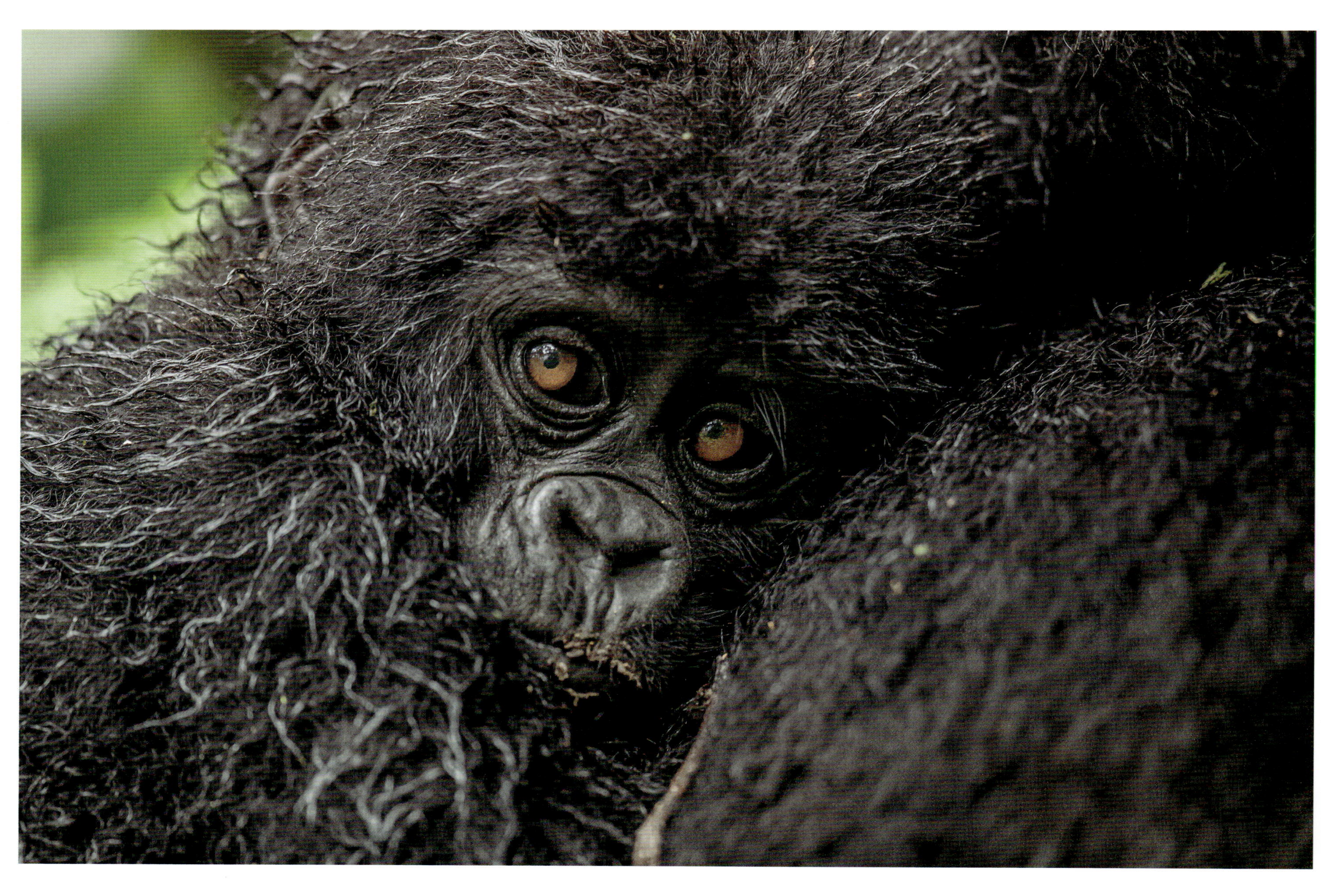

Paul Goldstein
Mountain Gorilla
Bwindi Impenetrable Forest, Uganda

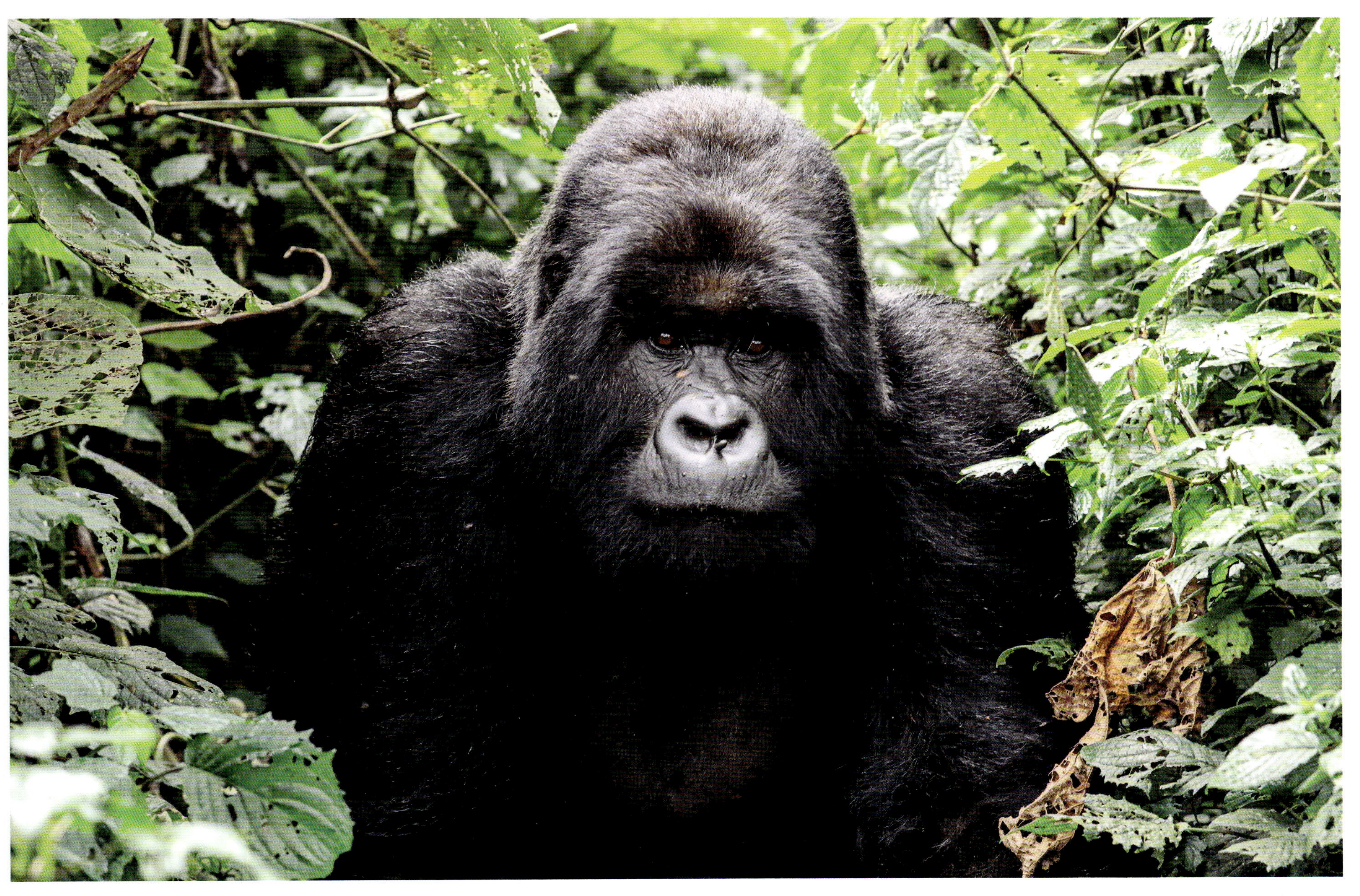

Graeme Green
Mountain Gorilla
Volcanoes National Park, Rwanda

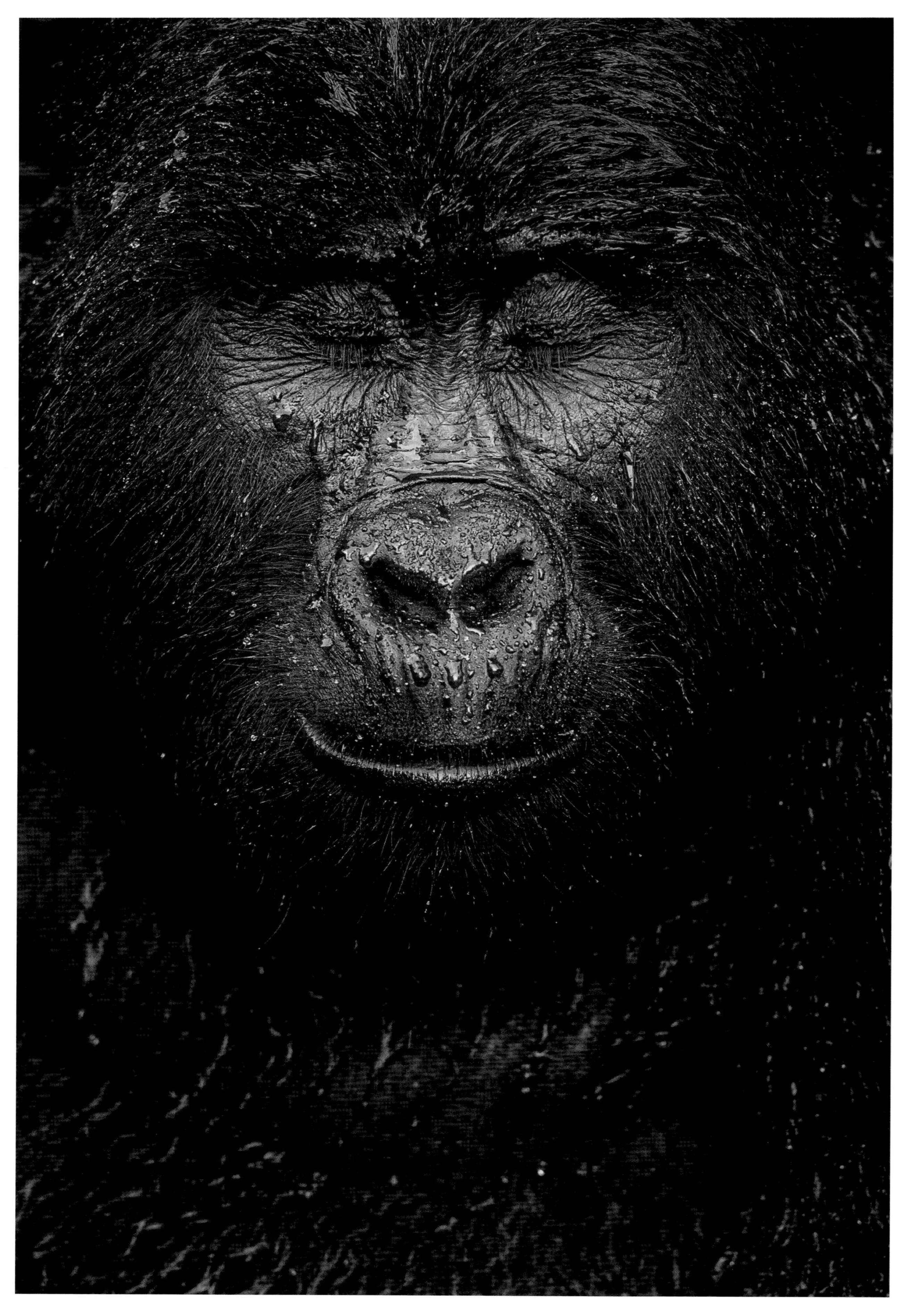

Majed Alzaabi
Mountain Gorilla
Bwindi Impenetrable Forest, Uganda

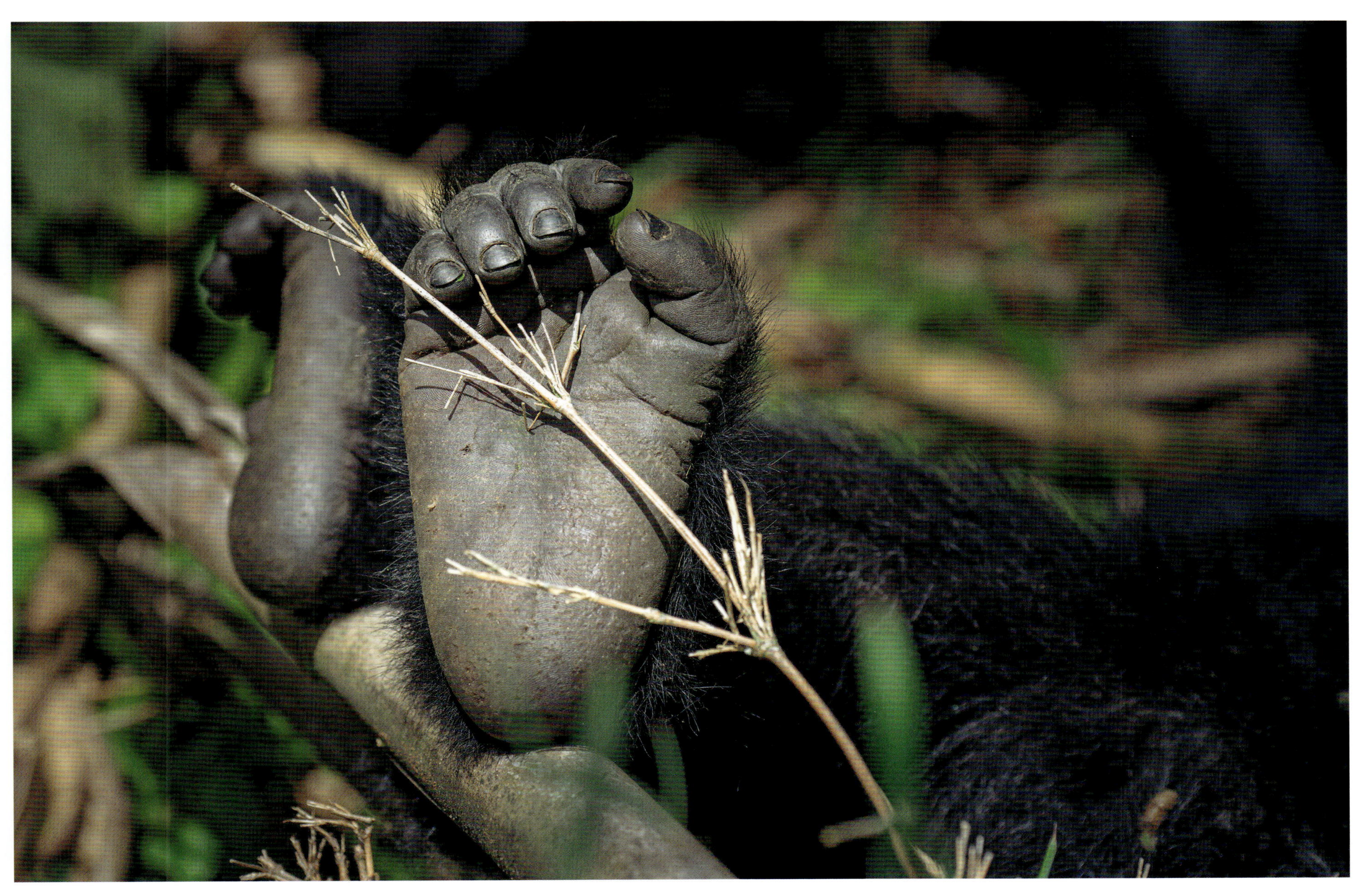

Ami Vitale
Mountain Gorilla
Volcanoes National Park, Rwanda

TIGERS

Tigers

Dr. Anish Andheria

President and CEO, Wildlife Conservation Trust

TIGERS EPITOMIZE POWER, GRACE, STEALTH, AND TENACITY. Wherever they are found, they are the top predators. Their brute strength, elusive nature, and interaction with humans conjured up the vision of a ruthless hunter, resulting in them getting lodged in Indian mythology and history. Durga, the goddess of power, rode a tiger. The tiger appears in rock paintings that are five to ten thousand years old. Nearly 4,500 years ago, long before the Indus Valley civilization arose, pictograms of tigers were regularly being used on ancient seals. The tiger is also mentioned in the two major Sanskrit epics of ancient India: the Mahabharata and Ramayana. Buddhism also has its share of tiger stories, the most popular being one from around the fifth century BCE in which Lord Buddha offers himself to a starving tigress to stop her from feeding on her own cubs.

Tigers are entwined in present-day Indian culture in the form of Waghoba, a deity worshipped by several tribes who continue to share their backyards with these magnificent large carnivores even today. This deity takes the form of a leopard or a tiger, or in some cases both. In the estuarine forests of Sundarbans that are contiguous across India and Bangladesh, where tigers have a reputation of attacking people, local communities offer prayers to Bonobibi, literally translated as *the lady of the forest*, whenever they enter the forest to collect honey, fish, or firewood. As the legend has it, Bonobini defeated Dakshin Rai, the ghostly tormentor, who then promised to prevent tigers from attacking humans. Thereafter, she became the ruler of mangrove forests.

There is a deep-rooted connection between people and tigers. However, the reverence for the species is not born out of culture or mythology. It simply grows in anybody who comes face to face with a tiger in the jungle. I've had countless fascinating interactions with tigers in Indian jungles over the last thirty years. Each incident is vividly etched in my mind. Such is the aura of the animal that it's almost impossible to not feel captivated by it.

This is also why the tiger has been adopted as a global icon of conservation. Project Tiger in India became an instant hit in the early 1970s, and is considered one of the most successful conservation programs on the planet. It achieved the impossible: aligning the government and local communities in a battle to bring a large carnivore back from the brink. Between 2006 and 2018, the tiger population in India doubled from just over 1,400 to nearly 3,000.

Against the odds, Indian culture has played a significant role in the resurgence of the tiger. Indian culture instills compassion in individuals for everything alive and establishes the connectedness between humans and other living beings. Although two hundred years of British rule managed to leave behind a culture of the hunting of wildlife for "sport," once the British left, India returned to her former self, which values wildlife.

Most other nations with tiger populations haven't fared that well. Until the 1950s, there were nine subspecies of tiger. Of these, the Caspian, Javan, and Balinese tigers disappeared between the 1950s and 1970s, and in all probability the South China tiger has met the same fate or is on the verge of extinction. Three of the thirteen countries where tigers were present—Laos, Cambodia, and Vietnam—have lost all their tigers. Two others—Myanmar and China—have very few left. Nepal and Bhutan have invested considerable effort in conserving tigers, but owing to their small size and undulating terrain, they have fewer than 300 individuals between them. Bangladesh has witnessed a sharp decline in its tiger population over the past decade. Fewer than 400 Sumatran tigers are estimated to remain in the wild, while Russia boasts fewer than 400 Siberian (or Amur) tigers, most of which inhabit the forests of the Russian Far East.

Five subspecies of tiger—the Bengal, Indochinese, Sumatran, Siberian, and Malayan—still roam the jungles of Asia. Of these, the Bengal tiger constitutes an overwhelming proportion of the 4,000 or so wild tigers that survive on our planet. Remarkably, about 3,000 tigers, more than 70 percent of the current world tiger population, are found in India, the country where they have their best chance at survival.

A male tiger requires around 5,500 pounds of meat each year, which translates to 40 to 50 large prey animals annually. An average adult male tiger in India weighs between 415 and 575 pounds, while an adult female seldom weighs more than 330 pounds.

Tigers need a large area to establish a stable population. The home range of a male tiger can be as large as 100 square miles. Tigers are highly territorial, with both adult males and females establishing territories that they guard ferociously from other tigers. Generally, a dominant territorial male will mate with three to four tigresses whose territories overlap with his own. Dominant tigresses hold on to fixed areas much longer than males, mating with the dominant male of the region. Mating generally results in three to four cubs, which stay with their mother for 18 to 24 months, learning pretty much everything from her, including defense, aggression, hunting, and hiding.

These characteristics formed the basis for choosing the tiger as a flagship species for conserving large tracts of forestland. The logic was simple: to save the tiger, one would have to safeguard large tracts of forests. In doing so, one would automatically save innumerable species of plants and animals that shared the space with the tiger, and, more importantly, protect the all-important catchment of rivers.

However, tigers' long-term survival can't be achieved by focusing on protected areas alone. Being large-ranging animals, their dispersal from one protected area to another through intervening forest patches or corridors is equally important. This isn't easy, as most corridors are peppered with a lot of people and the numerous threats that come with them, such as fragmentation due to roads, railroads, power lines, and canals, poaching of wild herbivores for bushmeat or to feed the international trade in tiger body parts, and retaliatory killing of tigers to avenge attacks on livestock. Lately, electrocution from people illegally tapping power lines has become one of the most potent causes of death for both wild herbivores and large carnivores, such as tigers and leopards.

In spite of the challenges and a whopping 1.4 billion people living amid an ever expanding economic and social disparity, India has done remarkably well in maintaining functional corridors for tigers.

However, the rise in inflation, coupled with crop raiding by wild herbivores and the loss of livestock to large carnivores, especially outside tiger reserves, is antagonizing local communities. Habitat degradation and deforestation are also forcing animals to forage across larger areas, exposing them to humans. Consequently, people have started taking the law into their own hands, killing both herbivores and carnivores in retaliation. Unless the growing strain between people and wildlife is addressed, community-based conservation programs will fail.

Many things can and should be done, but nothing will work better than restoring forest cover. India's forests could be doubled in size if only 50 percent of the country's subsistence farmers moved from traditional crops to agroforestry. This would be a win-win for both farmers and wildlife, as it would drastically reduce crop losses, increase biodiversity, and create an alternate source of income for villagers through wildlife tourism.

The Indian government may have defused the immediate threat to the tiger, but the species is far from secure. On one hand, there are advances in science, growing clarity about climate change, and the increased understanding of natural ecosystems, which together emphasize the need to prioritize natural resources over human-made assets. On the other hand, governments across the planet continue to liquidate natural wealth—forests, mountains, rivers, fresh air, and wildlife—for short-term, diminishing returns. There is a constant tug-of-war between the mindless pilferage of natural wealth and the will to protect the tiger.

However, the survival of the tiger well into the twenty-first century is a testimony to the ability of humans to turn the tide of devastation. In saving this supreme predator, we have managed to preserve an integral part of our own natural heritage that connects us humans with all other denizens of this beautiful blue planet. The tiger is the undisputed guardian of our rich past, one that will hopefully be with us long into the future. Whenever I listen to the roar of a tiger reverberating through the Indian jungle, something deep within reassures me that there is hope for life on this planet, despite us humans.

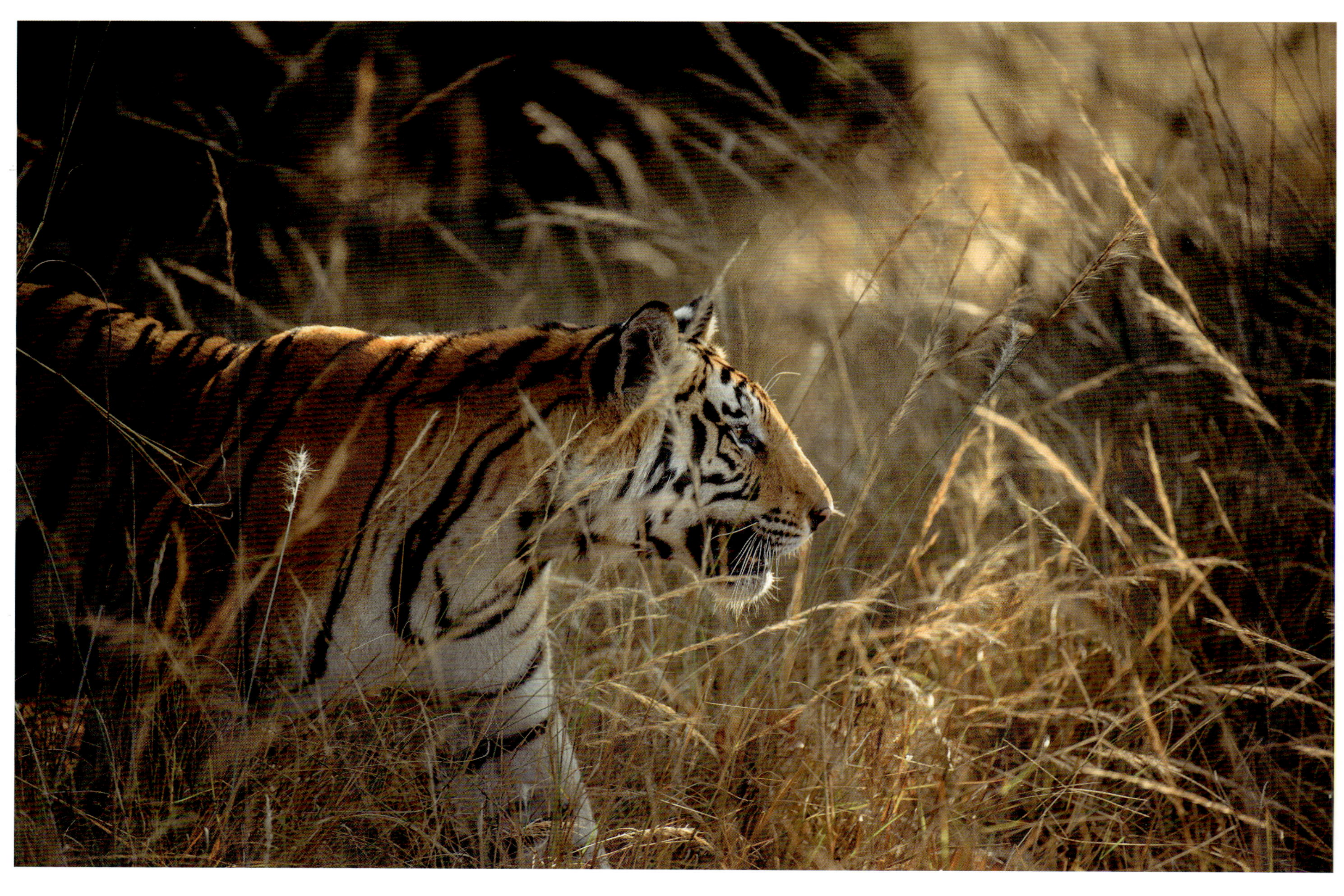

Andy Parkinson
Bengal Tiger
Bandhavgarh National Park, India

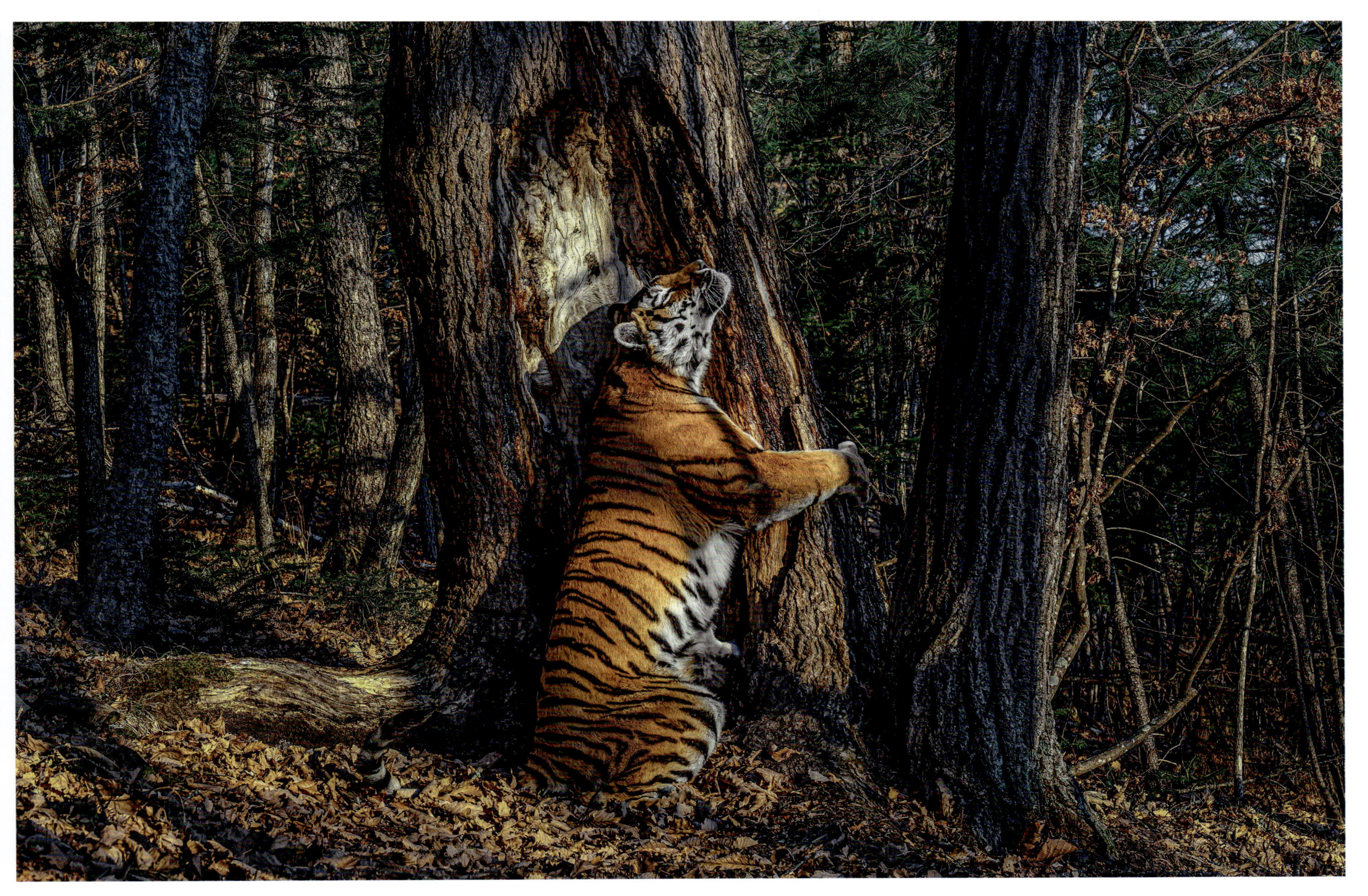

Sergey Gorshkov
Siberian Tiger
Land of the Leopard National Park, Russia

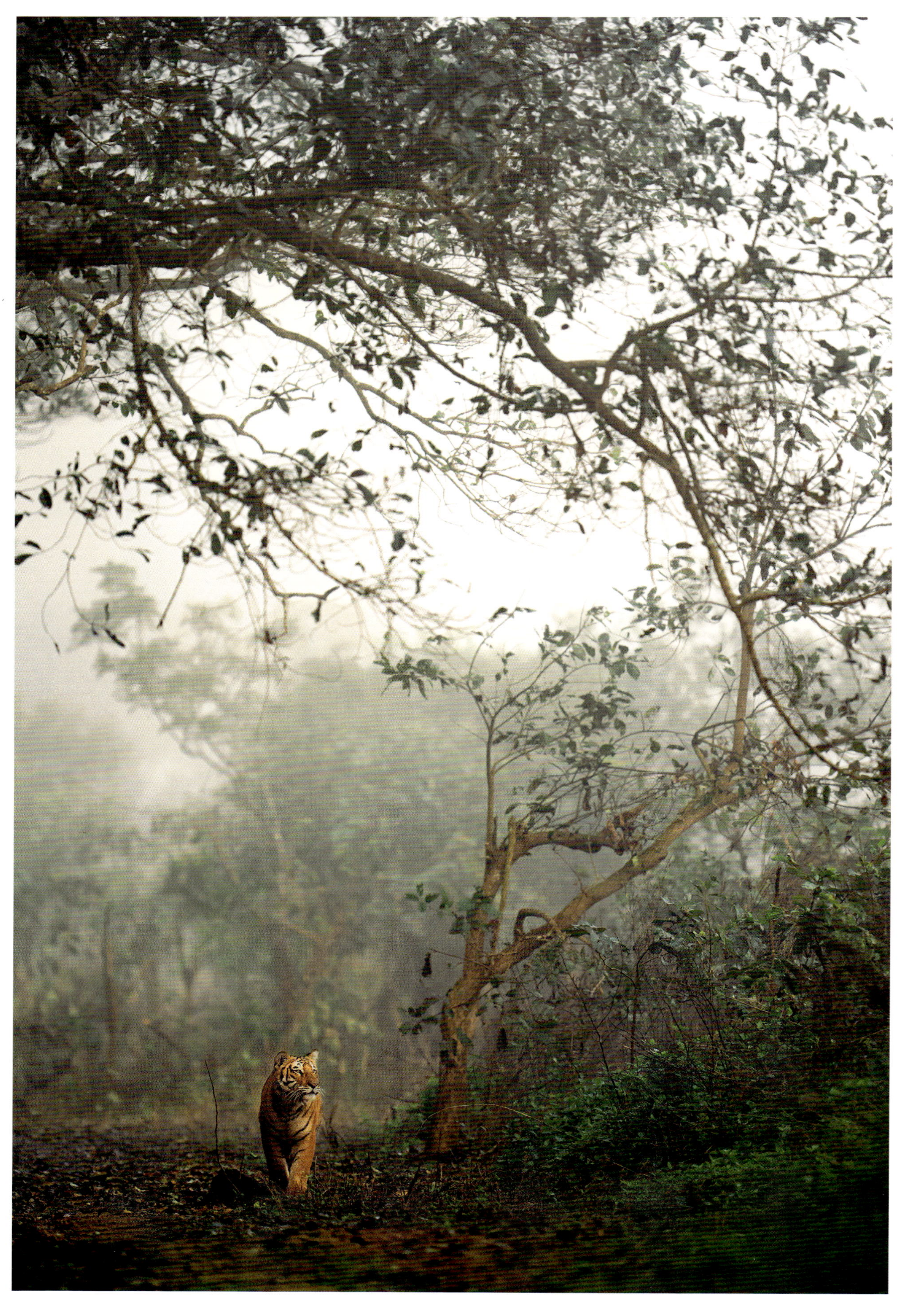

Aarzoo Khurana
Bengal Tiger
Jim Corbett National Park, India

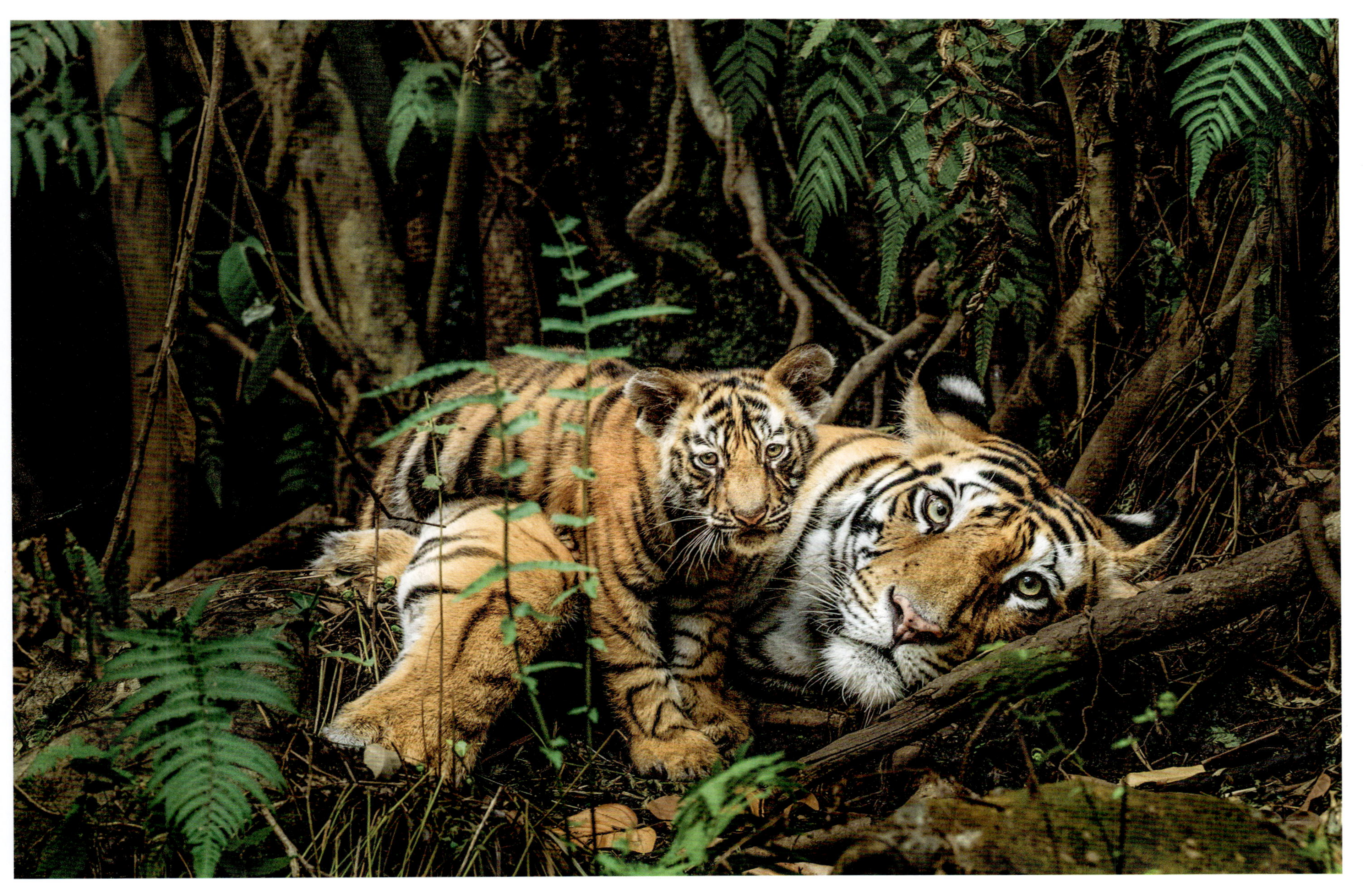

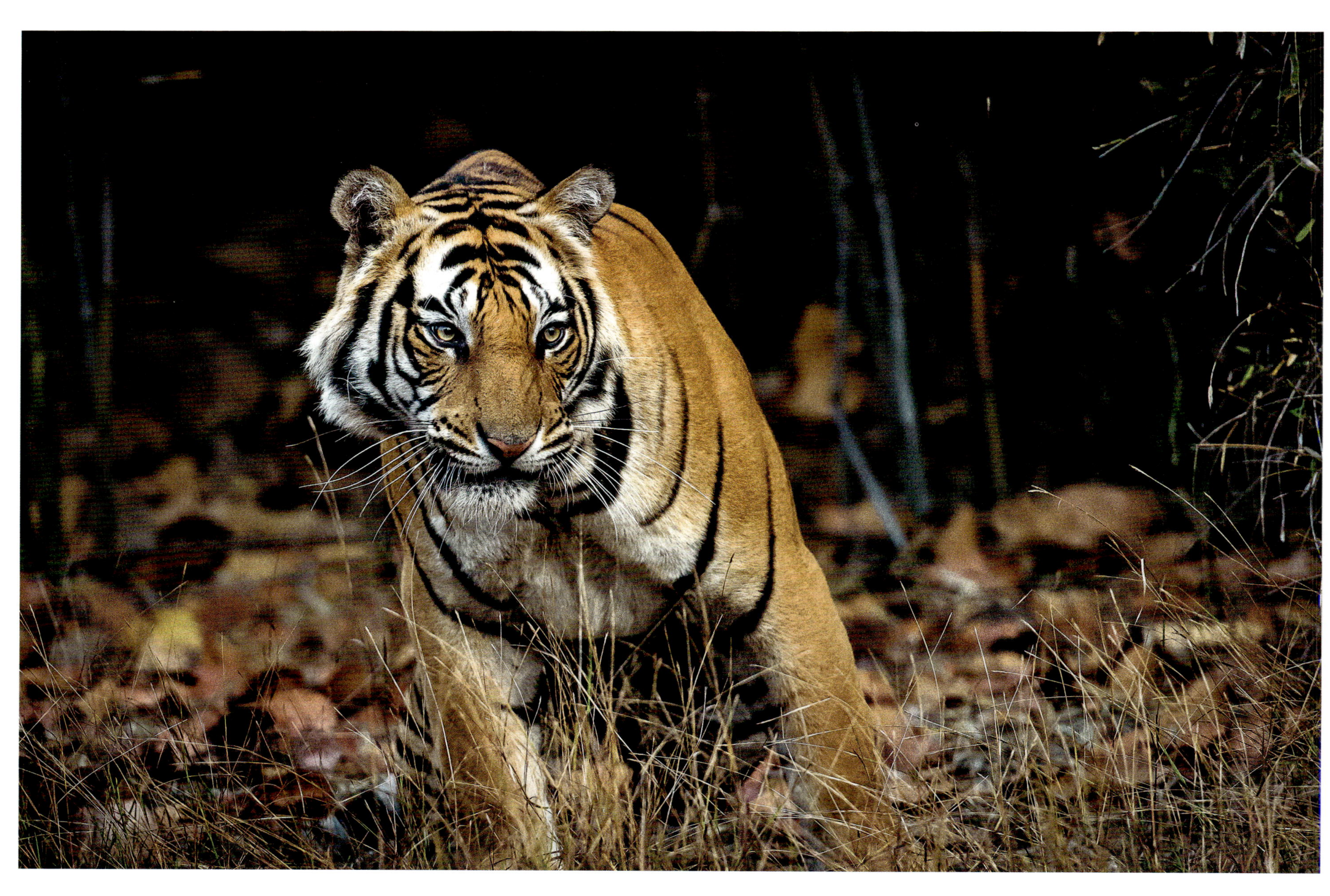

Richard I'Anson
Bengal Tiger
Bandhavgarh National Park, India

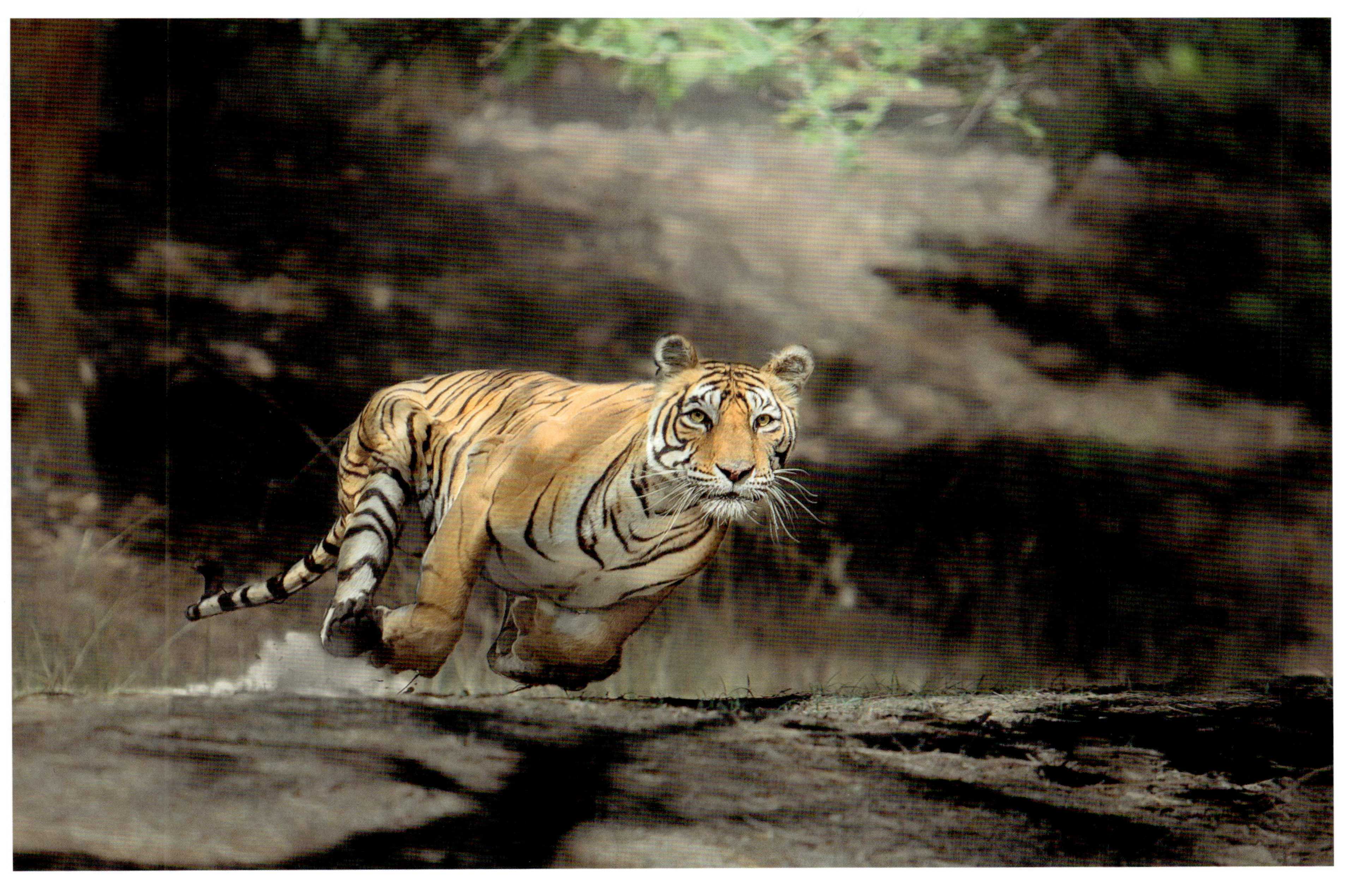

Thomas Vijayan
Bengal Tiger
Bandhavgarh National Park, India

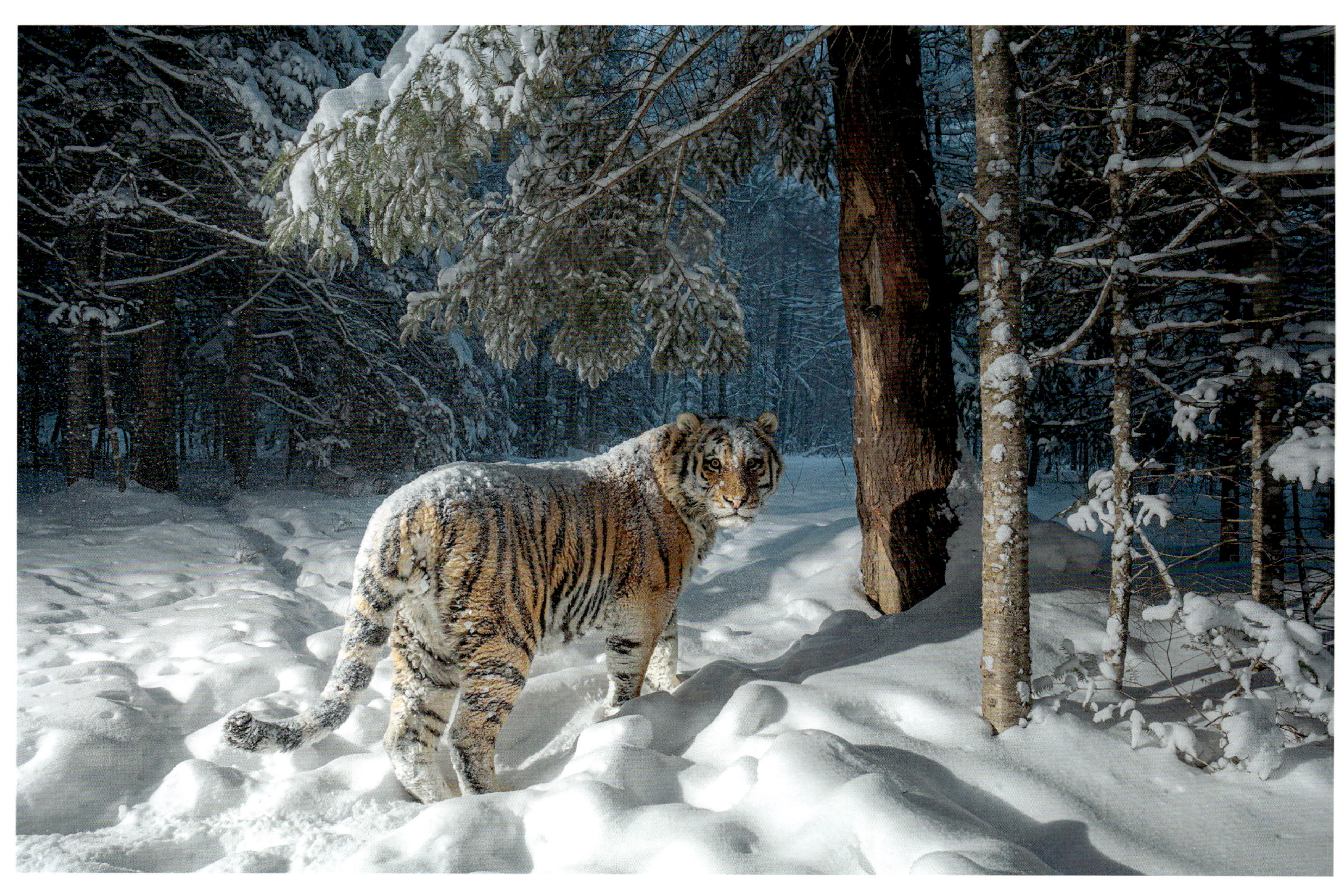

Sascha Fonseca
Siberian Tiger
Central Sikhote-Alin, Russia

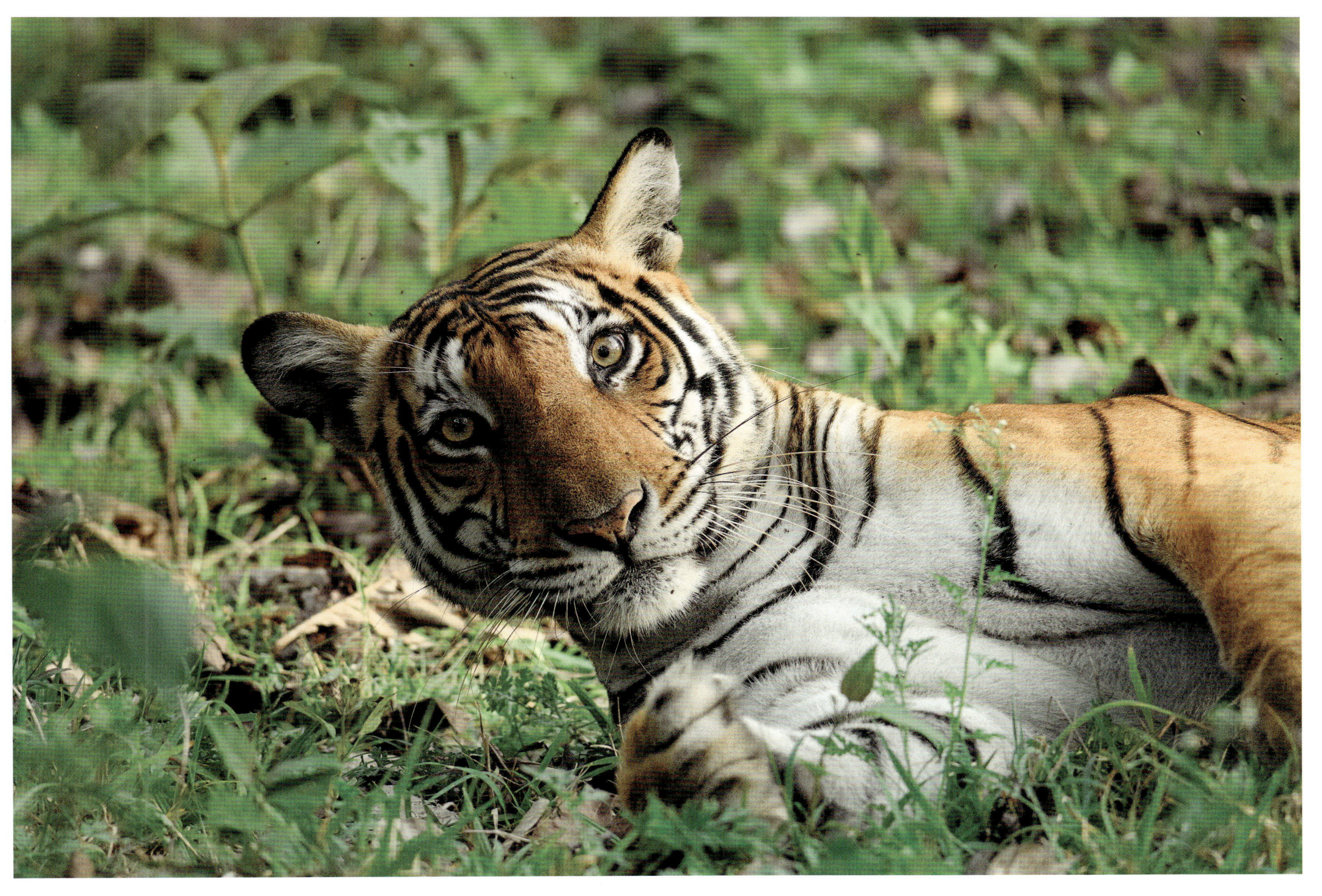

Ramakrishnan Aiyaswamy
Bengal Tiger
Nagarahole Tiger Reserve, India

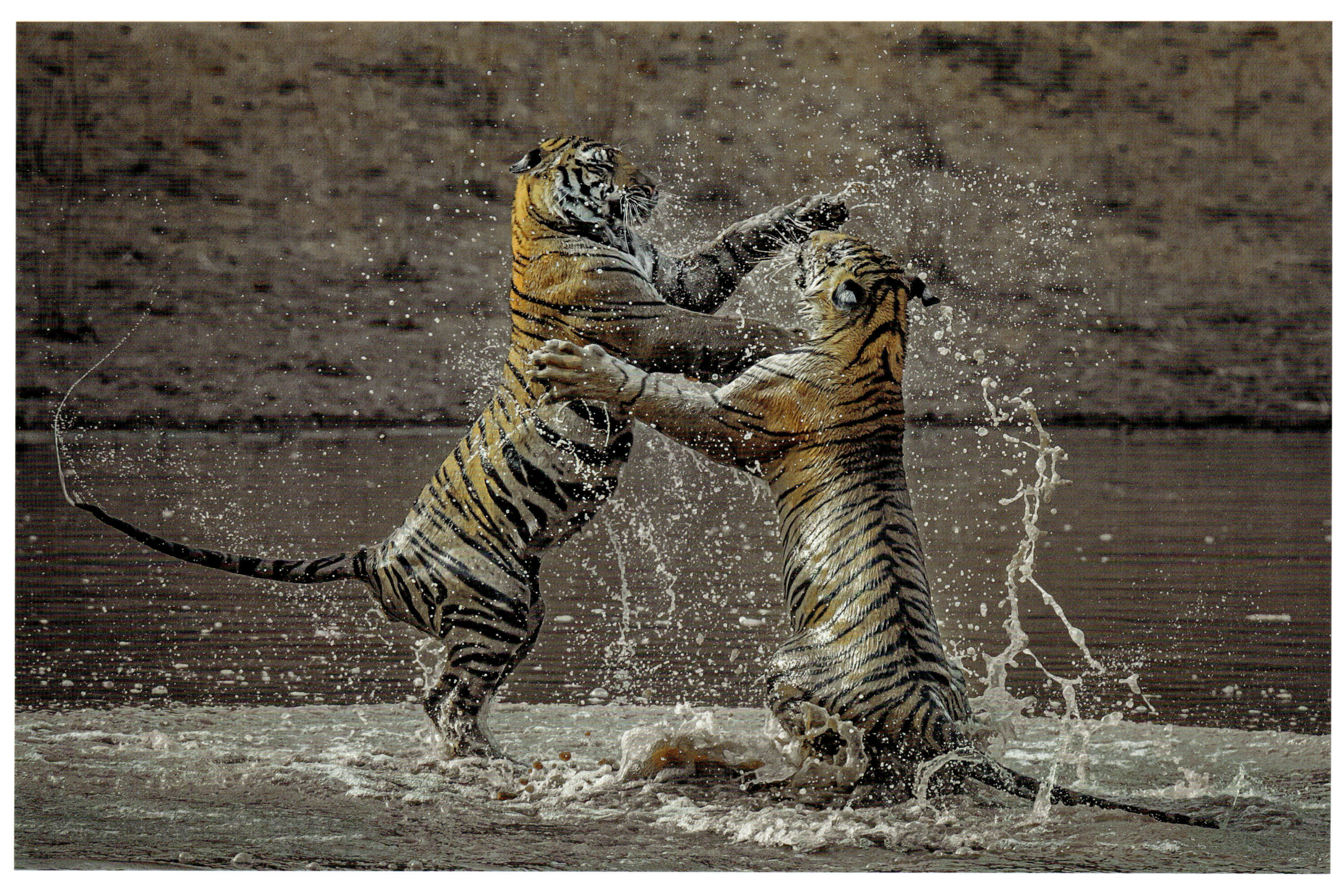

Paul Goldstein
Bengal Tigers
Bandhavgarh National Park, India

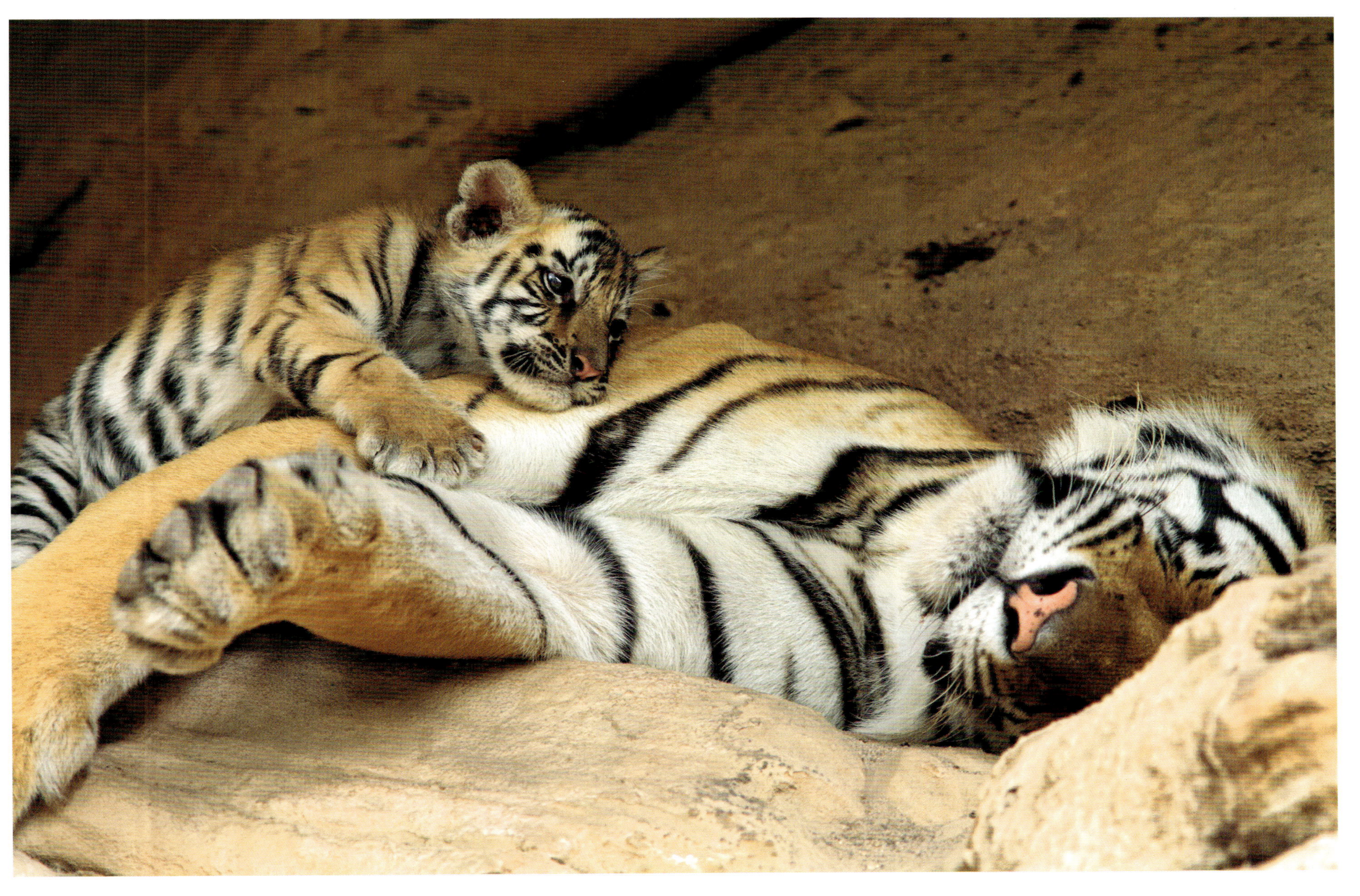

Suzi Eszterhas
Bengal Tigers
Bandhavgarh National Park, India

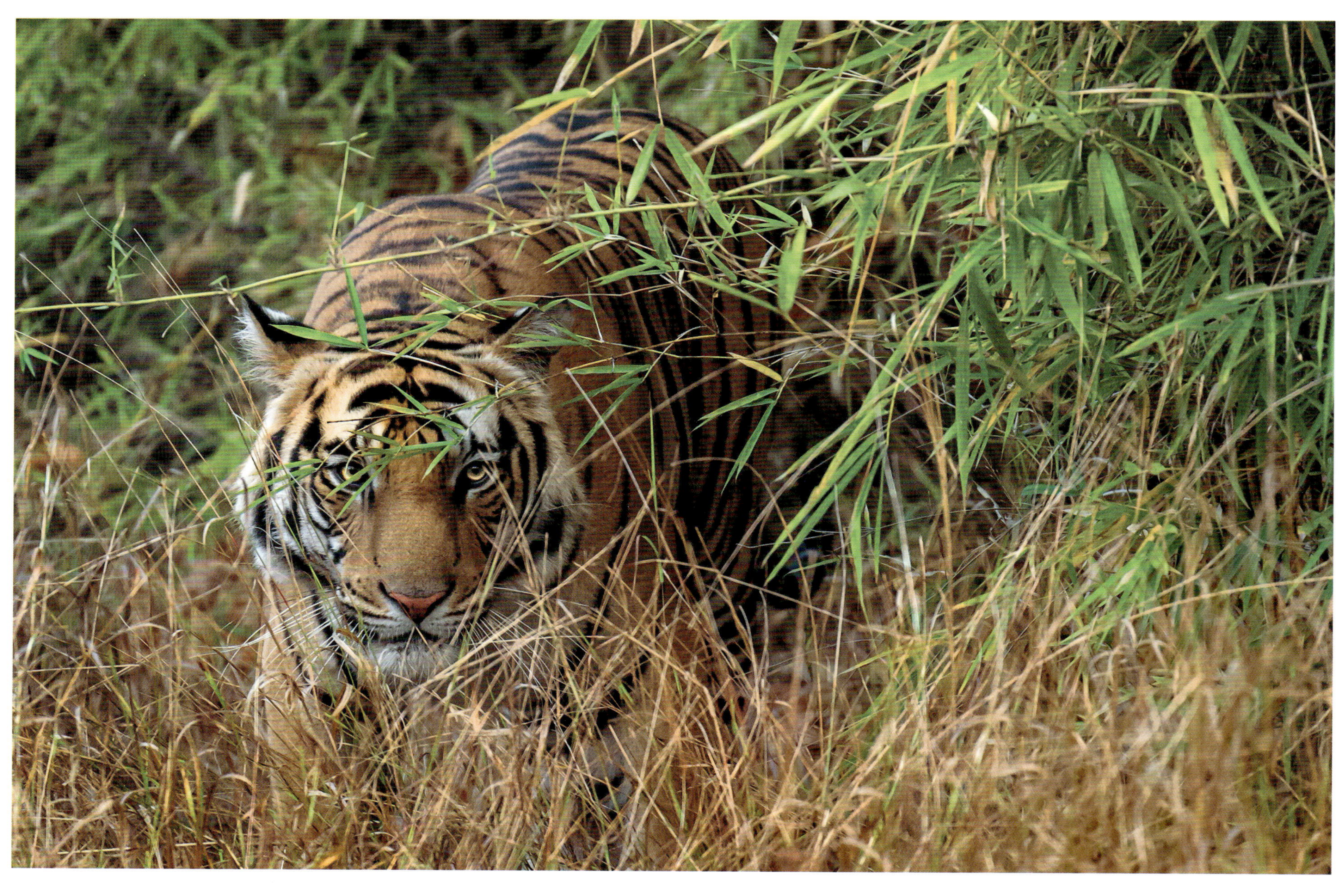

Art Wolfe
Bengal Tiger
Bandhavgarh National Park, India

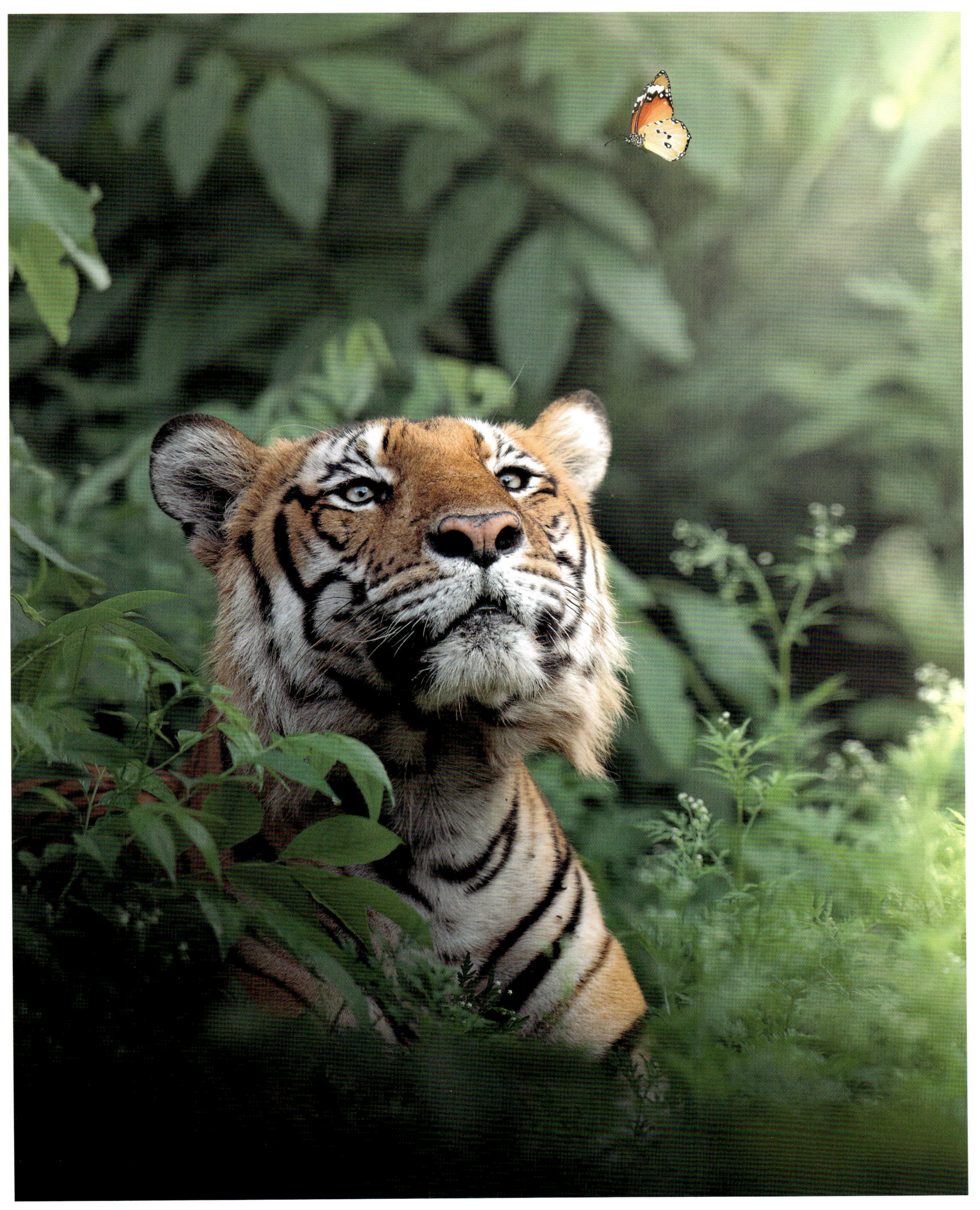

Sujuaan Gasim
Bengal Tiger
Nagarahole Tiger Reserve, India

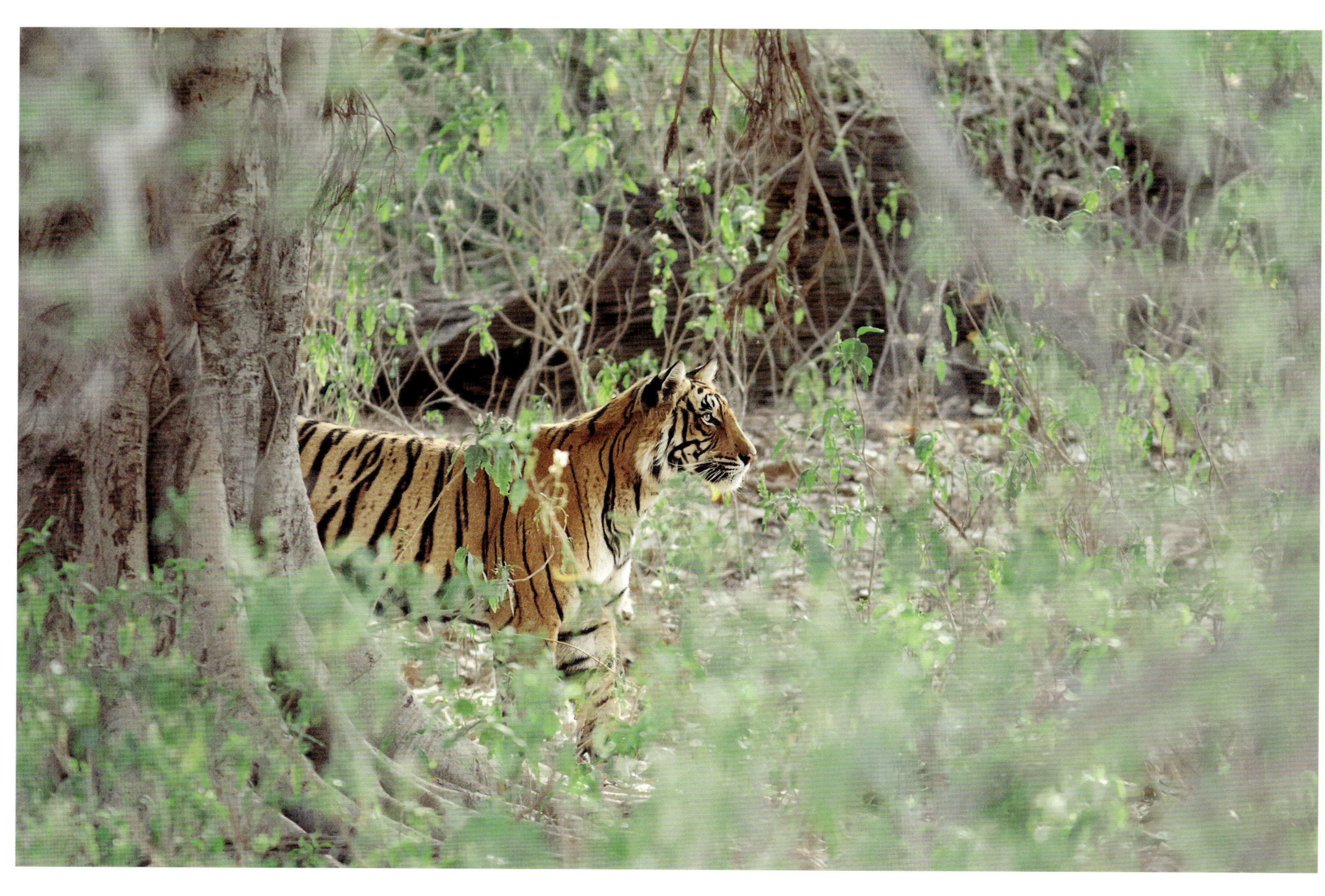

Anette Mossbacher
Bengal Tiger
Ranthambore National Park, India

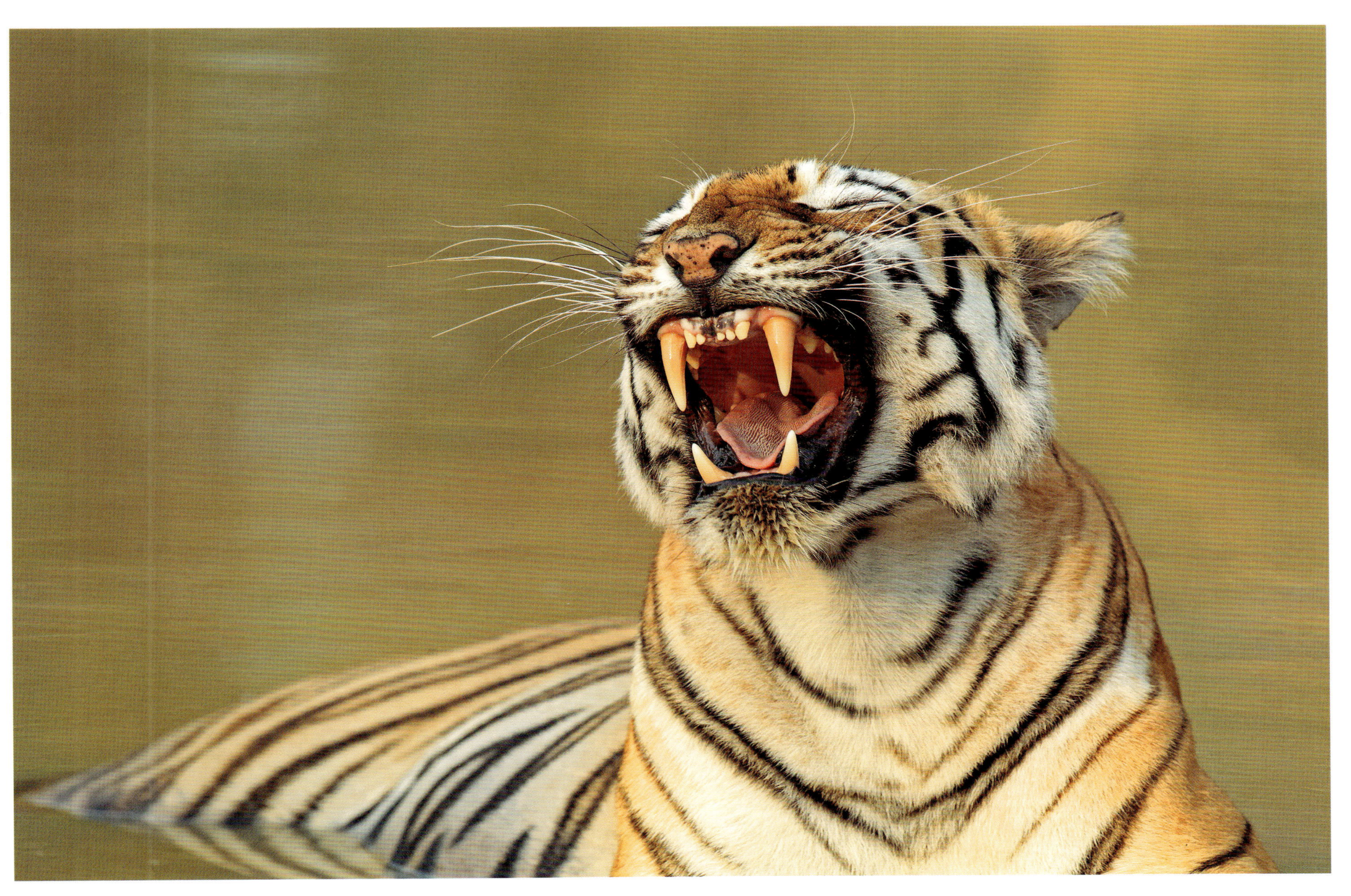

Aishwarya Sridhar
Bengal Tiger
Tadoba Andhari Tiger Reserve, India

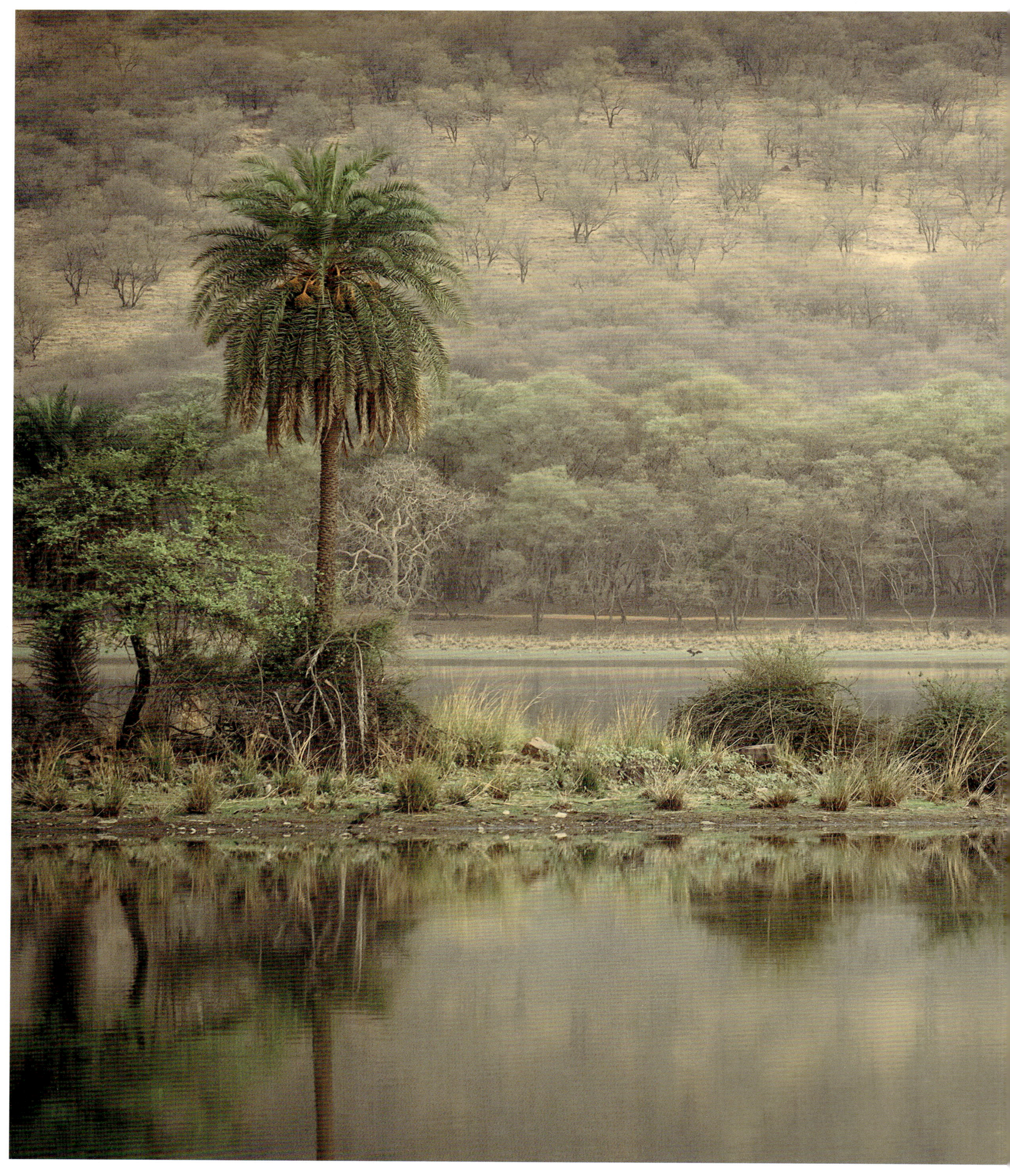

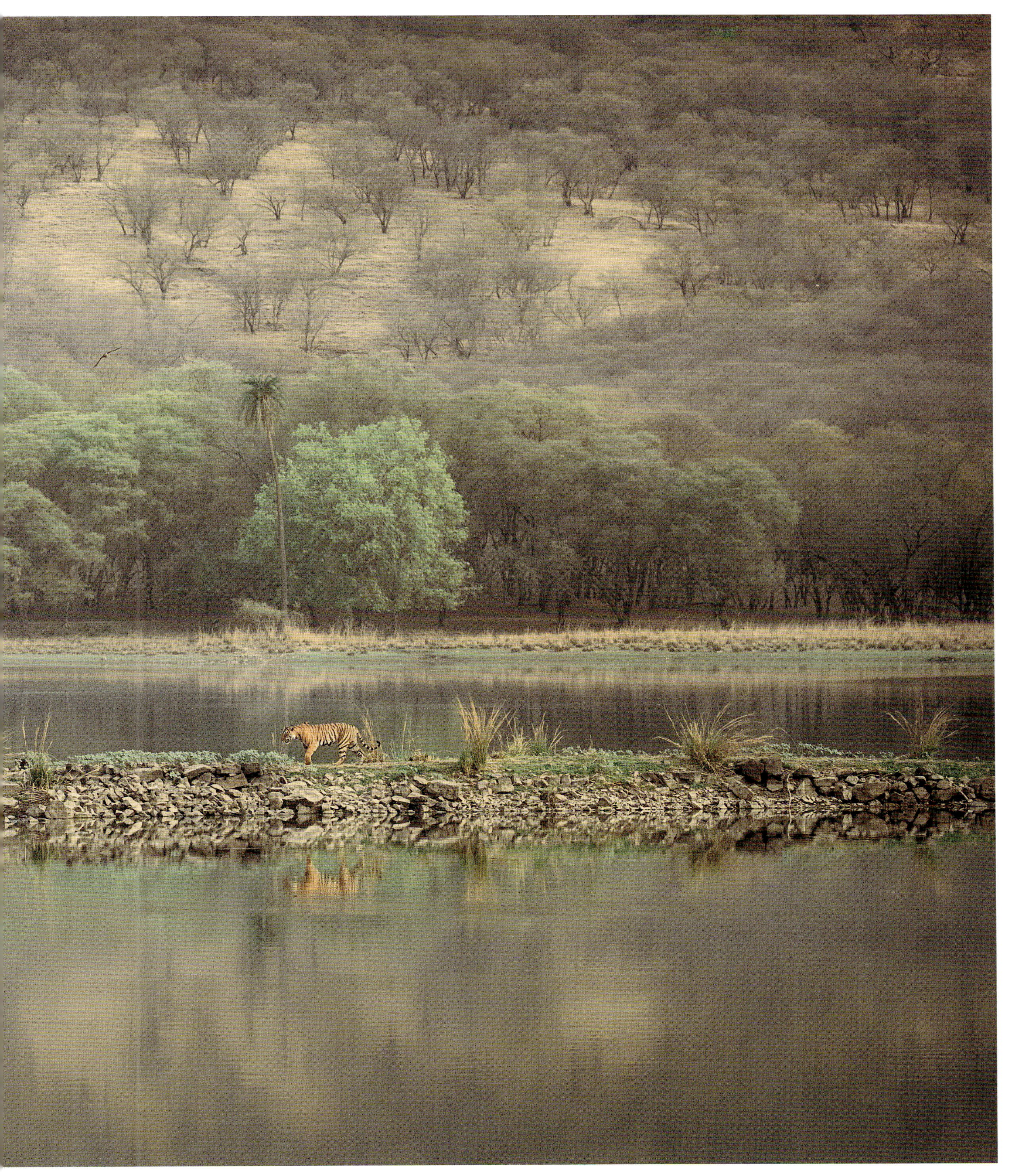

Vladimir Cech, Jr.
Bengal Tiger
Ranthambore National Park, India

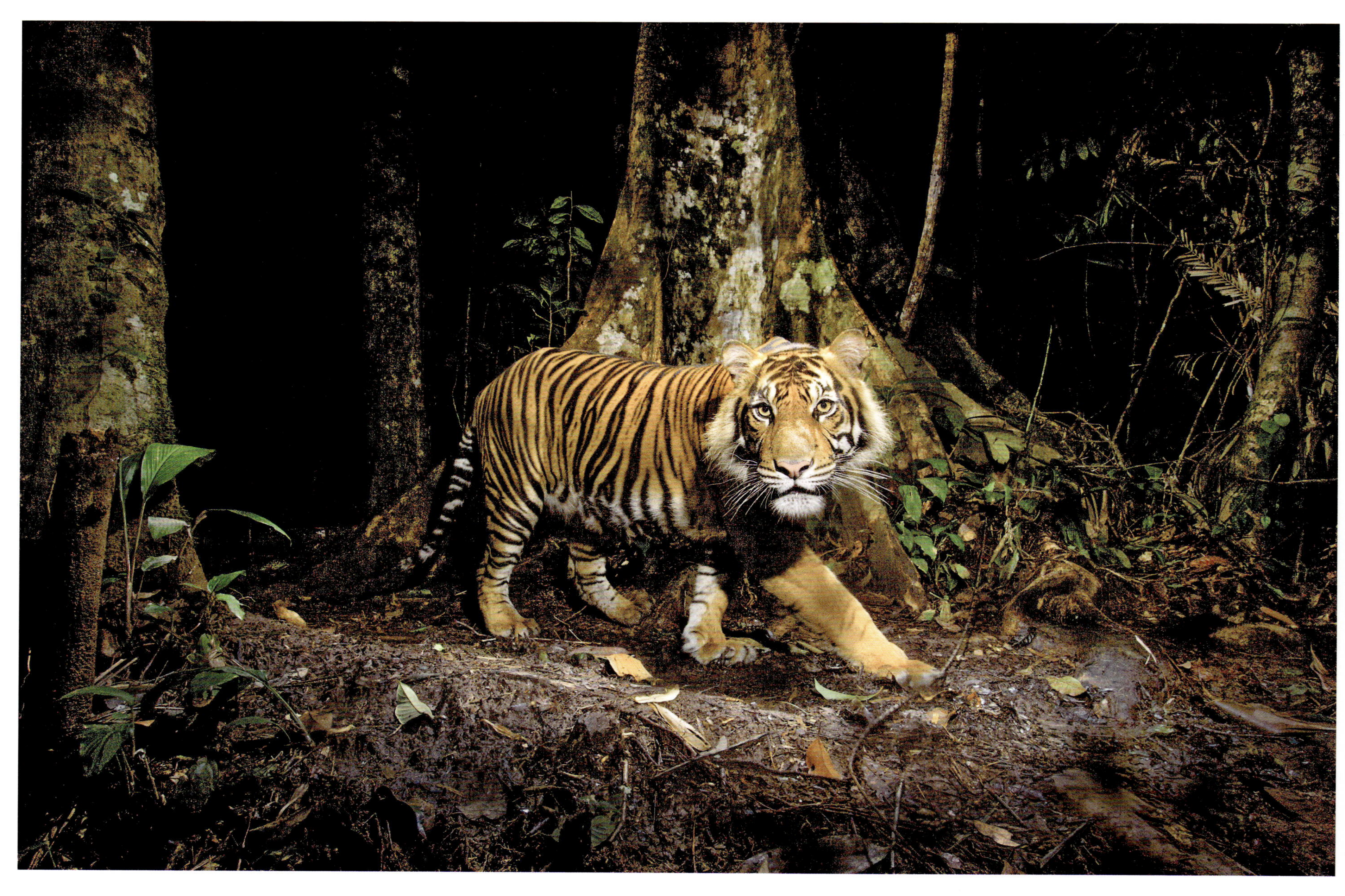

Steve Winter
Sumatran Tiger
Bandhavgarh National Park, India

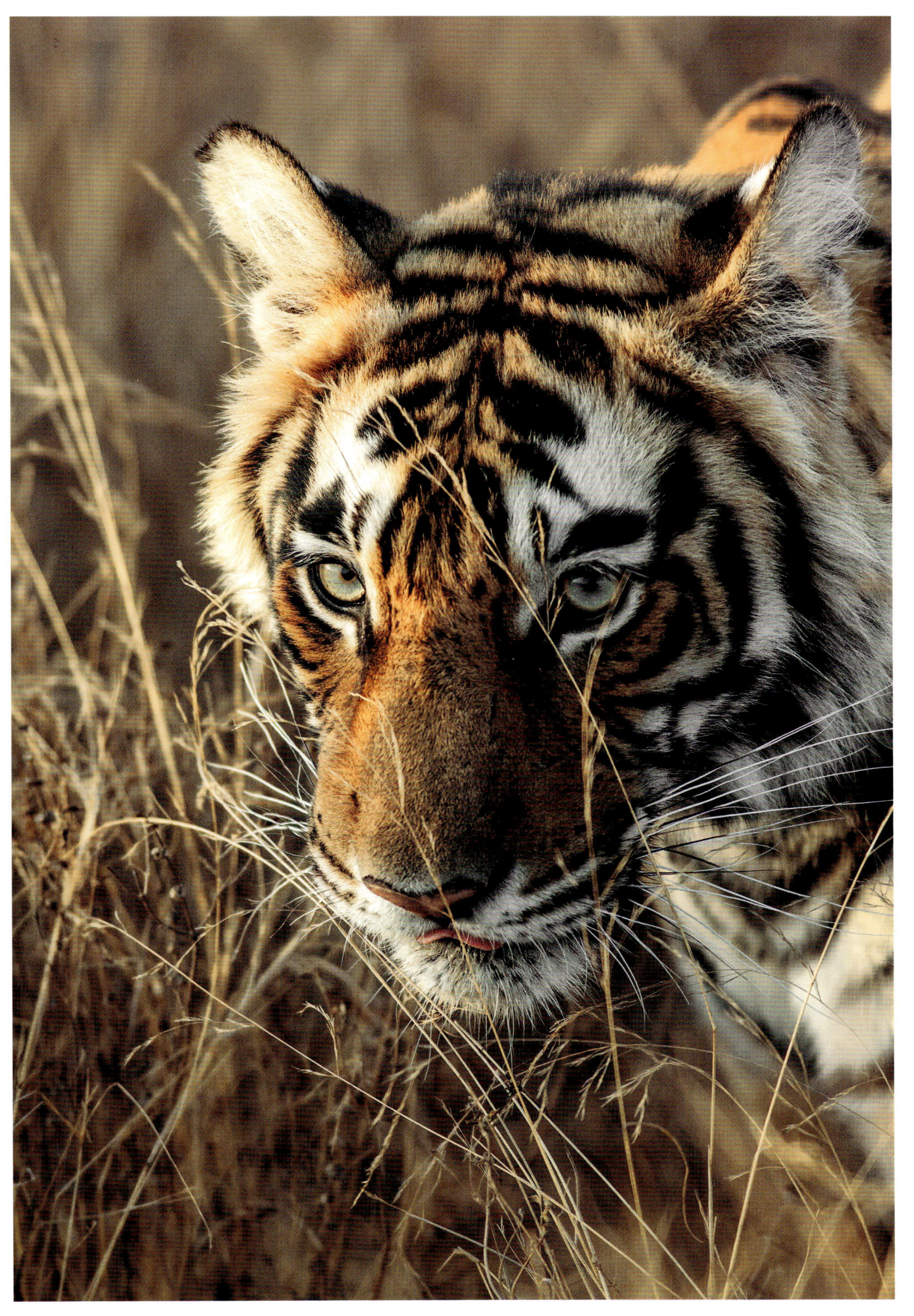

Brian W. Matthews
Bengal Tiger
Ranthambore National Park, India

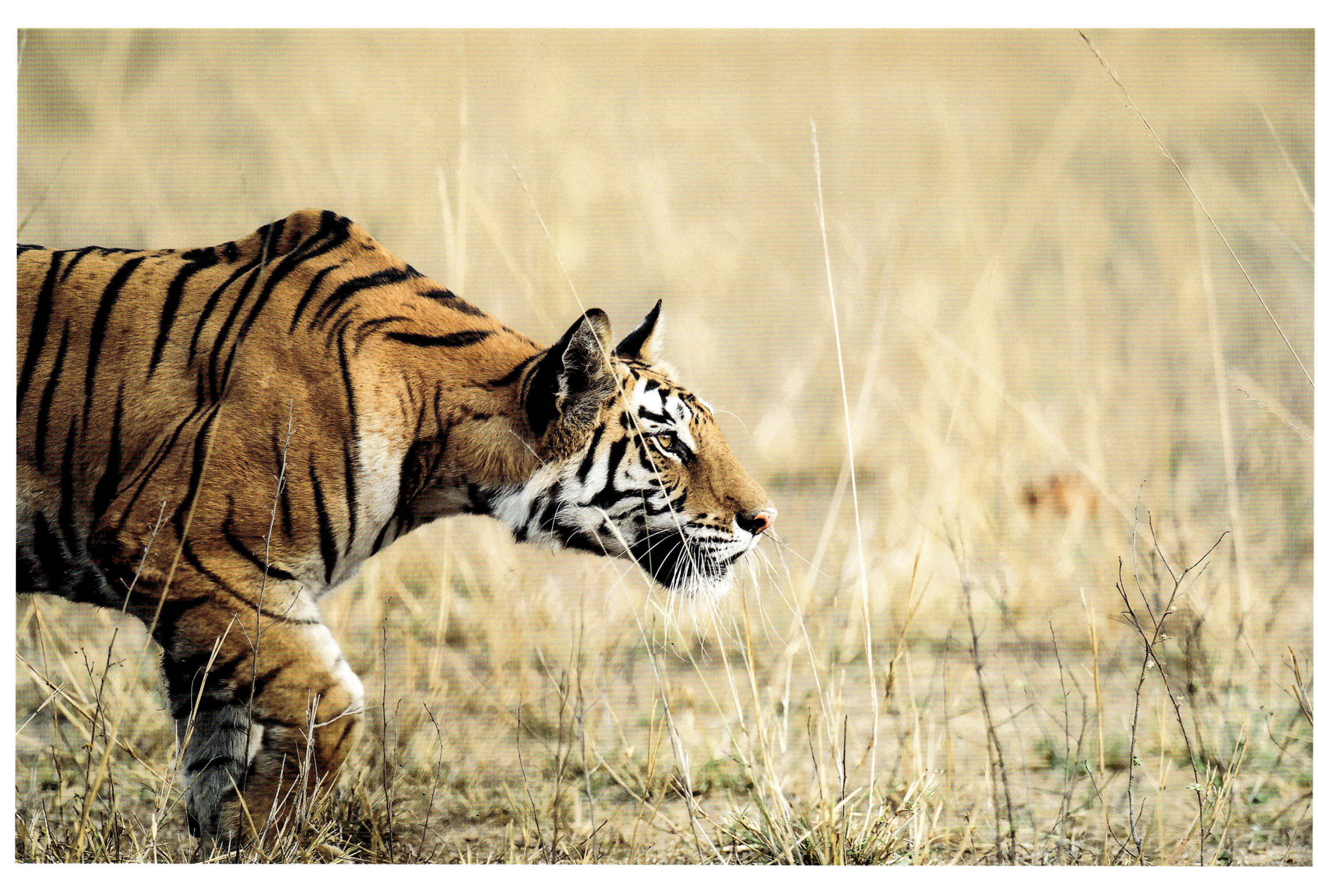

Latika Nath
Bengal Tiger
Bandhavgarh National Park, India

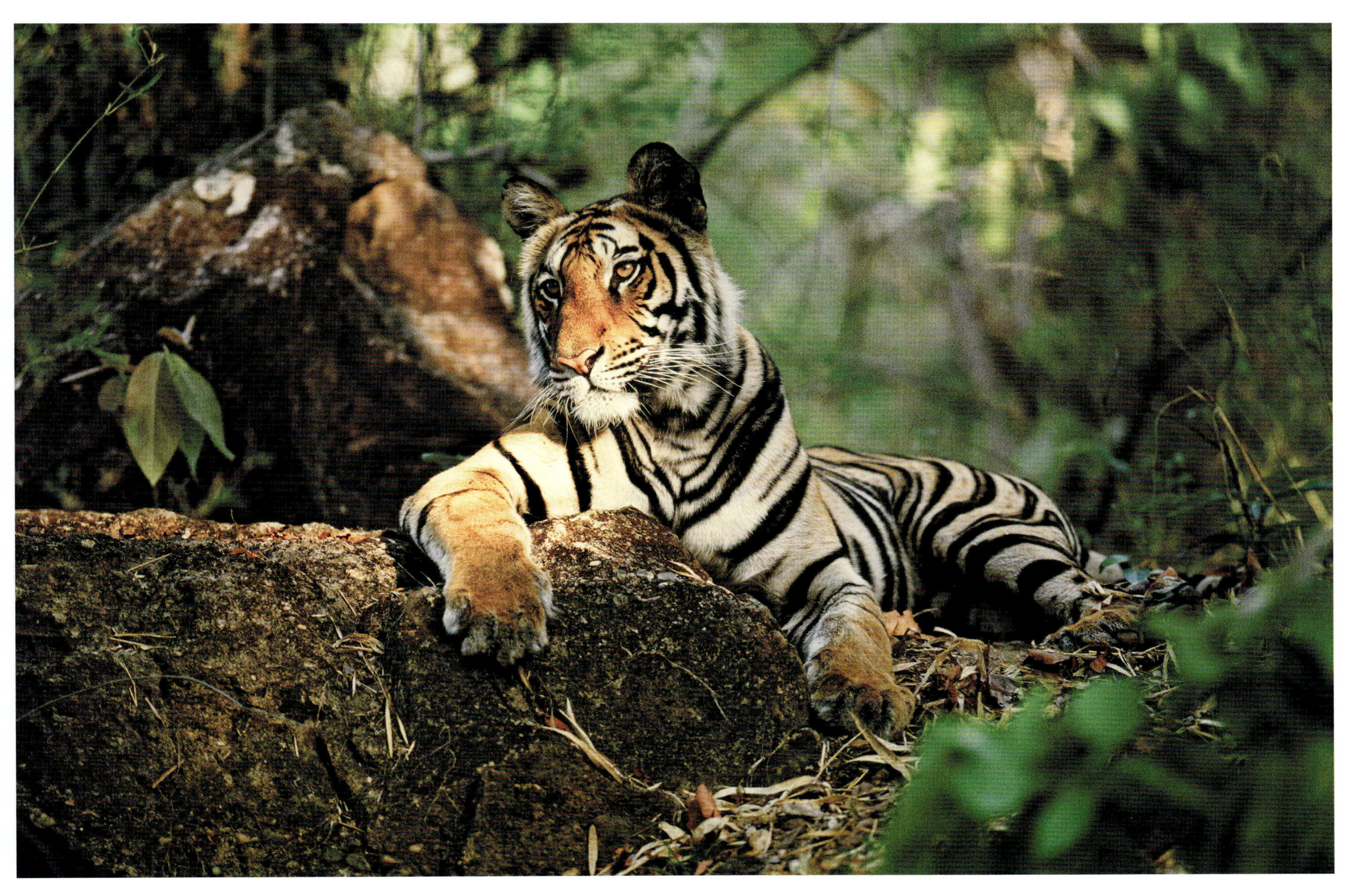
Thomas D. Mangelsen
Bengal Tiger
Bandhavgarh National Park, India

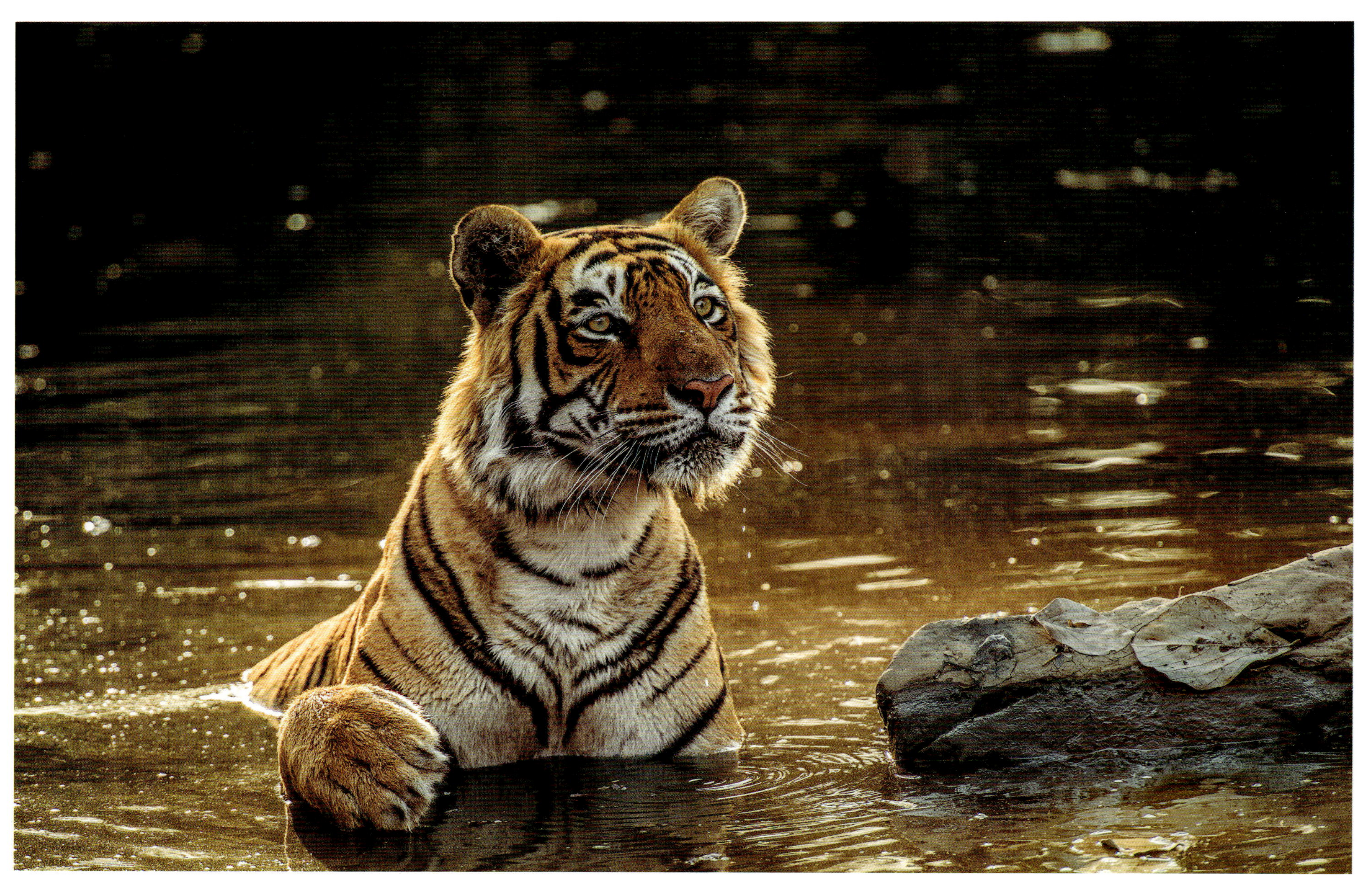

Teeku Patel
Bengal Tiger
Ranthambore National Park, India

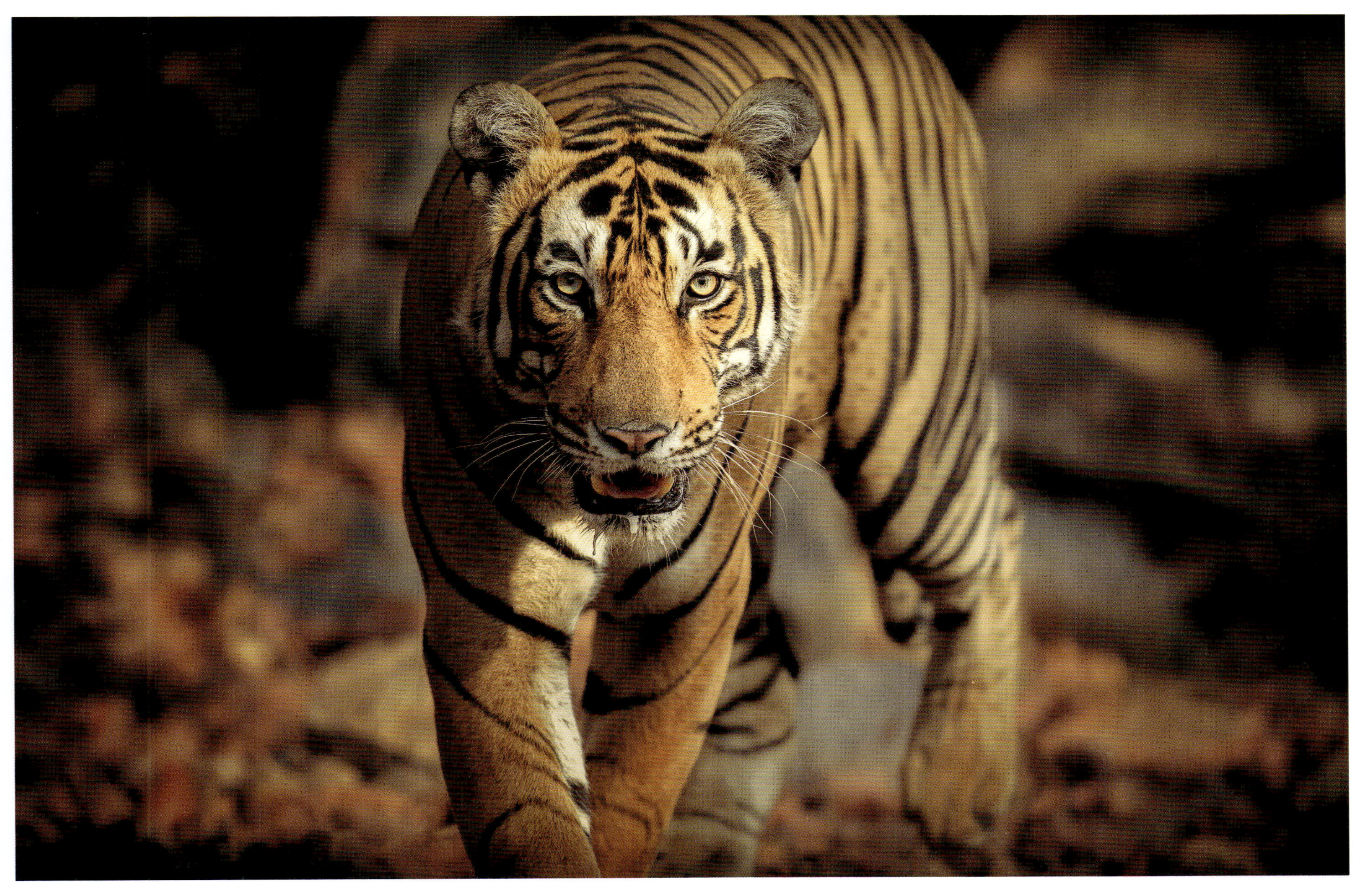

Vladimir Cech, Jr.
Bengal Tiger
Ranthambore National Park, India

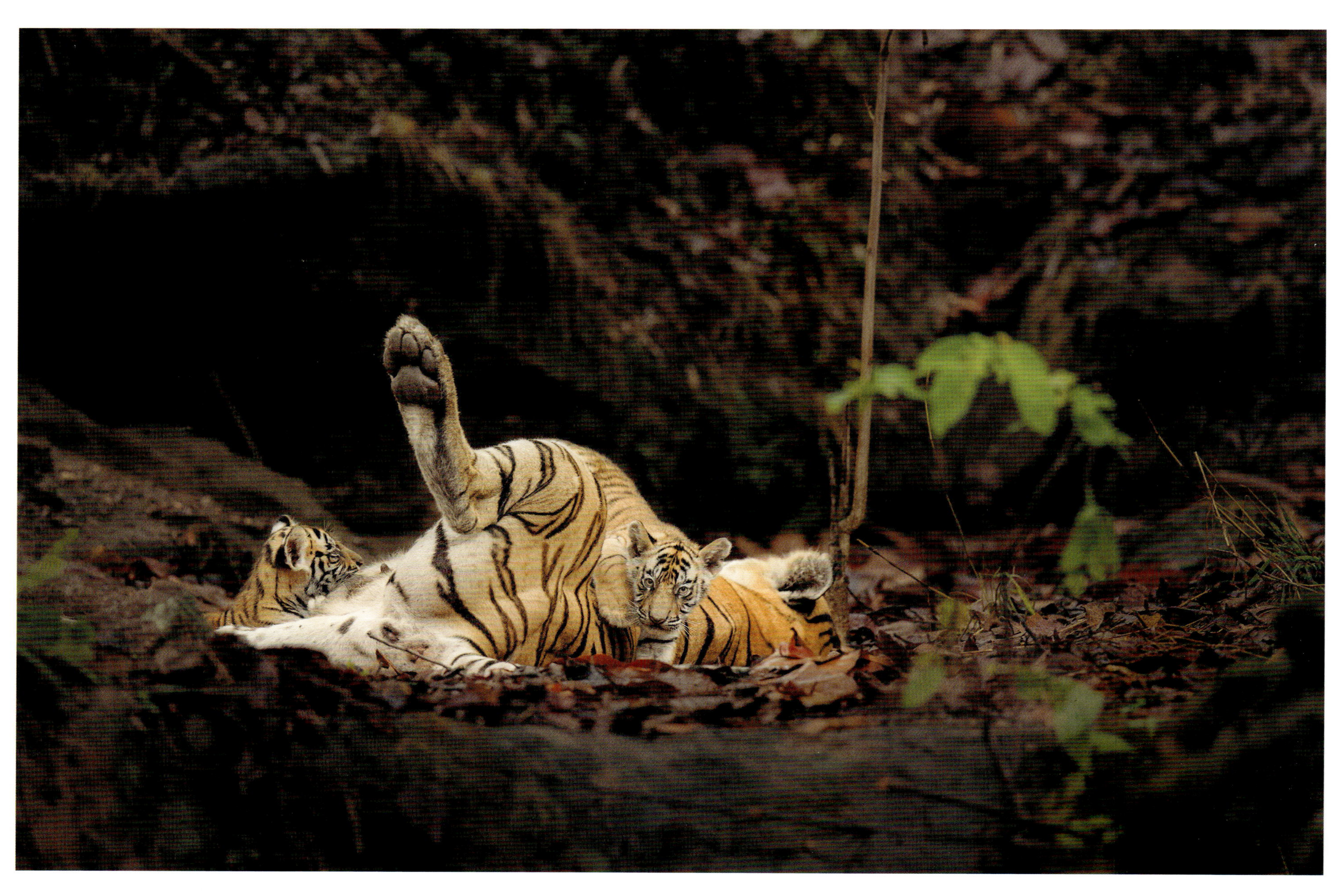

Thomas Vijayan
Bengal Tiger
Bandhavgarh National Park, India

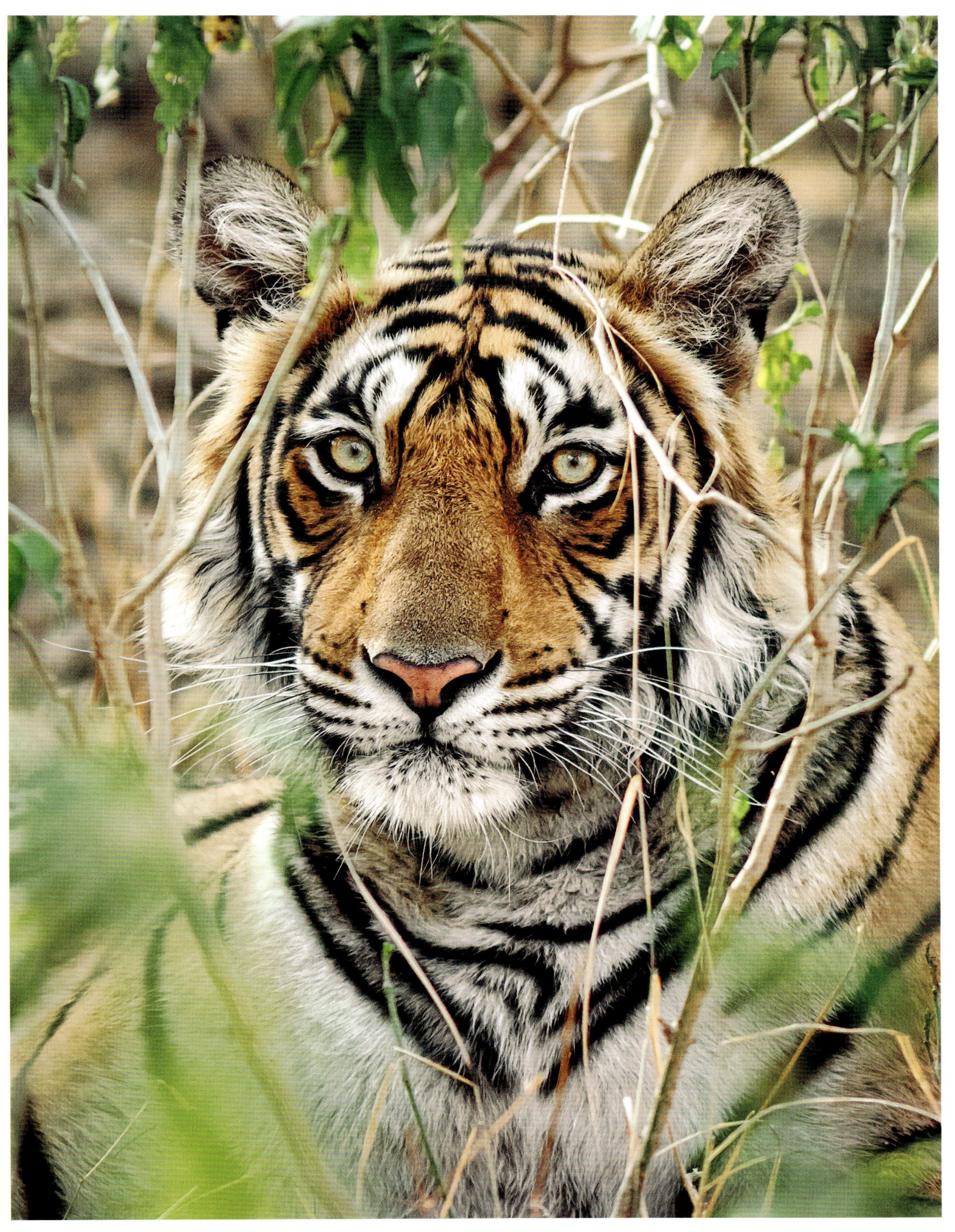

Anette Mossbacher
Bengal Tiger
Ranthambore National Park, India

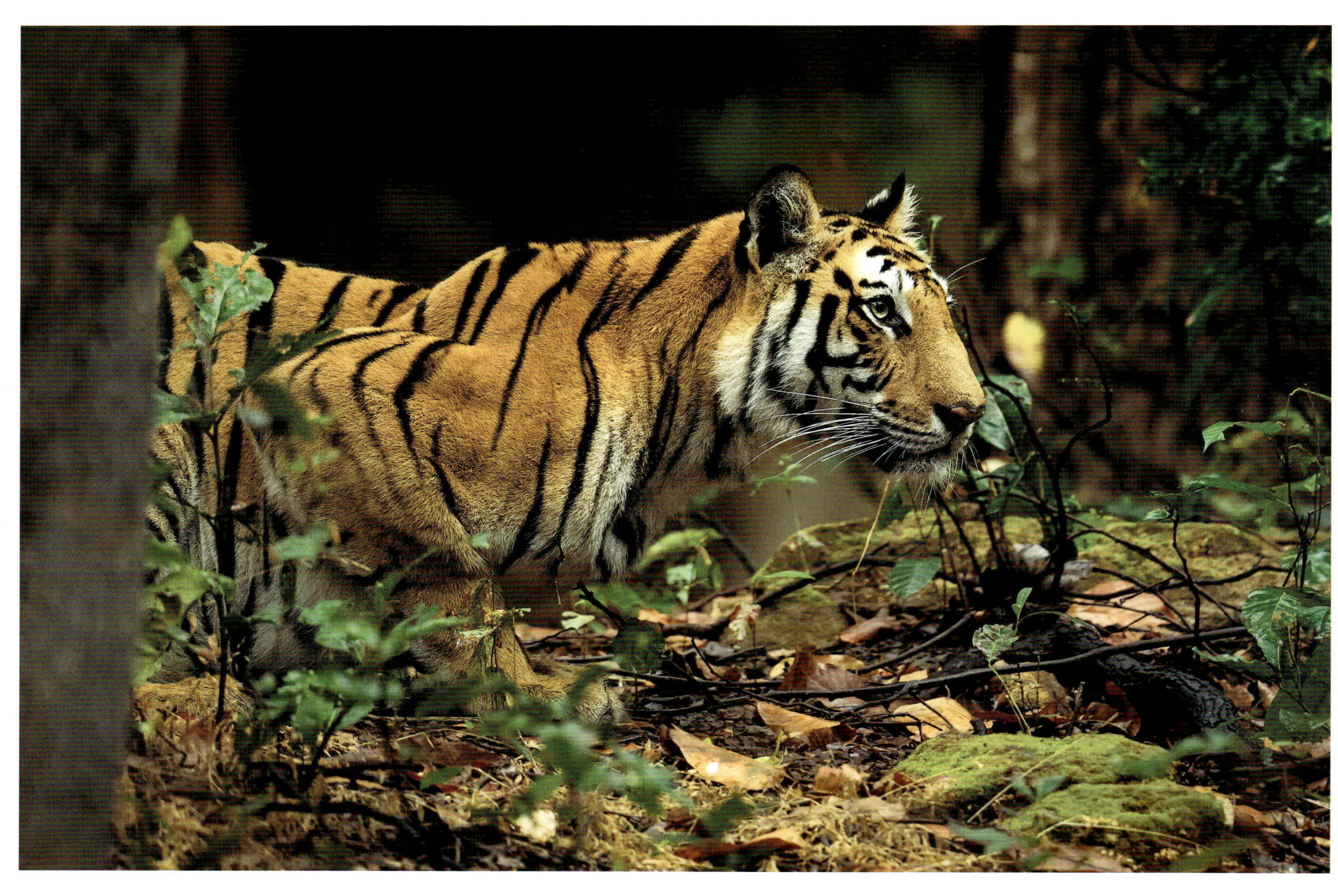

Mangesh R. Desai
Bengal Tiger
Tadoba Andhari Tiger Reserve, India

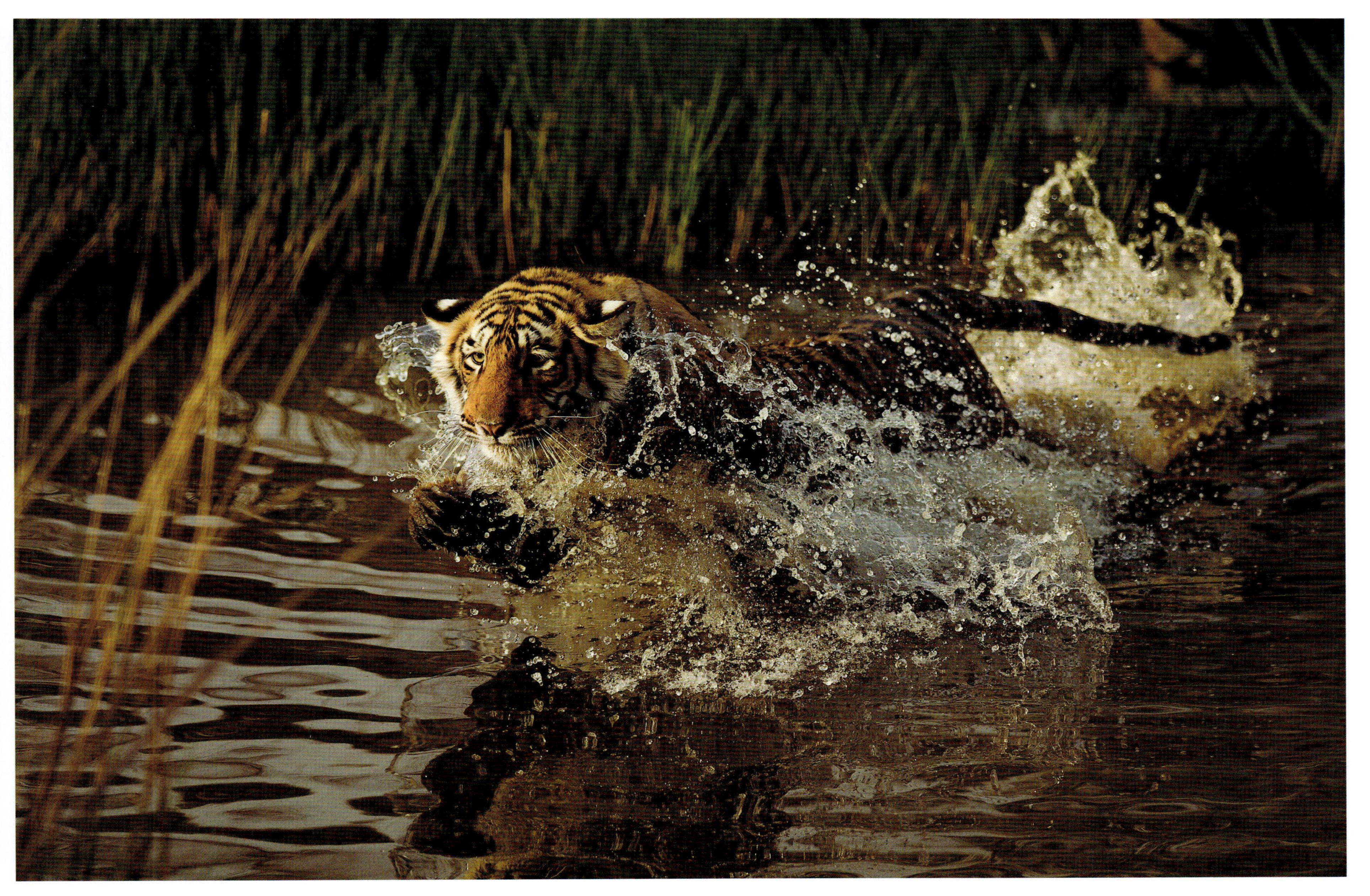

Sudhir Shivaram
Bengal Tiger
Ranthambore National Park, India

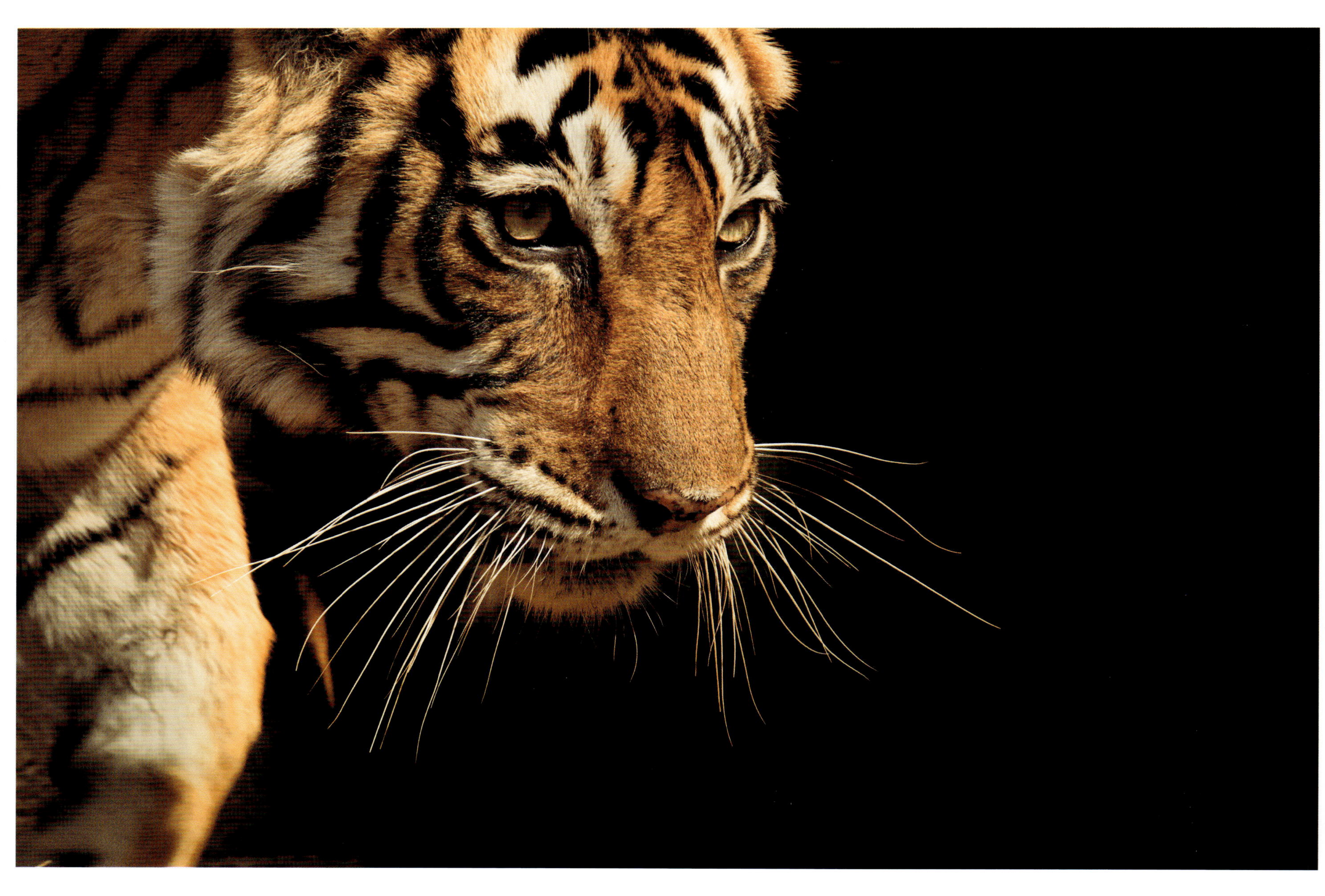

Piper Mackay
Bengal Tiger
Ranthambore National Park, India

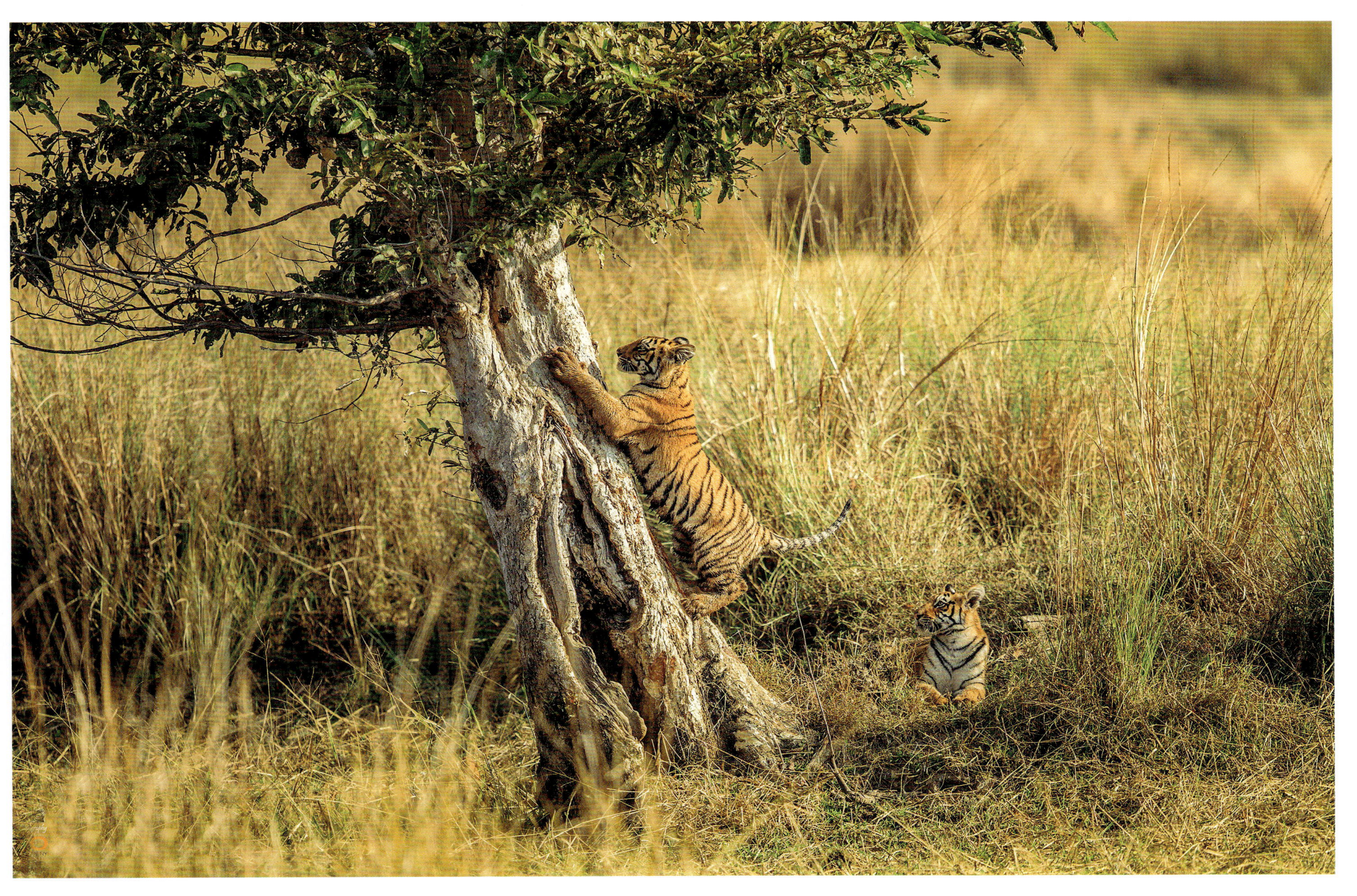

Shibu Preman
Bengal Tiger
Tadoba Andhari Tiger Reserve, India

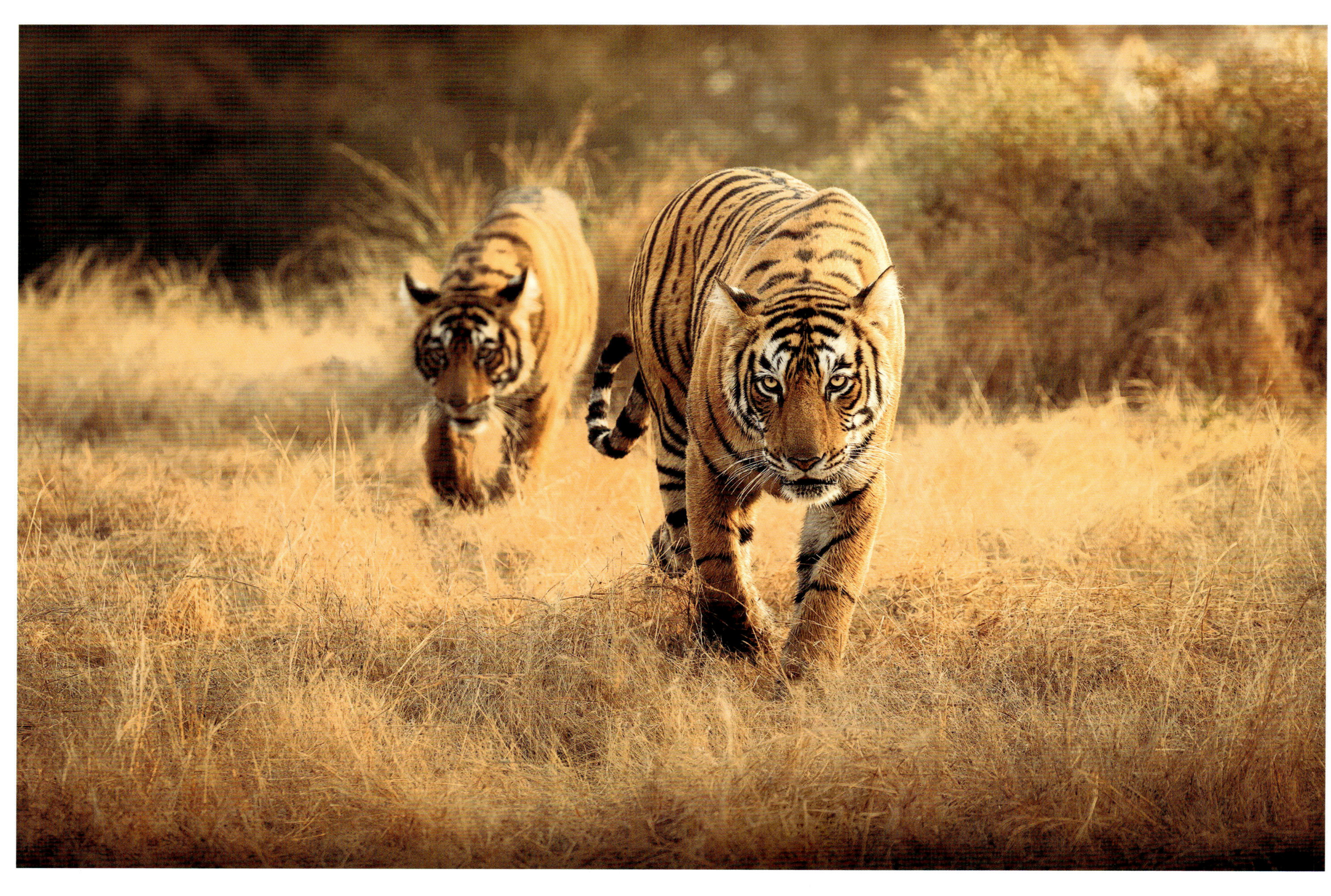

Vladimir Cech, Jr.
Bengal Tigers
Ranthambore National Park, India

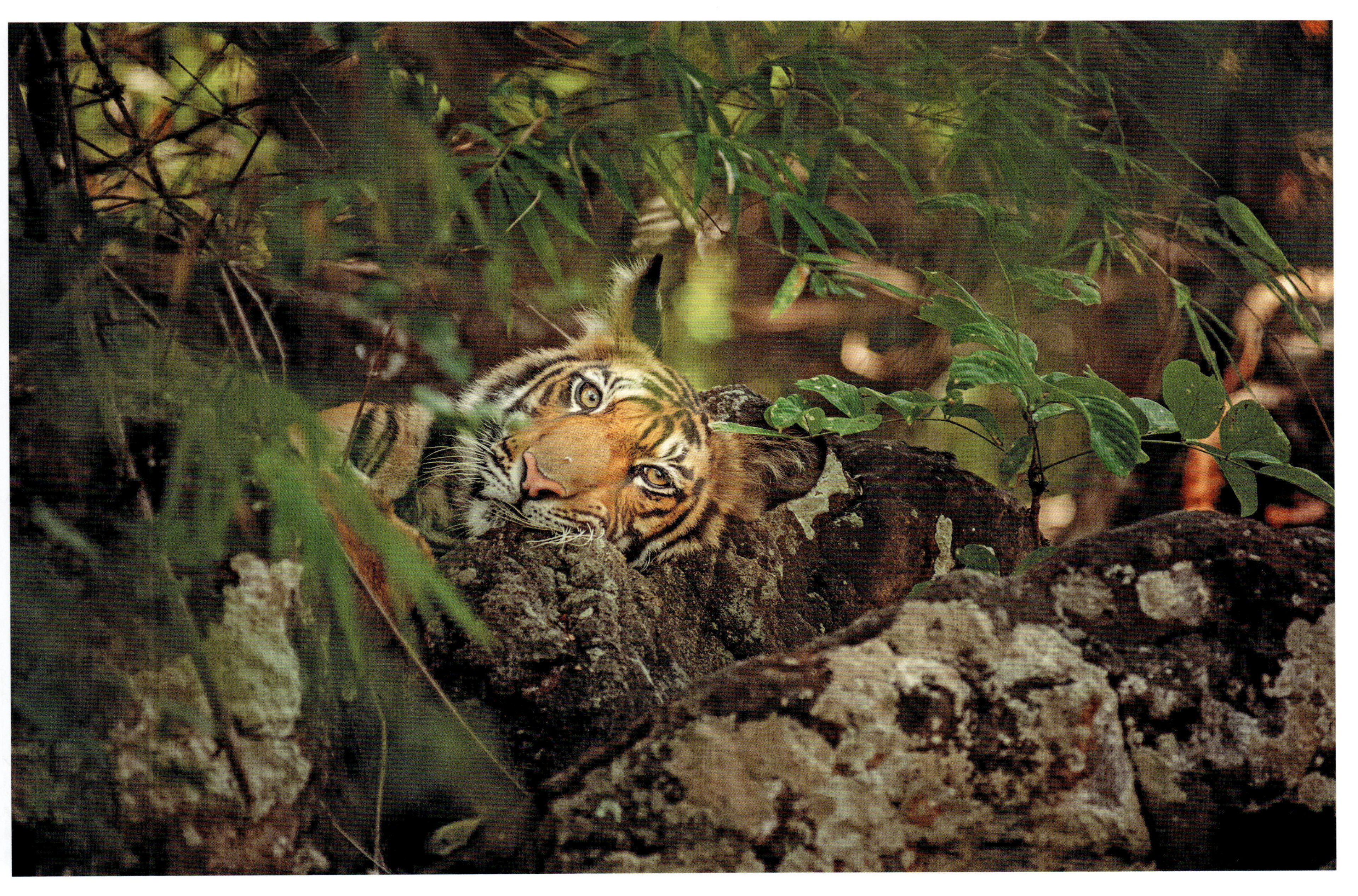

Andy Parkinson
Bengal Tiger
Bandhavgarh National Park, India

WHAT WE STAND TO LOSE

No Species Left Behind

Dr. Wes Sechrest

CEO and Chair, Re:wild

WE ALL GROW UP WITH WHAT THE LATE AMERICAN biologist and conservationist Professor E. O. Wilson called biophilia, an innate tendency to seek connections with other forms of life and with nature. While social media, technology, and other modern-world distractions often risk moving us gradually away from this love of animals and other living organisms, many people retain a strong desire to understand and protect the life on our planet.

I lived some of my early childhood years in Florida, spending time in the Everglades, the Florida Keys, and on the Atlantic Ocean. My father, a US Air Force fighter pilot, moved the family to suburban Massachusetts when I was seven, and my mother, a botanist, continued to bring our family out into nature. As I grew up, I learned more about wildlife and ecosystems, and saw firsthand what it looked like when forests were bulldozed for housing developments in my hometown of Acton. I read stories about pollution in Boston Harbor and learned more about the many environmental crises accelerating across the planet. The more I learned about the state of the planet, the more committed I became to help protect nature.

I've been fortunate to connect with nature throughout my life, knowing that it is fraught with what humans might consider paradoxical states of being. The wild is both beautiful and treacherous. It is sometimes loud, sometimes quiet. The wild is vulnerable to threats from human development, such as oil and gas drilling and animal agriculture, while also being the most powerful force on Earth. Nature is an ancient technology that's so advanced it created elephants and moths, vultures and sharks, and us.

I have always believed that all biodiversity matters, that we must work to save species and ecosystems to maintain a livable planet, which is critical to addressing the interconnected crises of climate, biodiversity, and human well-being. In 2017, Re:wild and partners launched the Search for Lost Species, which set out to find species around the world that had been lost to science for a minimum of ten years, making conservation success stories out of rediscoveries of forgotten animals, plants,

and fungi, like the Fernandina Galápagos tortoise in Ecuador, Wallace's giant bee in Indonesia, and Jackson's climbing salamander in Guatemala.

At the time of the launch, Jackson's climbing salamander had been lost to science since 1975. It was found again in 2017 by Ramos León, a local guard at the Finca San Isidro Amphibian Reserve in Guatemala, who, while sitting down for his lunch break, spotted the salamander at the edge of the reserve. León's discovery started a chain reaction of conservation initiatives that culminated in the expansion of the Finca Reserve and increased protection for other threatened species, including the Yucatán black howler monkey, highland guan, and yellow-blotched palm pit viper.

In an assessment of global biodiversity and ecosystem services released in 2019, the United Nations and the Intergovernmental Science-Policy Platform on Biodiversity and Ecosystem Service (IPBES) reported that over one million animal and plant species are at risk of extinction. One million is an unfathomable number, though you don't need to be a mathematician to understand that the loss of a million wild species would create an avalanche of consequences for the continuation of life on Earth as we know it.

In 2021, IPBES and the Intergovernmental Panel on Climate Change produced the first joint report showing that the world needs to treat climate change and biodiversity loss as two parts of the same problem. We know that these two crises tie directly to human well-being, from dealing with the impacts of floods, hurricanes, droughts, and megafires to emerging infectious diseases. We have recently seen the last of these issues play out on the world stage for over two years, with much of human society locked in the grip of a coronavirus that found its way out of the wild into a human host, very likely because of the industrial hunting, capture, and trade of wild animals. One of the many benefits of biodiversity, of a wild that is intact, is protection from new pathogens. The natural checks and balances of healthy ecosystems help to prevent pathogens from spreading from wildlife to humans, maintain a stable climate, and increase human well-being.

One of the ways we can help each other understand what's happening in our world is through the telling of stories. For thousands of years, Indigenous peoples have used the power of storytelling to explain natural phenomena and our connection to nature. Storytelling is an old and universal tool that humans developed to make sense of the Earth and our place in it. Similar to the way that biodiversity ties the wild together, storytelling creates webs of meaning that bind us to one another. It is through storytelling that we can begin to reconnect to the natural world.

We can and should harness stories as a tool to rewild ourselves. In fact, the collapse of most ancient civilizations has been linked directly or indirectly to human-induced changes in our environment, from the Mayans to the Indus Valley Civilization to Easter Island. We are now repeating this mistake on a global scale. However, a major part of the solution is protecting and restoring nature, saving the vital biodiversity that underlies healthy ecosystems. A healthy ecosystem in turn provides resilience against storms, mitigates climate change, creates clean water and air, and keeps nature's medicine cabinet available to humanity.

As scientists glean more about the secrets of our world, old theories are replaced by new ones, hypotheses are adjusted, and the stories we tell about life on our planet evolve. In a similar way, the discovery of a new species, rediscovery of a lost species, or extinction of a species demands a shift in our collective understanding about the makeup of our planet's biodiversity.

Consider the Galápagos giant tortoise complex, for example. A species complex describes a group of species that share so many similar characteristics that it can be difficult even for scientists to tell the difference between them. In the case of the tortoises of the Galápagos, we know of at least fifteen distinct giant tortoise species, thirteen of which survive today scattered throughout the archipelago. Scientists believe these species evolved on the Galápagos Islands over the course of two to three million years, after dispersing from South America, likely washed out in a river and pushed across the Eastern Pacific by the Humboldt Current. The arrival of the first tortoises to the Galápagos was completely random and changed the islands forever.

The giant tortoise has long been a symbol of the global importance of conserving endangered species. Once a total population of 300,000 strong, giant tortoises thrived in the Galápagos until pirates and whalers learned these species can survive for up to a year without food and water. Because of this special adaptation, which enabled giant tortoises to survive long journeys across the ocean, they were kept on board ships for fresh meat during long voyages. Today, giant tortoise populations have been reduced to 10 to 15 percent of their original numbers.

Fernandina Island is the youngest island in the Galápagos and has no human settlements, but the endemic tortoise was thought to be long extinct due to human hunting. The island is also an active shield volcano with regular eruptions. Lava flows across Fernandina in thick ropes of pahoehoe and 'a'a, which harden into rock armor around the island, making it both difficult to explore and a hotbed for the continuation and creation of life. It's too easy to consider volcanoes only destructive. They're not. Without them, the Galápagos Islands wouldn't exist and neither would the species native to those islands.

This takes us back to the concept of paradox in the wild. On an expedition to Fernandina Island in 2019, a team of scientists from the Galápagos National Park Directorate and other groups found a single female giant tortoise at the edge of a volcano. Two years later, genetic testing at Yale University confirmed a match between this lonely, hundred-year-old female (called Fernanda, or Fern) and DNA from a Fernandina Galápagos giant tortoise collected in 1906, the same year this species was previously considered lost to science. Traces of giant tortoise scat and other tracks observed on the expedition suggest Fernanda might not be alone. As part of restoration and rewilding efforts in the Galápagos, I'm optimistic that future expeditions will uncover the presence of more individual Fernandina Galápagos giant tortoises, enabling the start of a conservation breeding program. Nature is resilient, and life, given a chance, always finds a way.

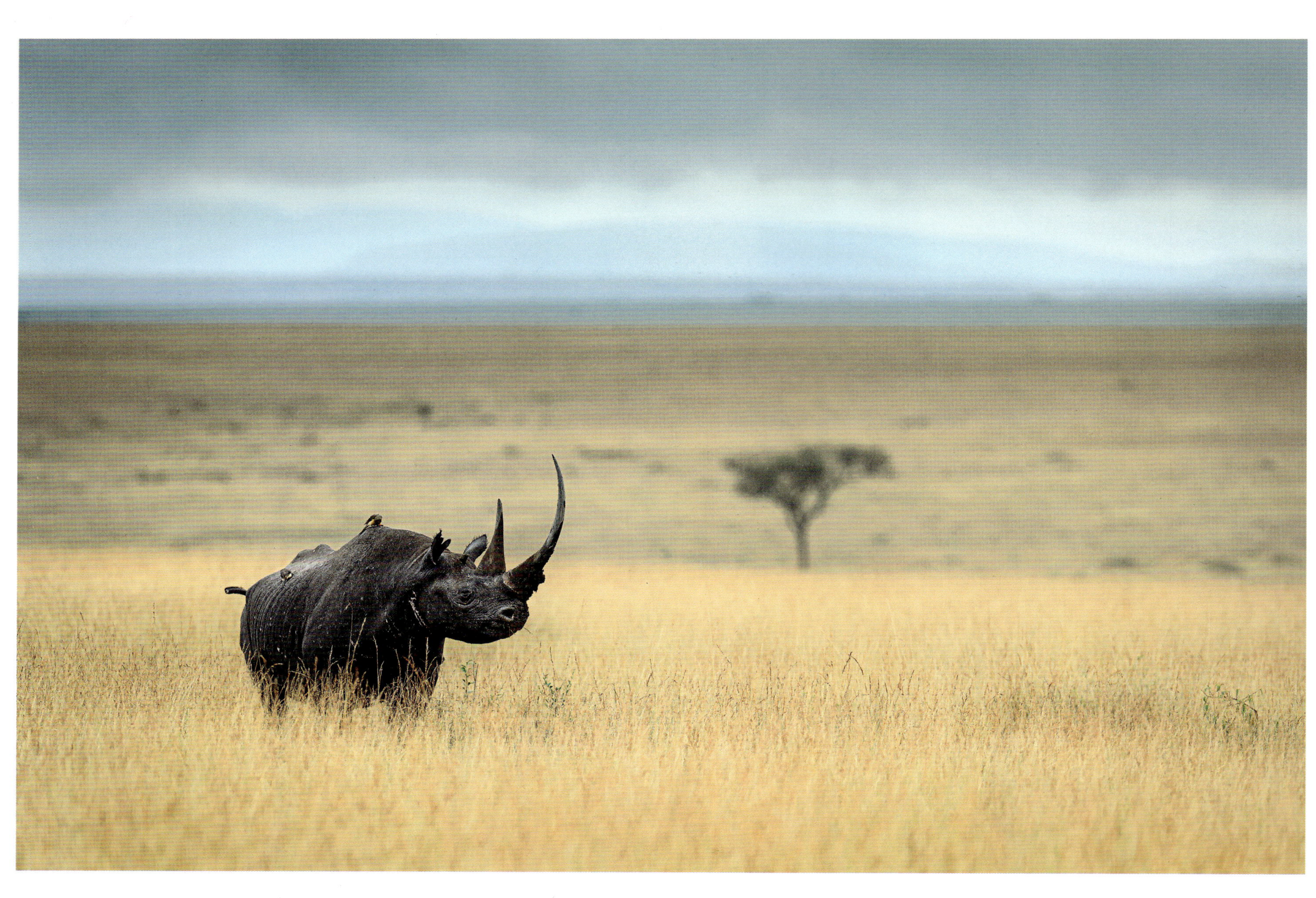

David Lloyd
Black Rhinoceros
STATUS: CRITICALLY ENDANGERED
Maasai Mara National Reserve, Kenya

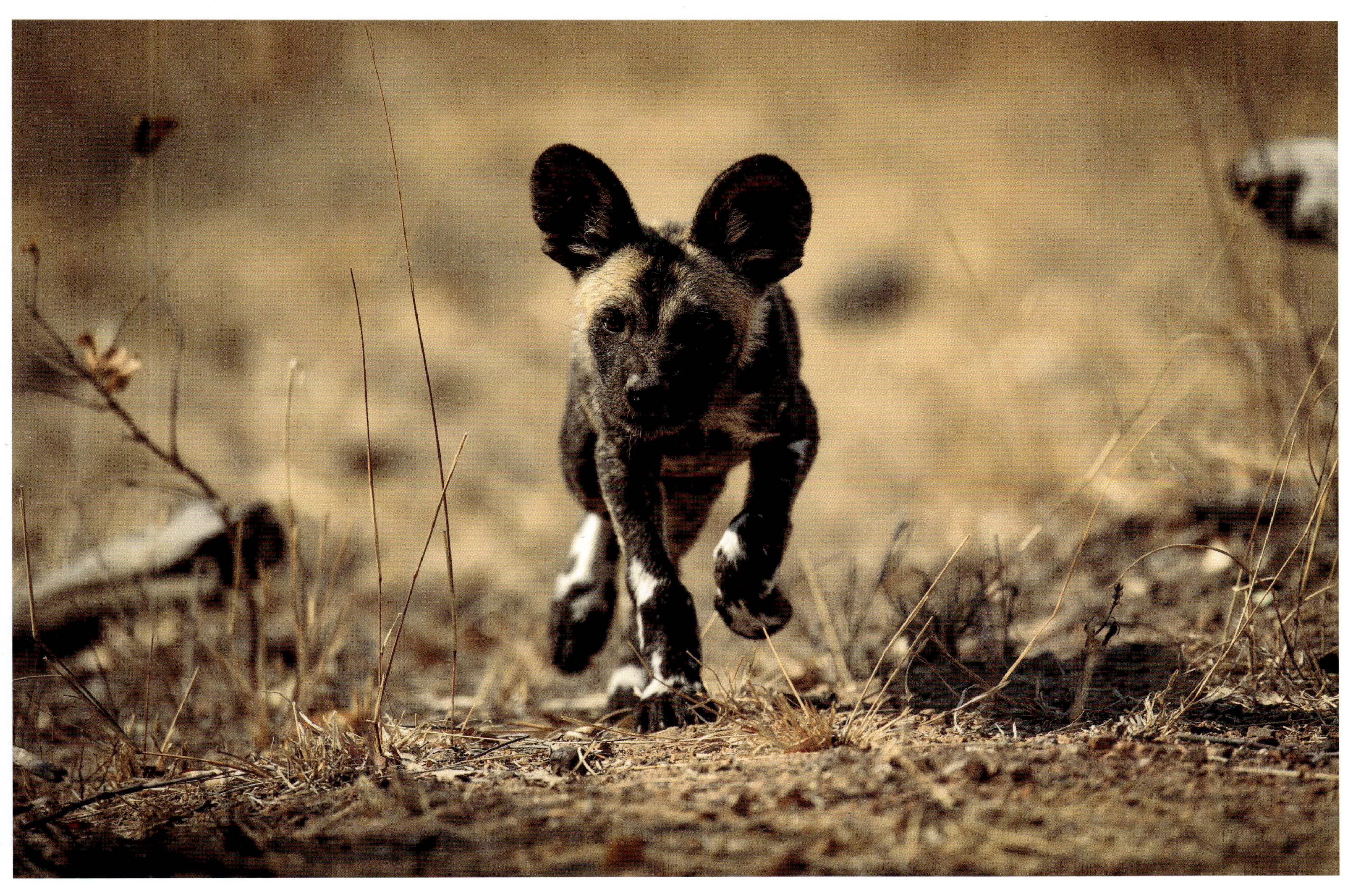

Alessandro Beconi
Wild Dog
STATUS: ENDANGERED
Kruger National Park, South Africa

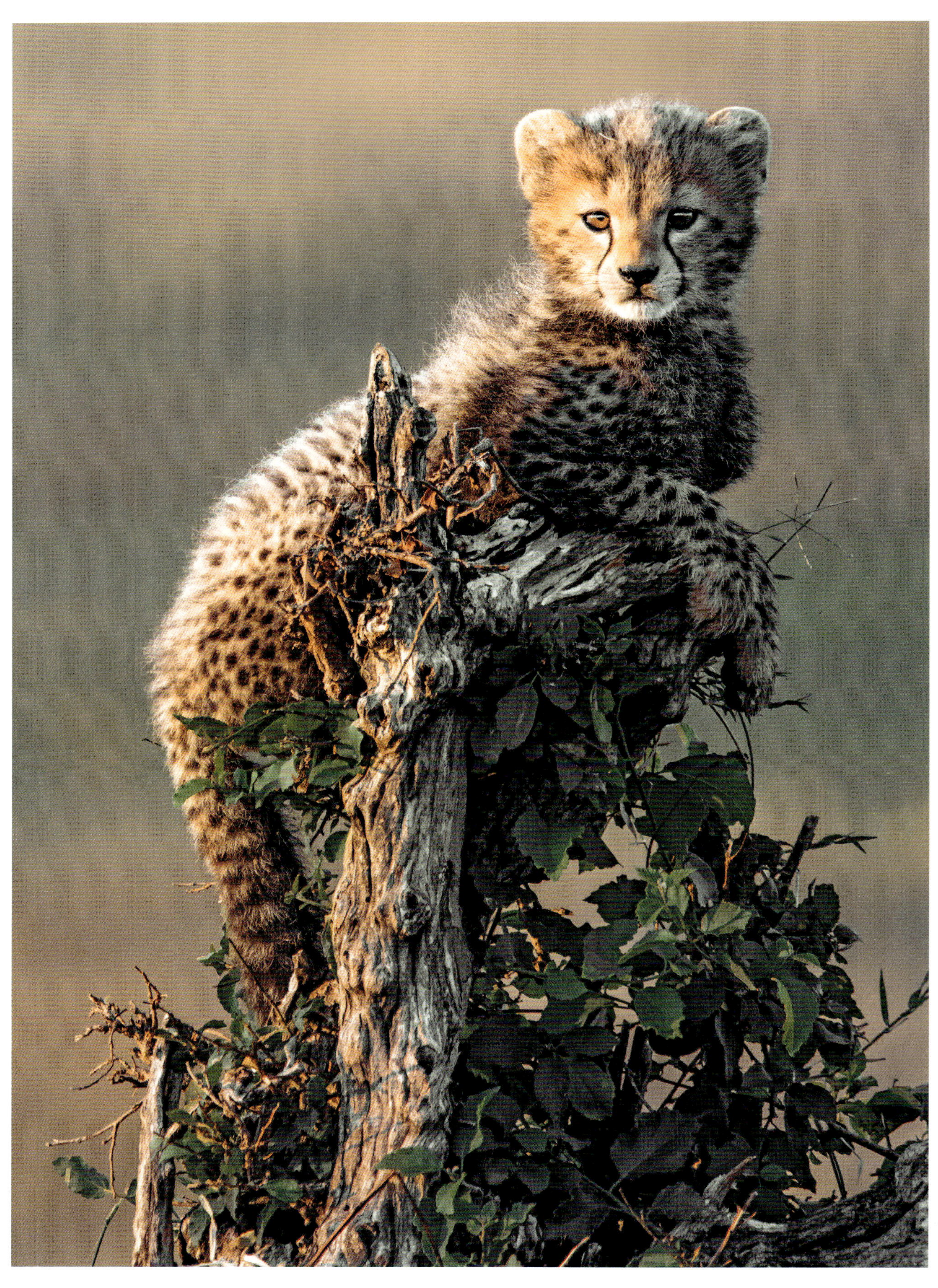

Nili Mahendra Gudhka
Cheetah
STATUS: VULNERABLE
Maasai Mara National Reserve, Kenya

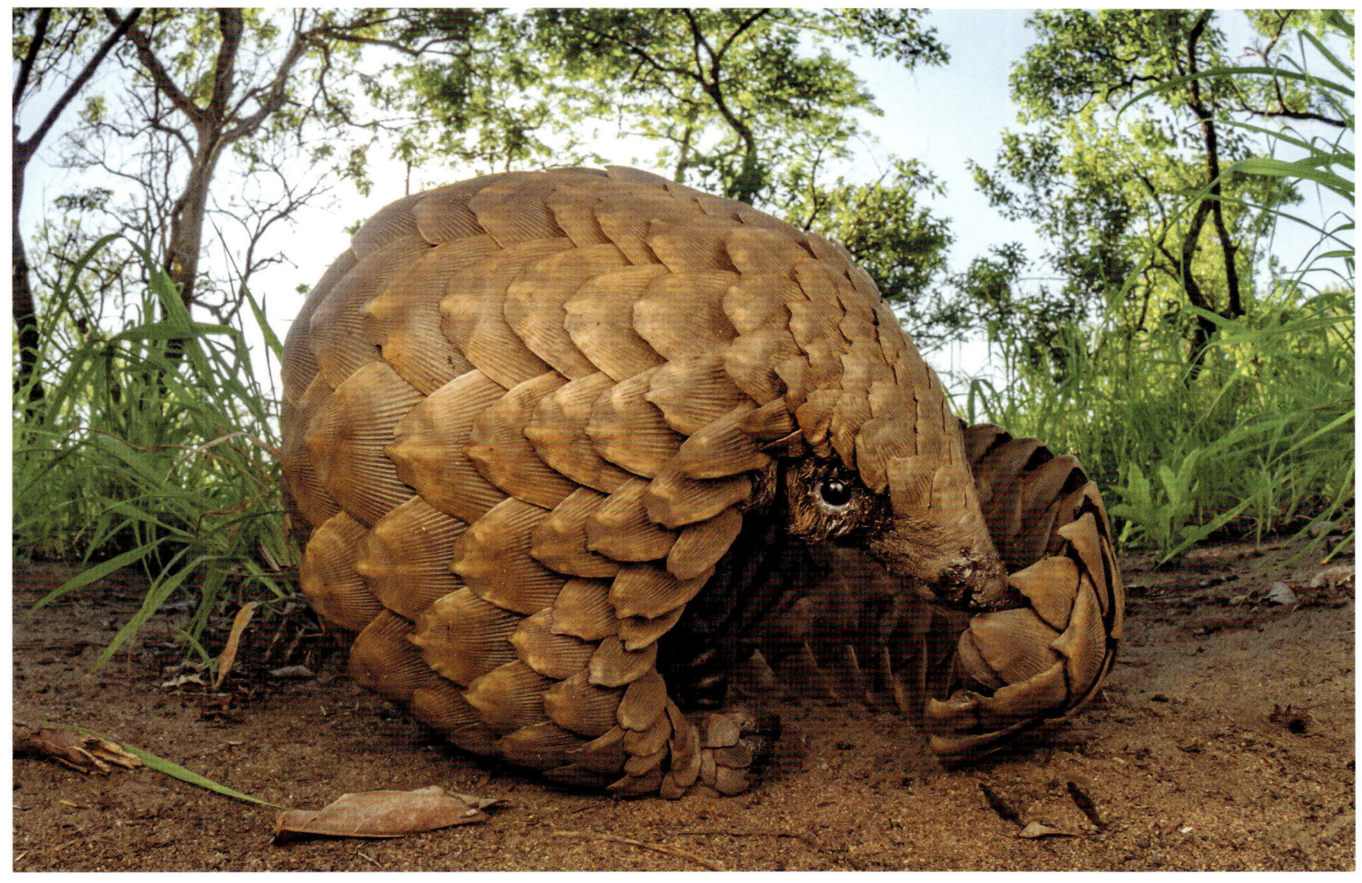

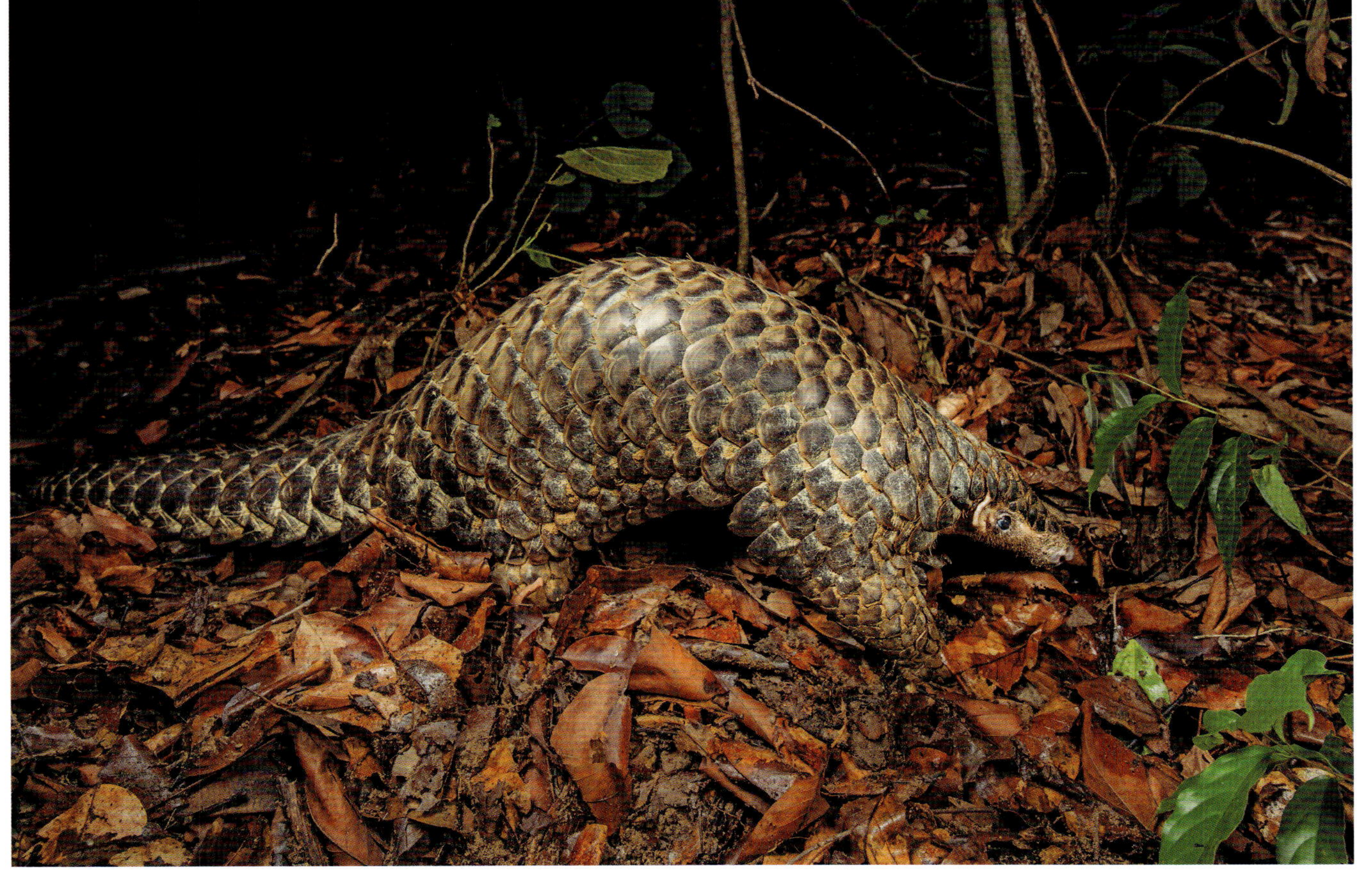

Jen Guyton
Cape Pangolin
STATUS: VULNERABLE
Gorongosa National Park,
Mozambique

Scott Trageser
Chinese Pangolin
STATUS: CRITICALLY
ENDANGERED
Lawachara National Park,
Bangladesh

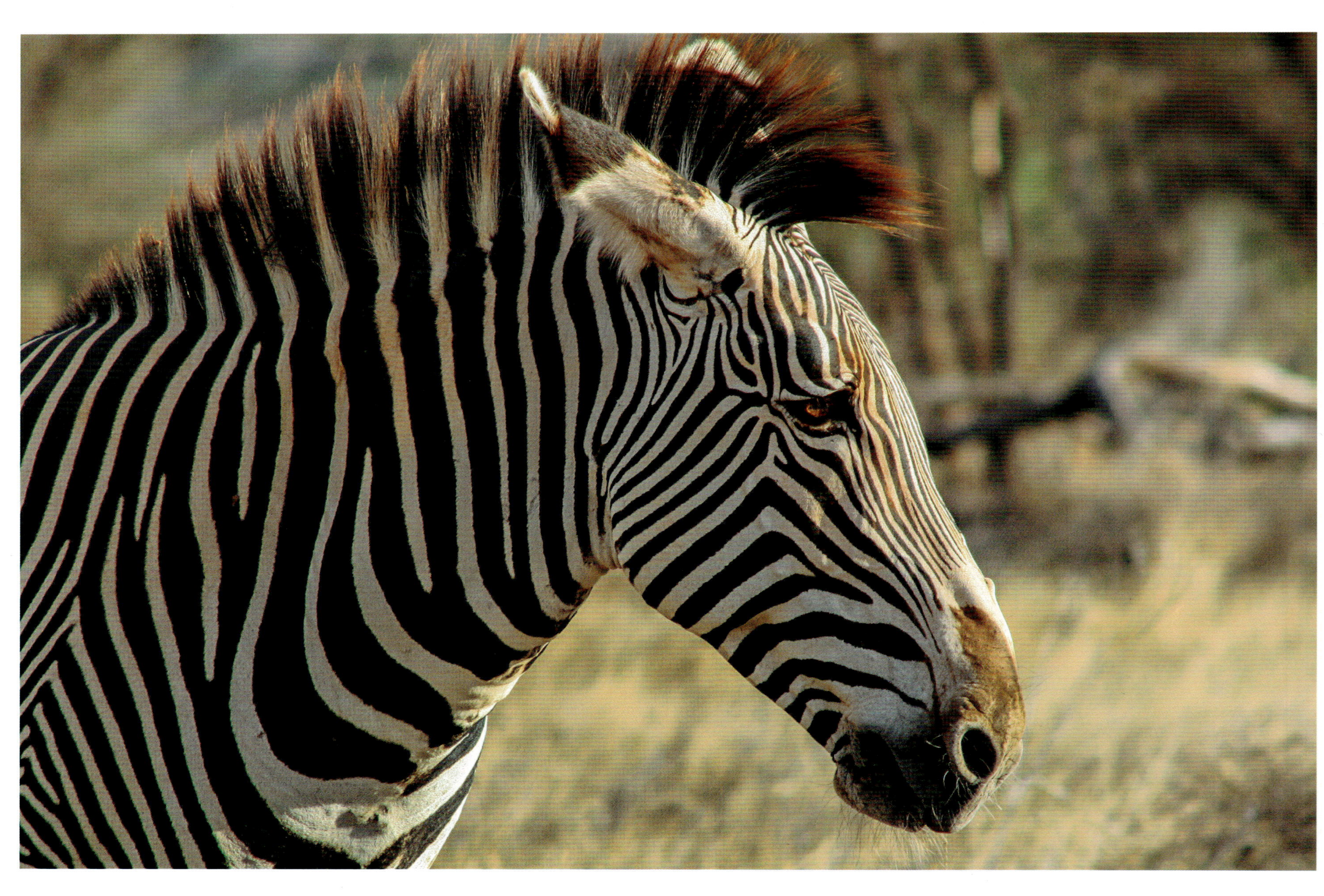

Graeme Green
Grevy's Zebra
STATUS: ENDANGERED
Samburu National Reserve, Kenya

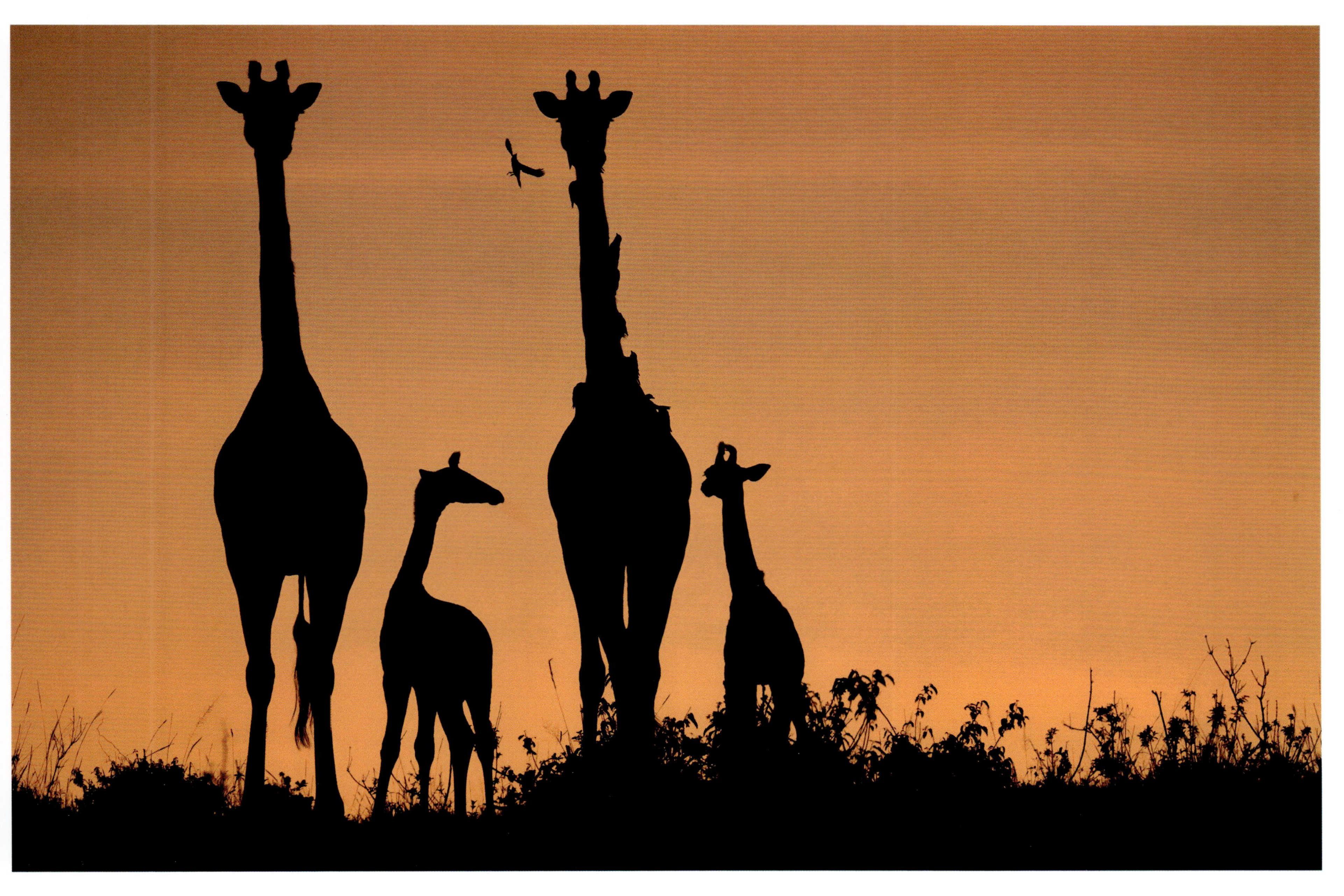

Antonio Liebana
Maasai Giraffes
STATUS: ENDANGERED
Ngorongoro Conservation Area, Tanzania

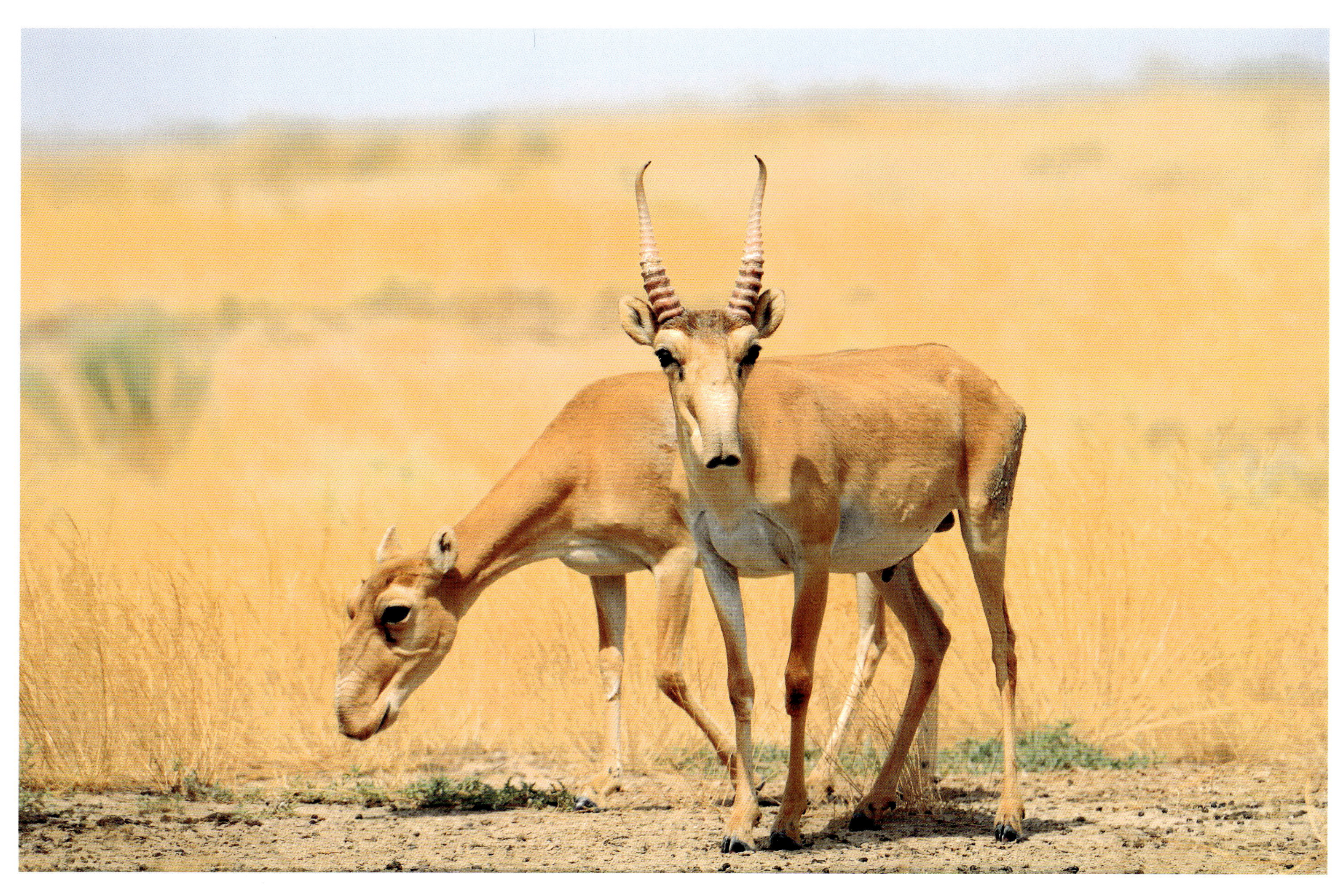

Victor Tyakht
Saigas
STATUS: CRITICALLY ENDANGERED
Chyornye Zemli Nature Reserve, Russia

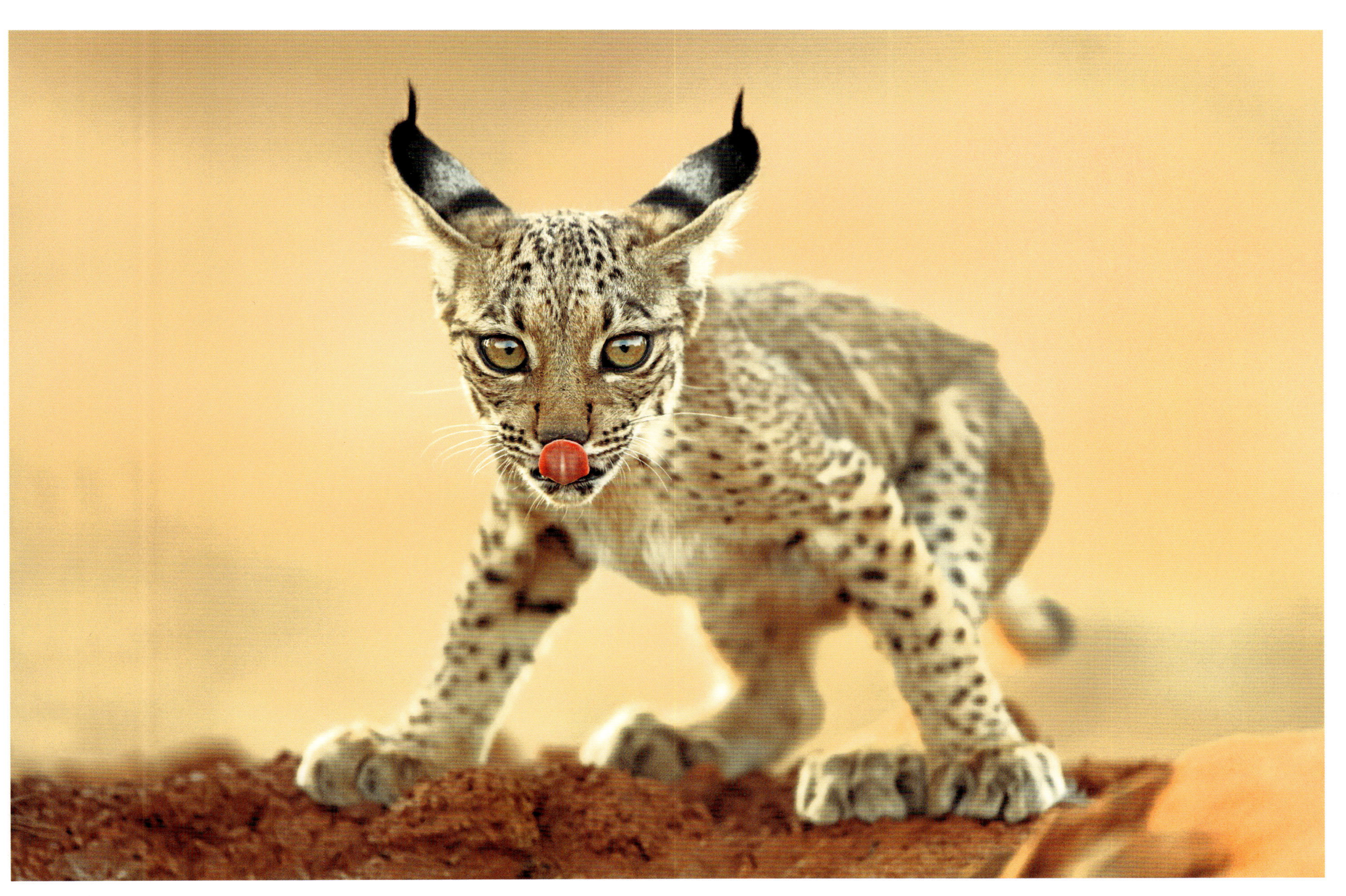

Antonio Liebana
Iberian Lynx
STATUS: ENDANGERED
Peñalajo, Ciudad Real, Spain

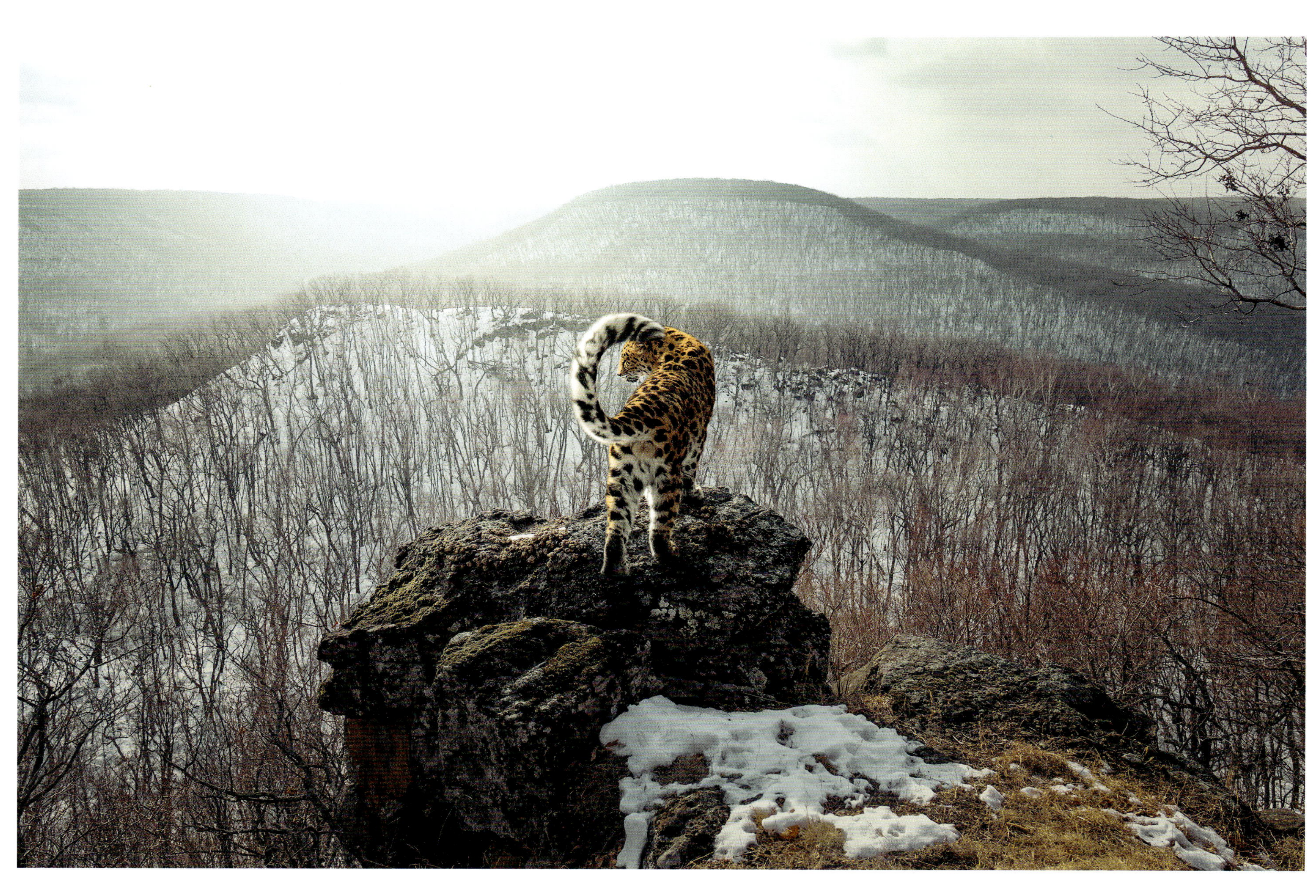

Thomas Vijayan
Amur Leopard
STATUS: CRITICALLY ENDANGERED
Land of the Leopard National Park, Russia

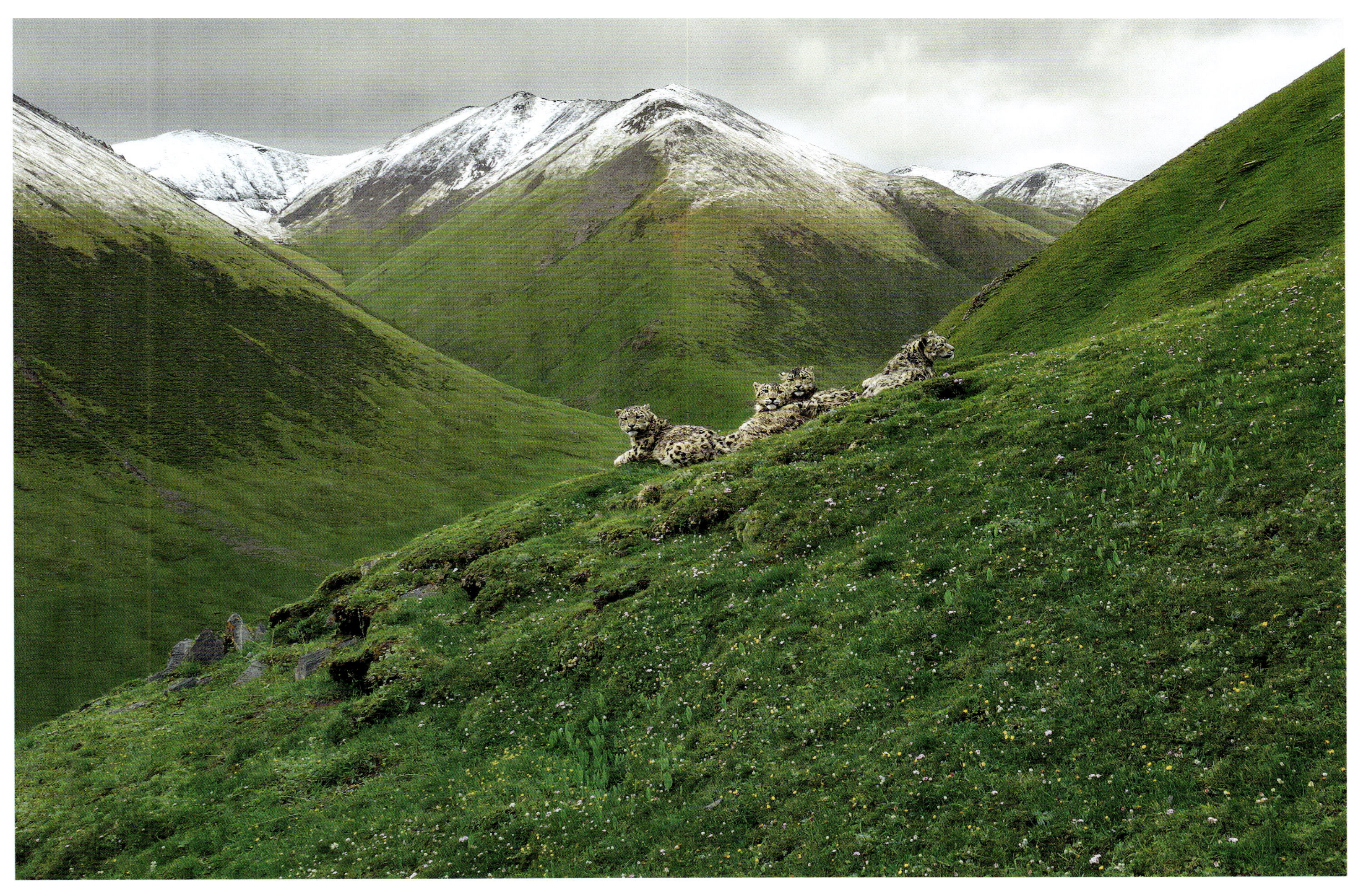

Xiaoyun Luo
Snow Leopards
STATUS: VULNERABLE
Shiqu, China

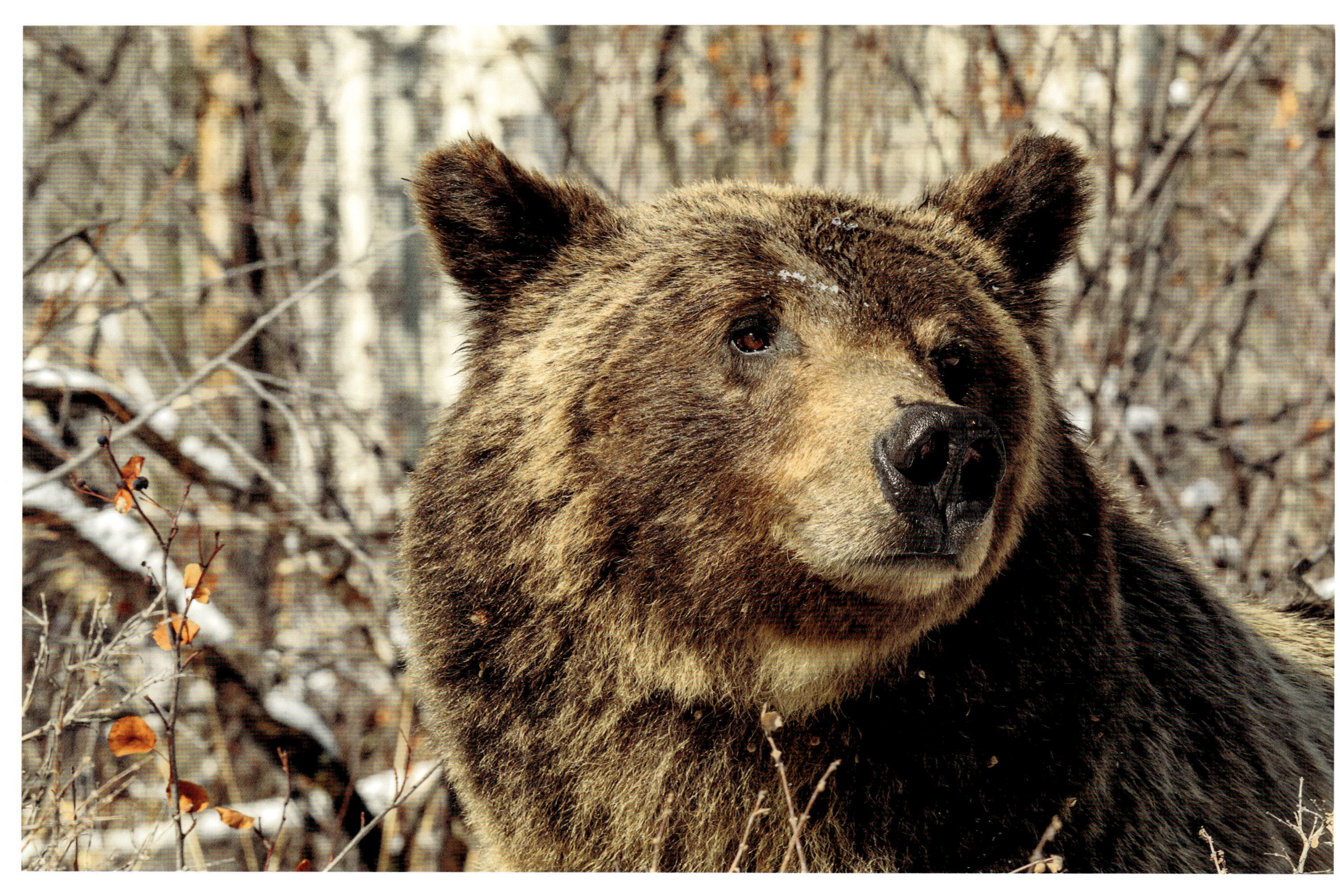

Thomas D. Mangelsen
Grizzly Bear
STATUS: THREATENED IN THE LOWER 48 STATES
(UNDER THE ENDANGERED SPECIES ACT)
Jackson Hole, Wyoming, United States

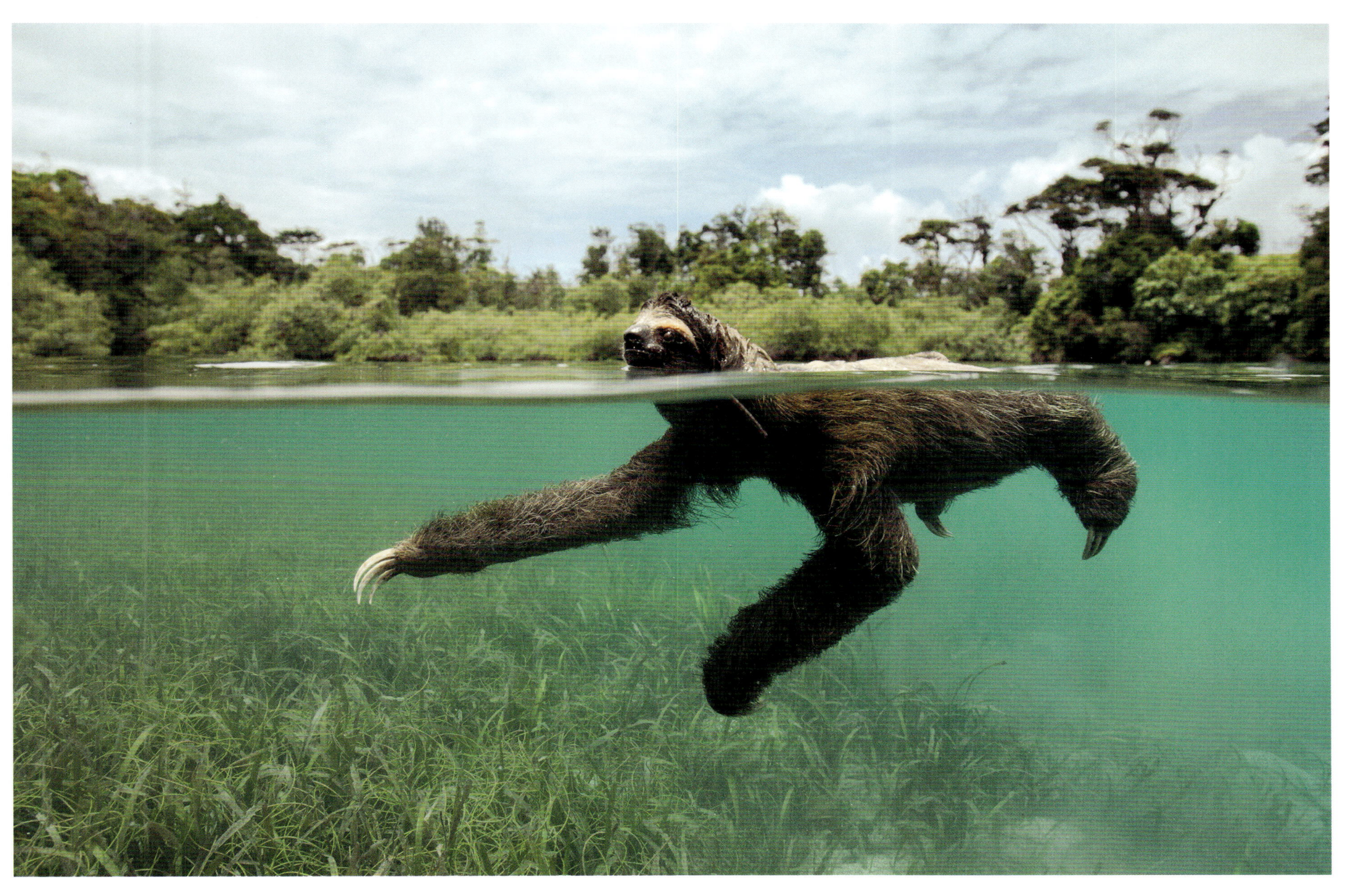

Suzi Eszterhas
Pygmy Three-toed Sloth
STATUS: CRITICALLY ENDANGERED
Isla Escudo de Veraguas, Panama

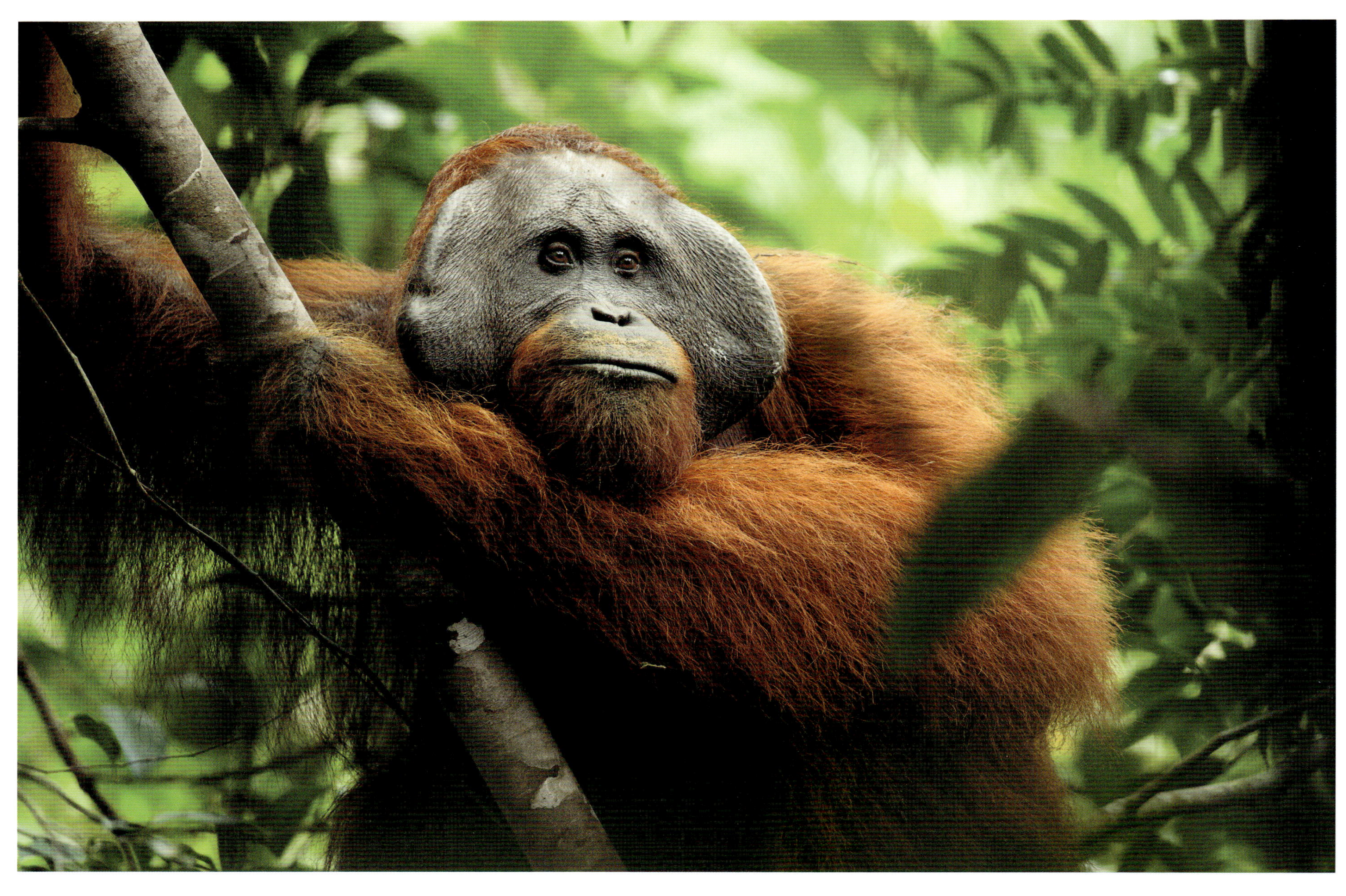

Tim Laman
Bornean Orangutan
STATUS: CRITICALLY ENDANGERED
Mount Palung National Park, Indonesia

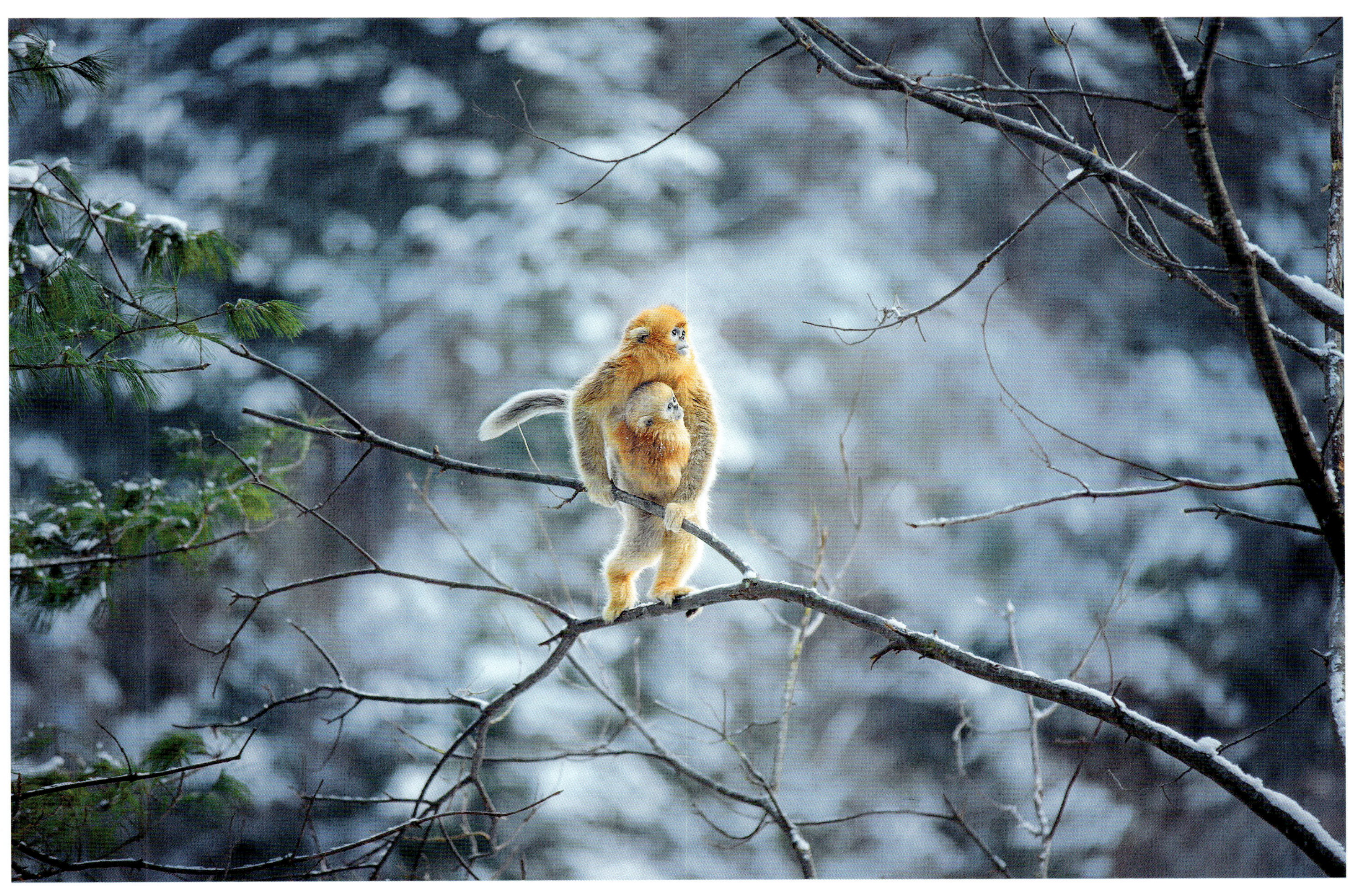

Qiang Zhang
Golden Snub-nosed Monkey
STATUS: ENDANGERED
Foping National Nature Reserve, China

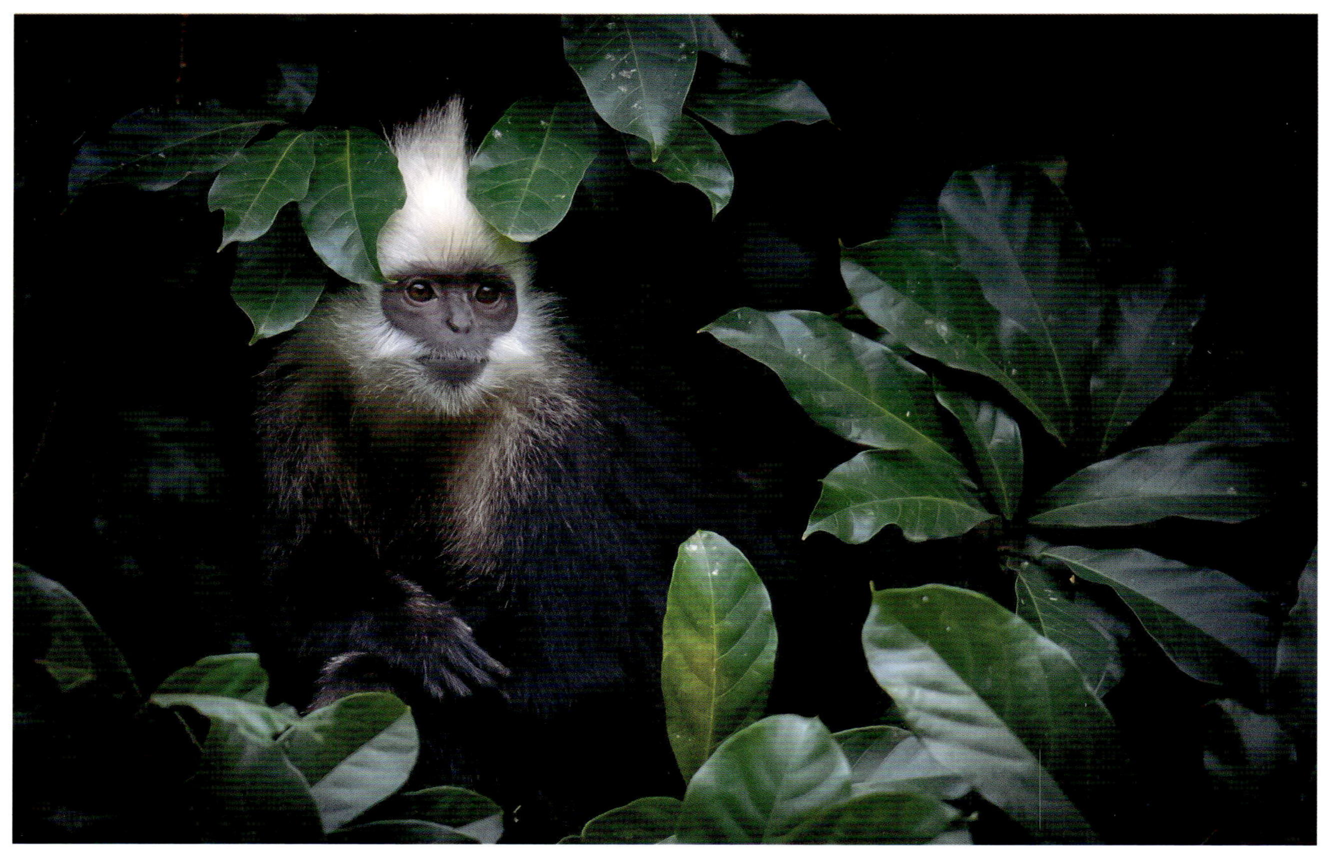

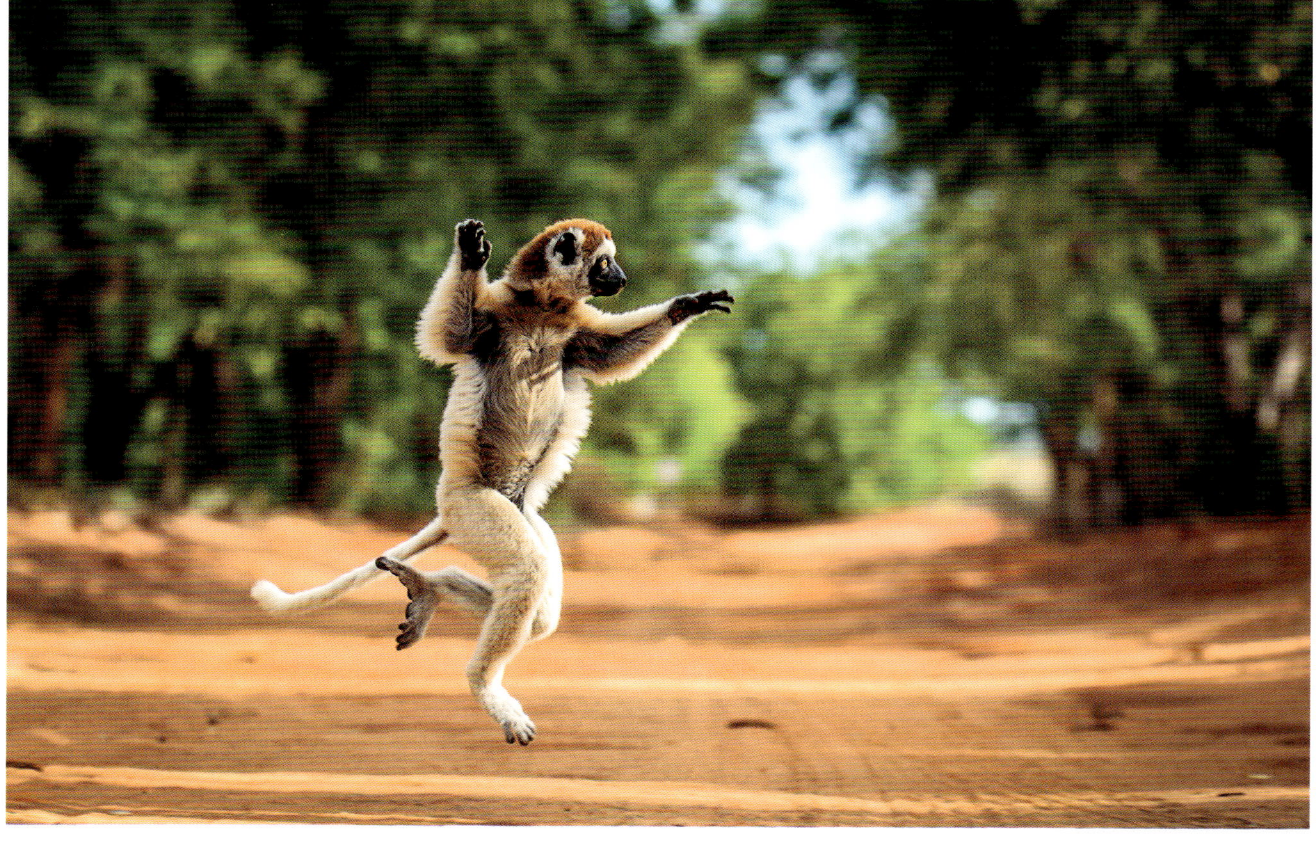

Xingchao Zhu
White-headed Black Langur
STATUS: CRITICALLY ENDANGERED
Chongzuo National Nature
Reserve, China

Shannon Wild
Verreaux's Sifaka
STATUS: CRITICALLY ENDANGERED
Berenty Reserve, Madagascar

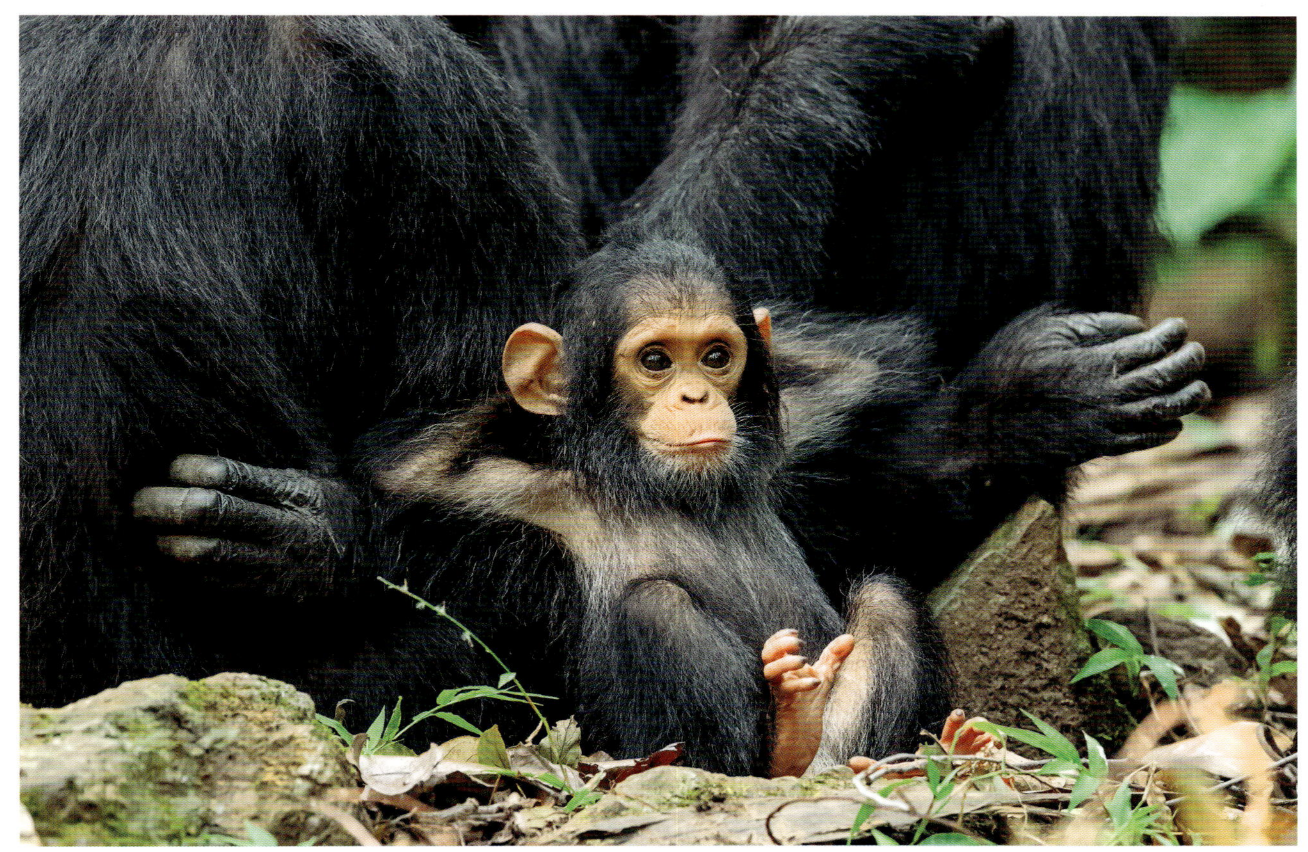

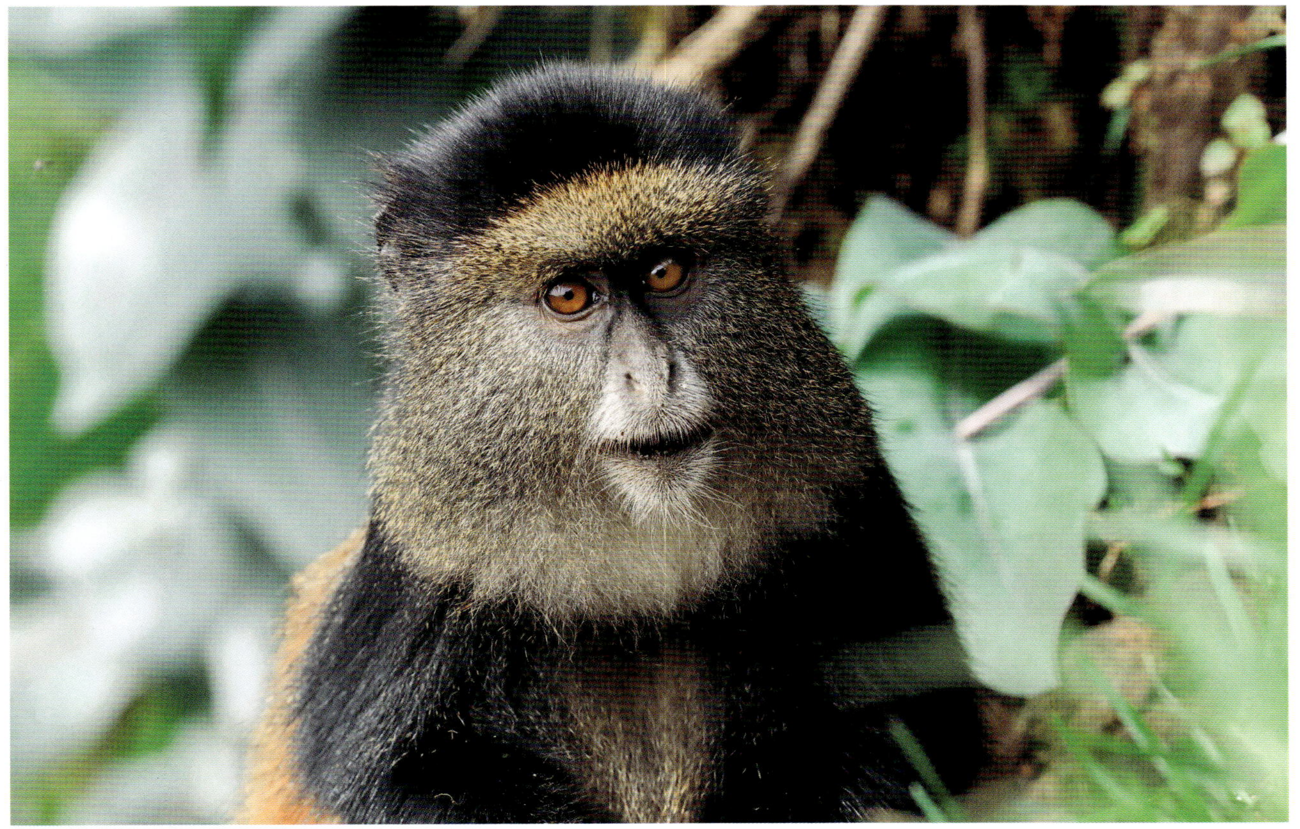

Thomas D. Mangelsen
Chimpanzees
STATUS: ENDANGERED
Gombe Stream National Park, Tanzania

Graeme Green
Golden Monkey
STATUS: ENDANGERED
Volcanoes National Park, Rwanda

225

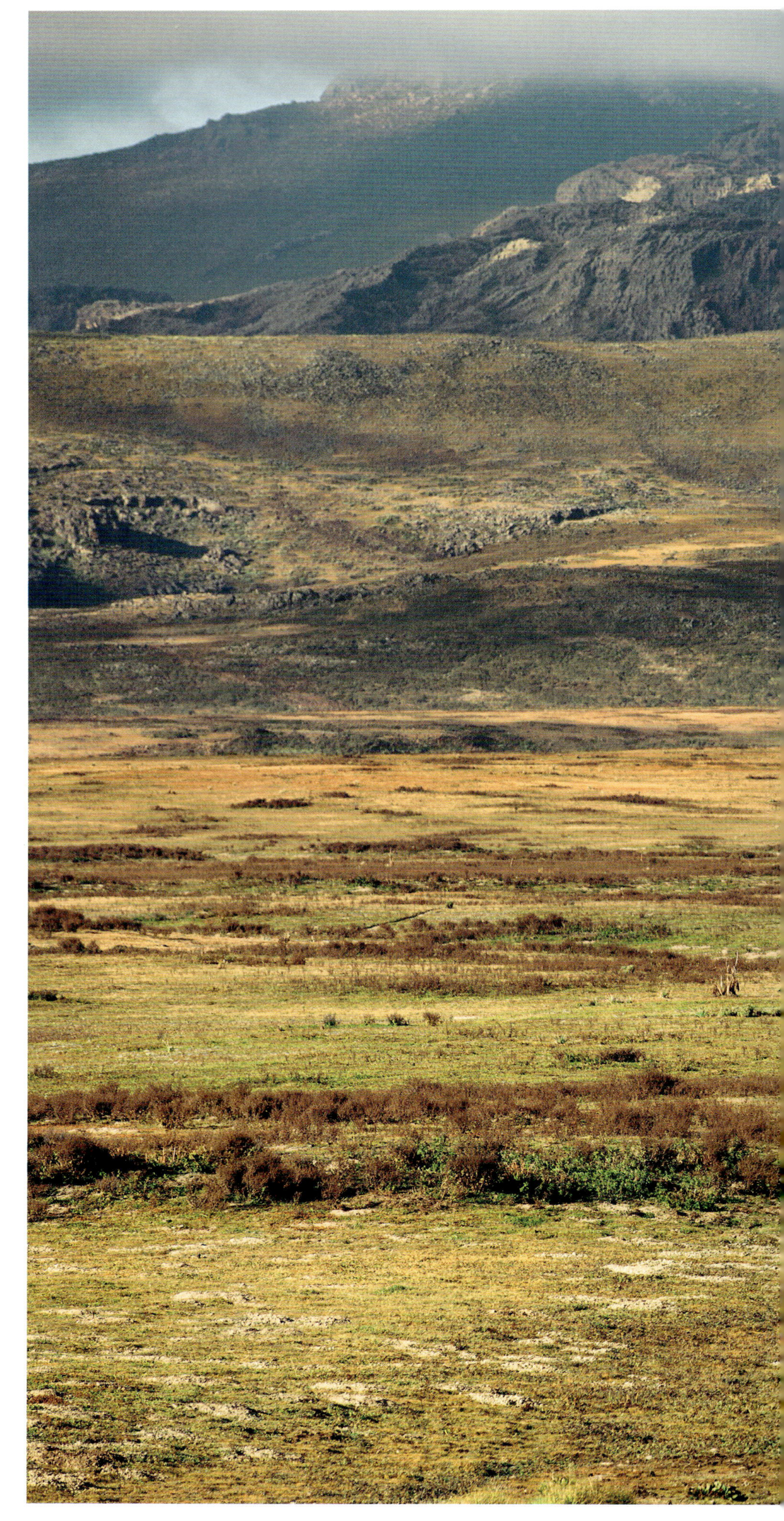

Will Burrard-Lucas
Ethiopian Wolf
STATUS: ENDANGERED
Bale Mountains National Park, Ethiopia

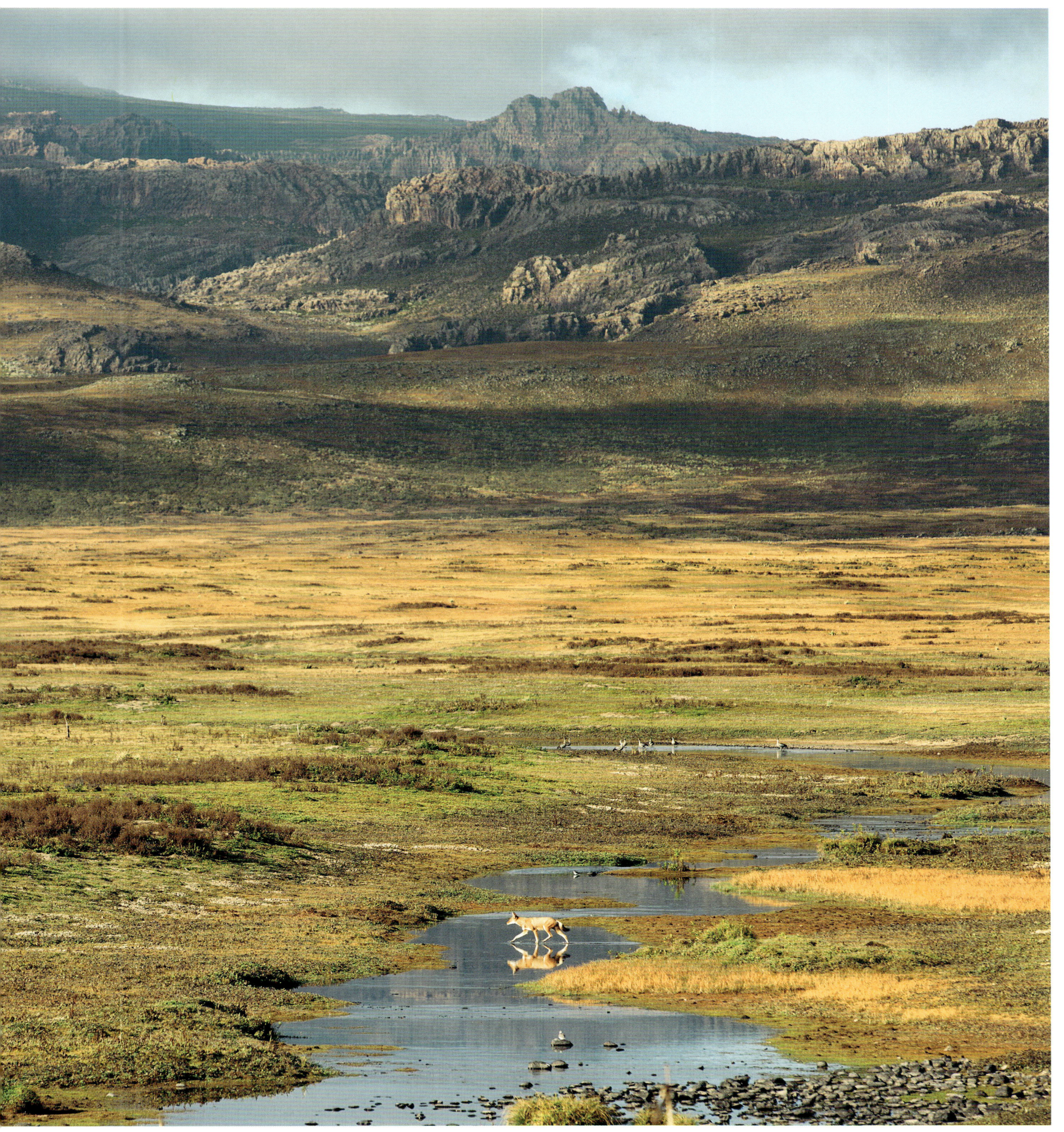

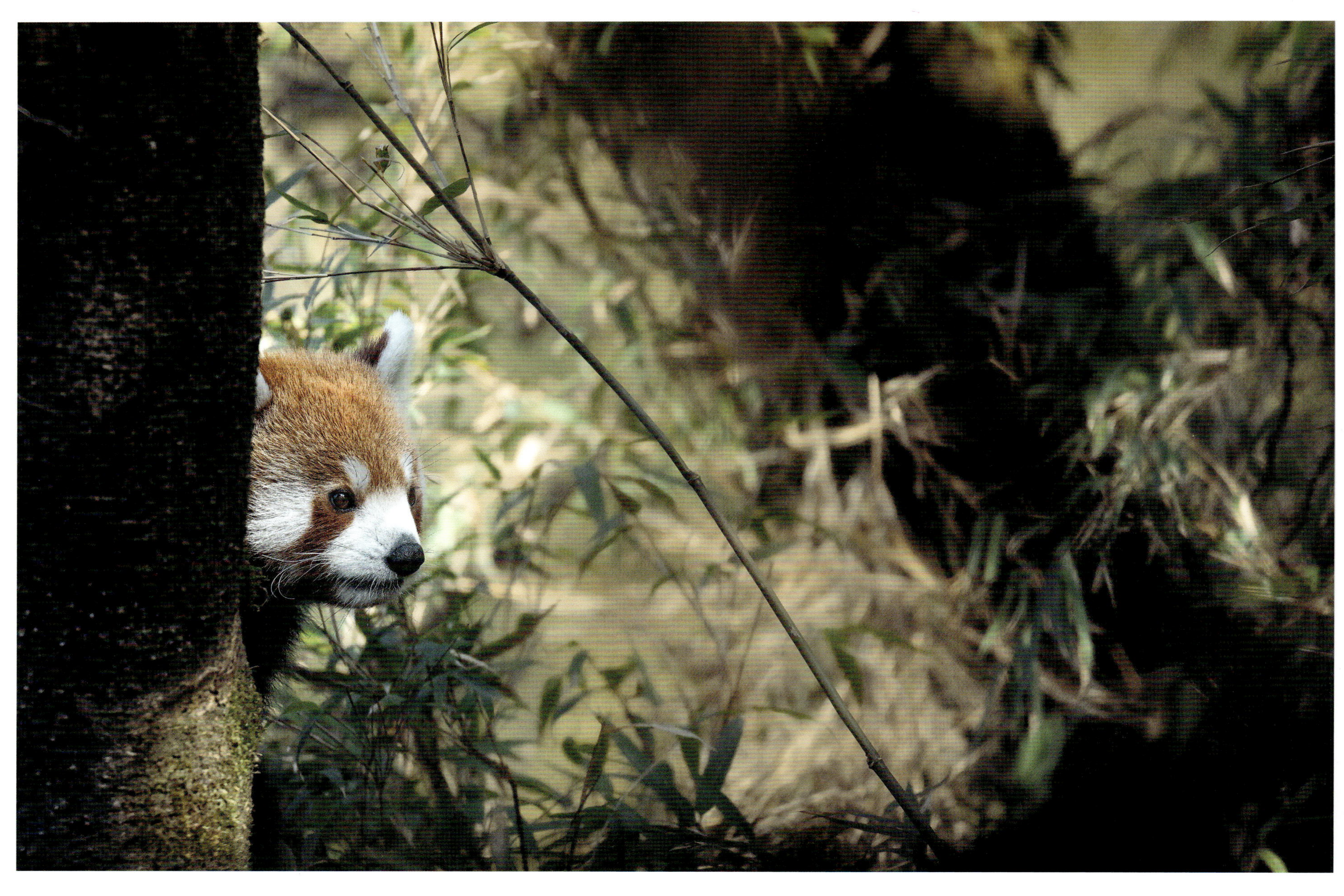

Shivang Mehta
Red Panda
STATUS: ENDANGERED
Singalila National Park, India

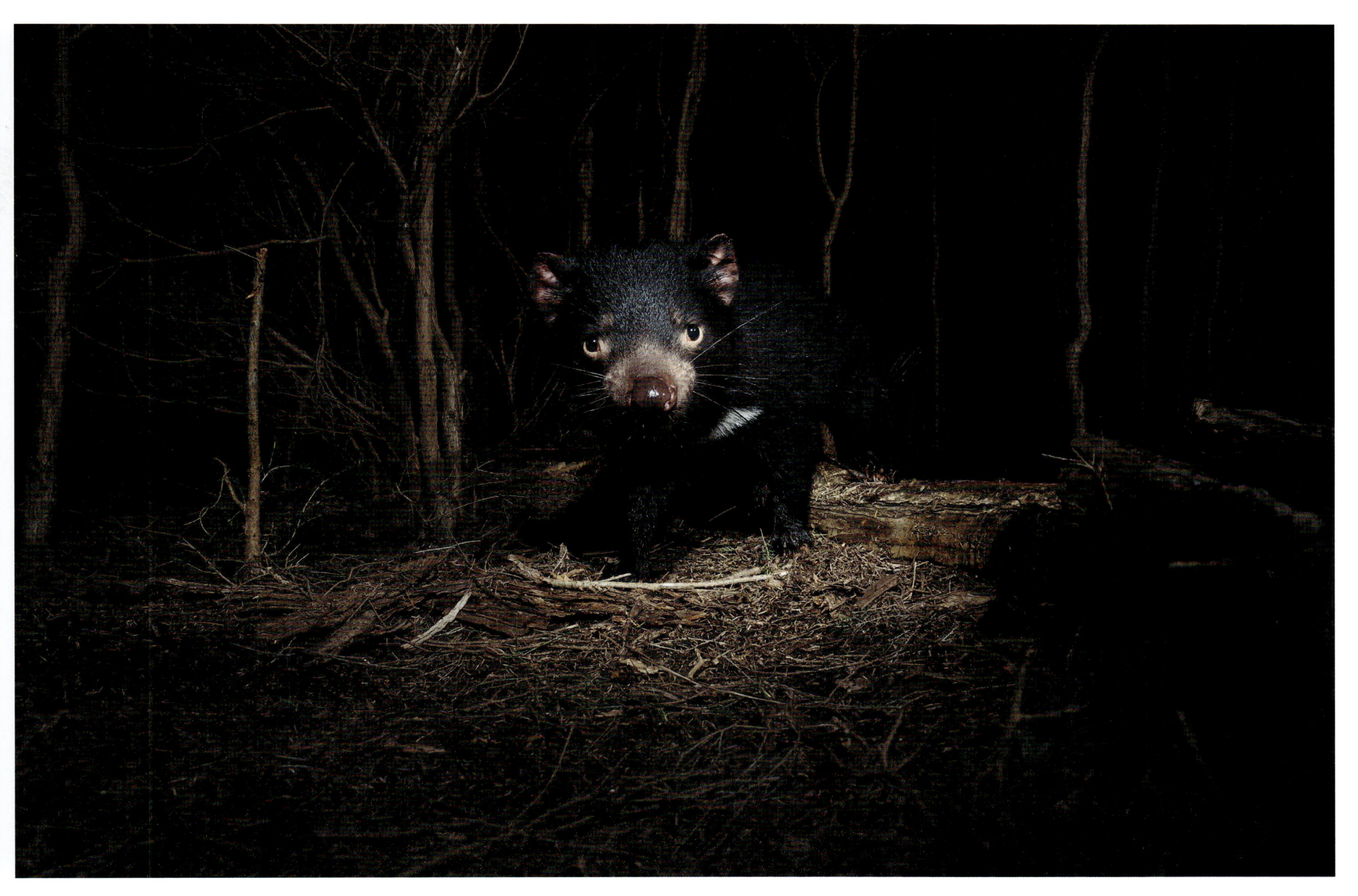

Heath Holden
Tasmanian Devil
STATUS: ENDANGERED
Narawntapu National Park, Australia

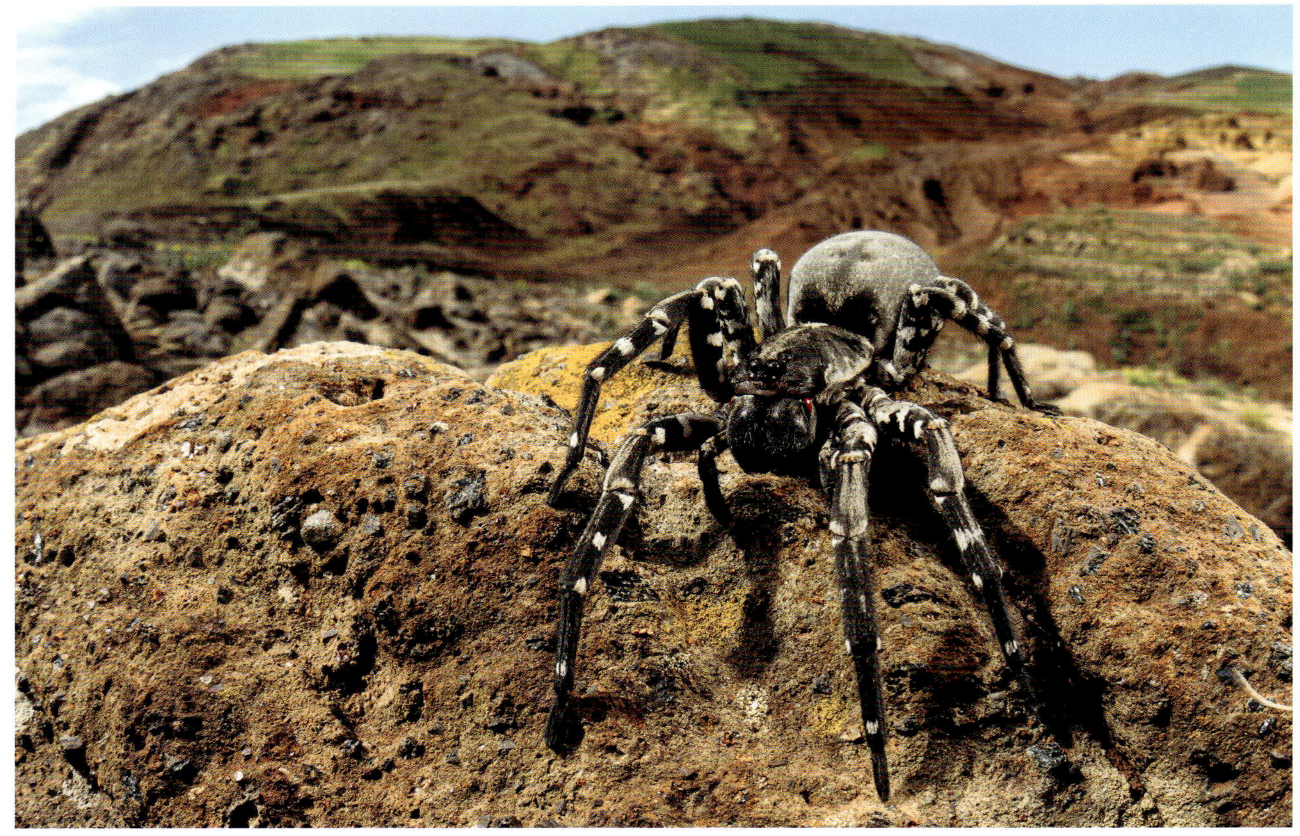

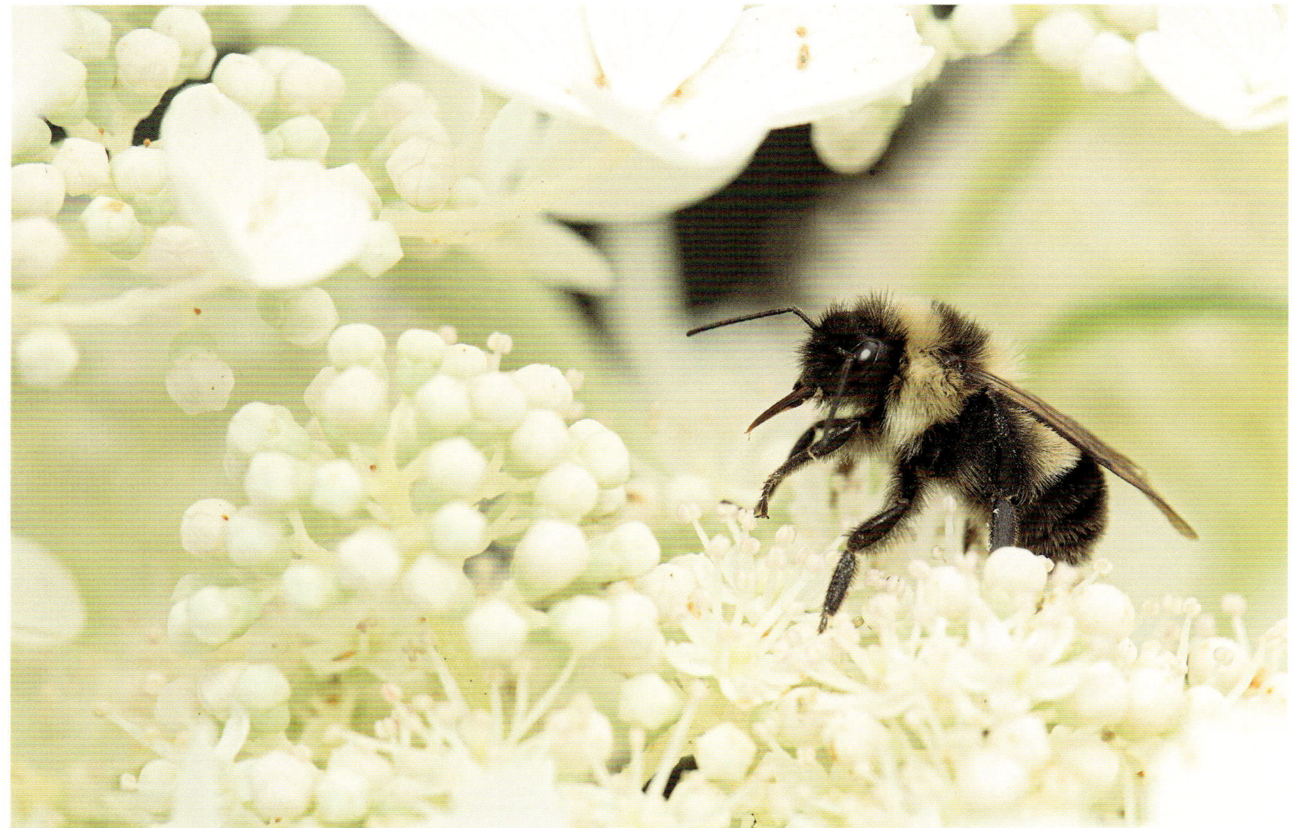

Emanuele Biggi
Deserta Grande Wolf Spider
STATUS: CRITICALLY
ENDANGERED
Desertas Islands, Madeira
Archipelago, Portugal

Clay Bolt
Rusty Patched Bumble Bee
STATUS: CRITICALLY
ENDANGERED
University of Wisconsin-
Madison Arboretum,
Wisconsin, United States

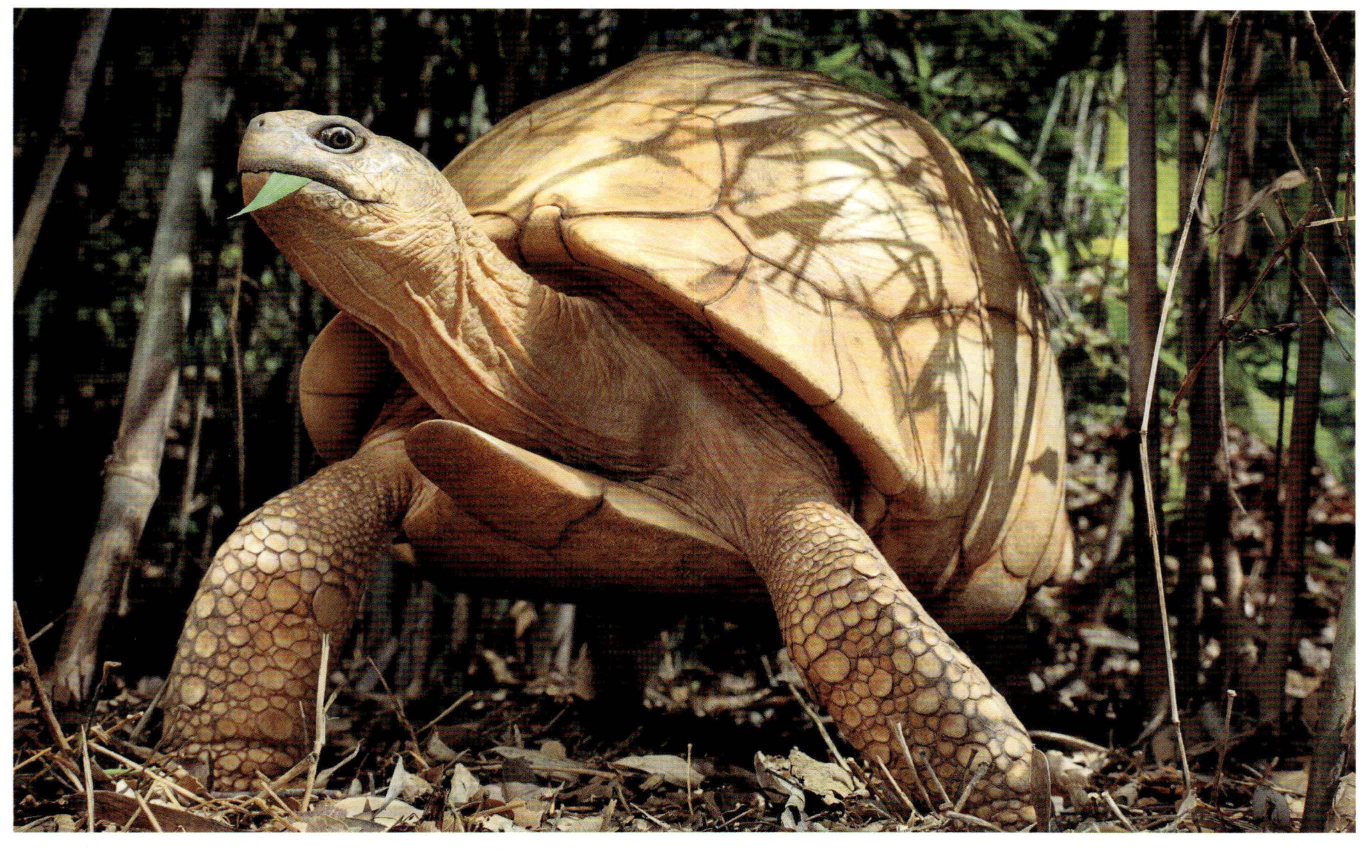

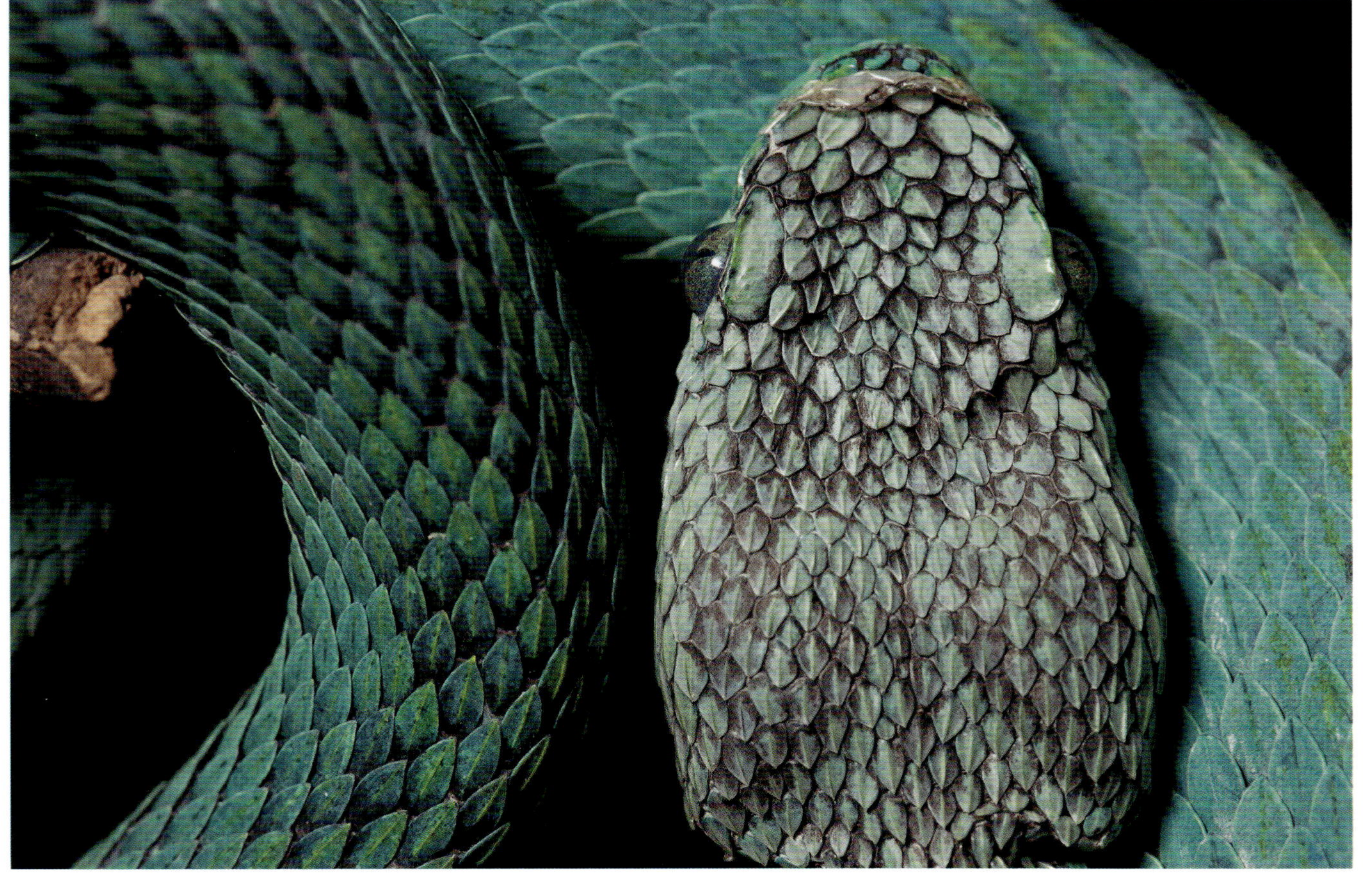

Tim Flach
Ploughshare Tortoise
STATUS: CRITICALLY
ENDANGERED
Baie de Baly National Park,
Madagascar

Robin Moore
Merendon Palm Pit Viper
STATUS: ENDANGERED
Sierra Caral Reserve,
Guatemala

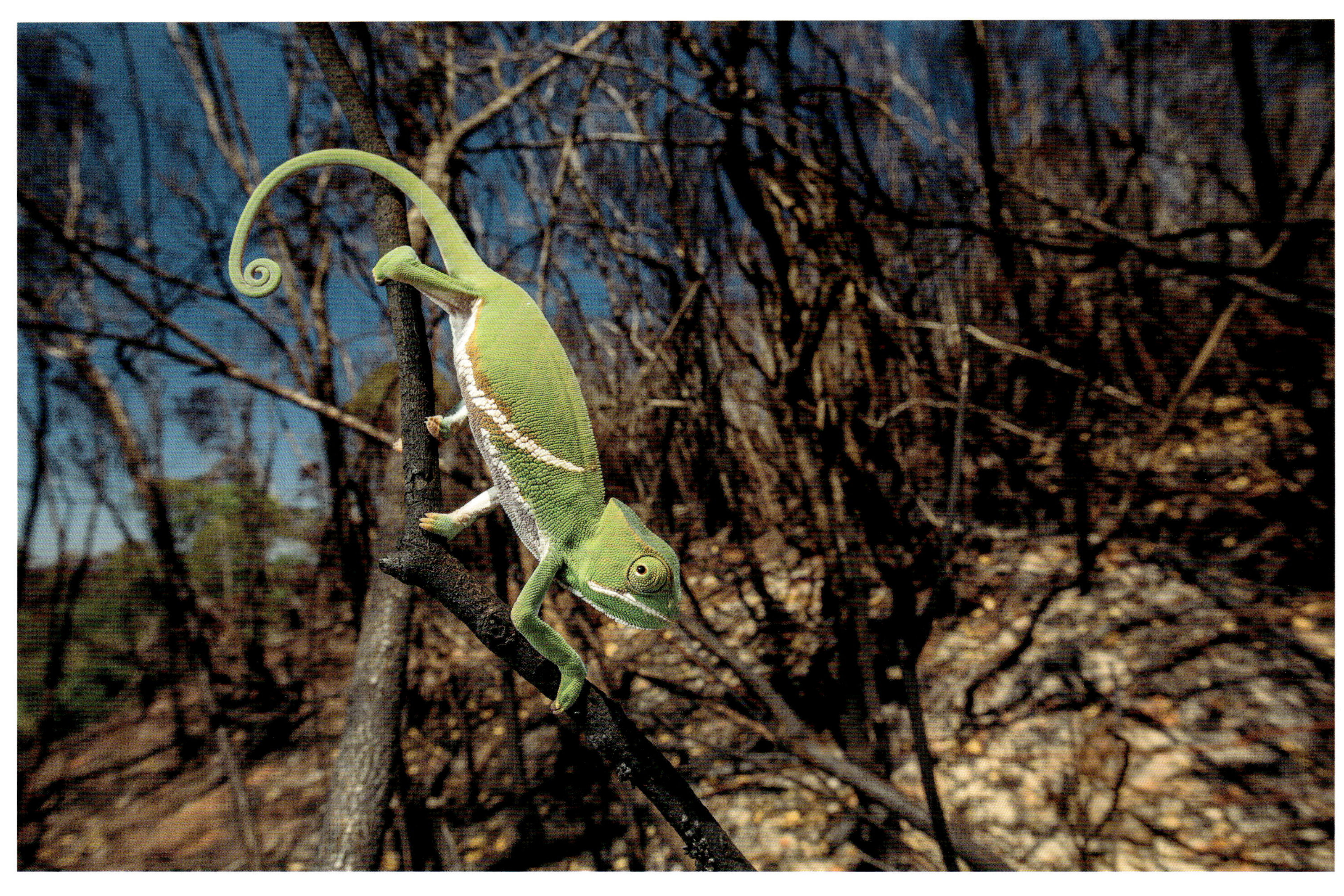

Christian Ziegler
Two-banded Chameleon
STATUS: ENDANGERED
Ranomafana National Park, Madagascar

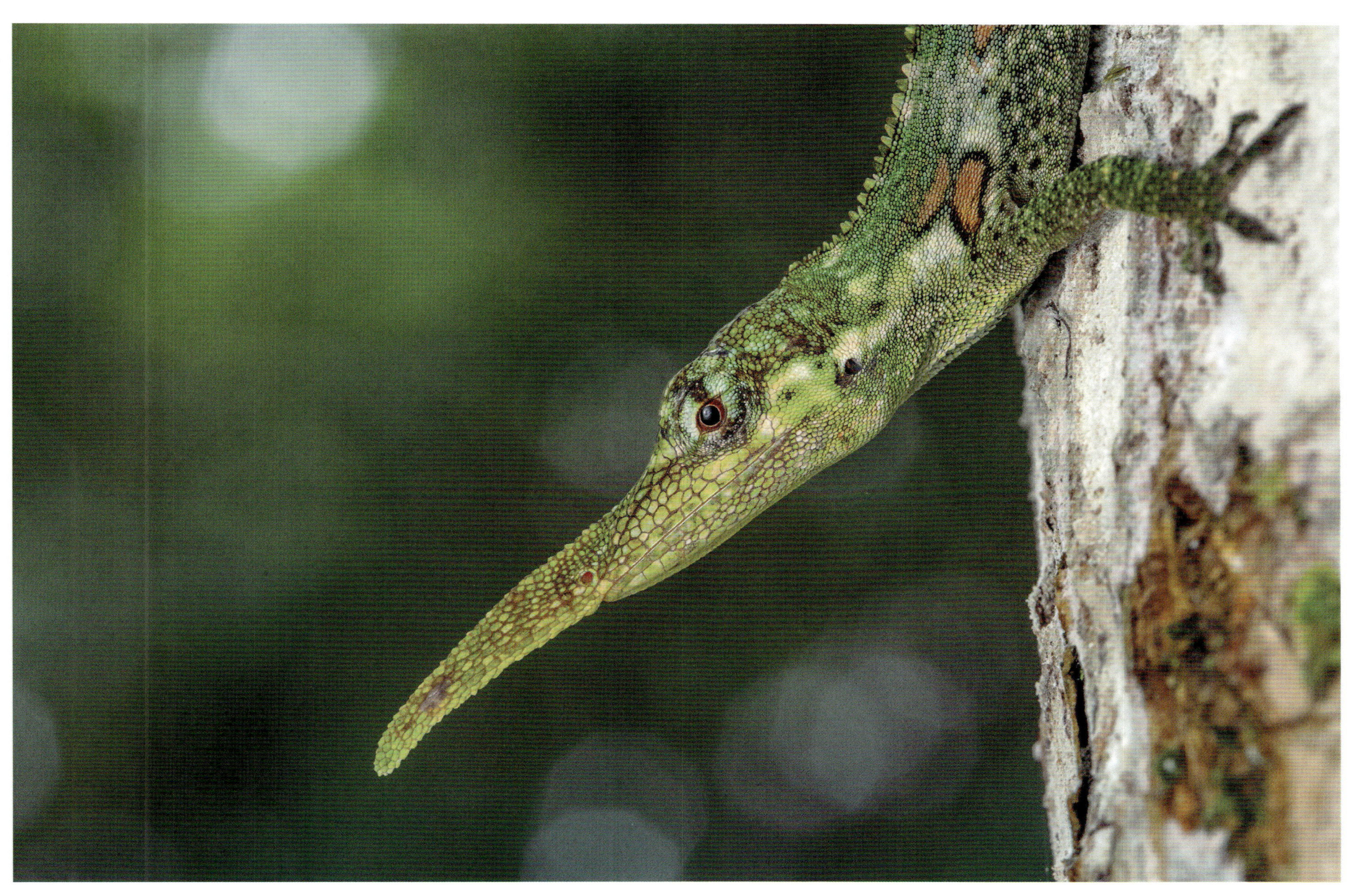

Jaime Culebras
Pinocchio Lizard
STATUS: ENDANGERED
Chocó Andino de Pichincha
Biosphere Reserve, Ecuador

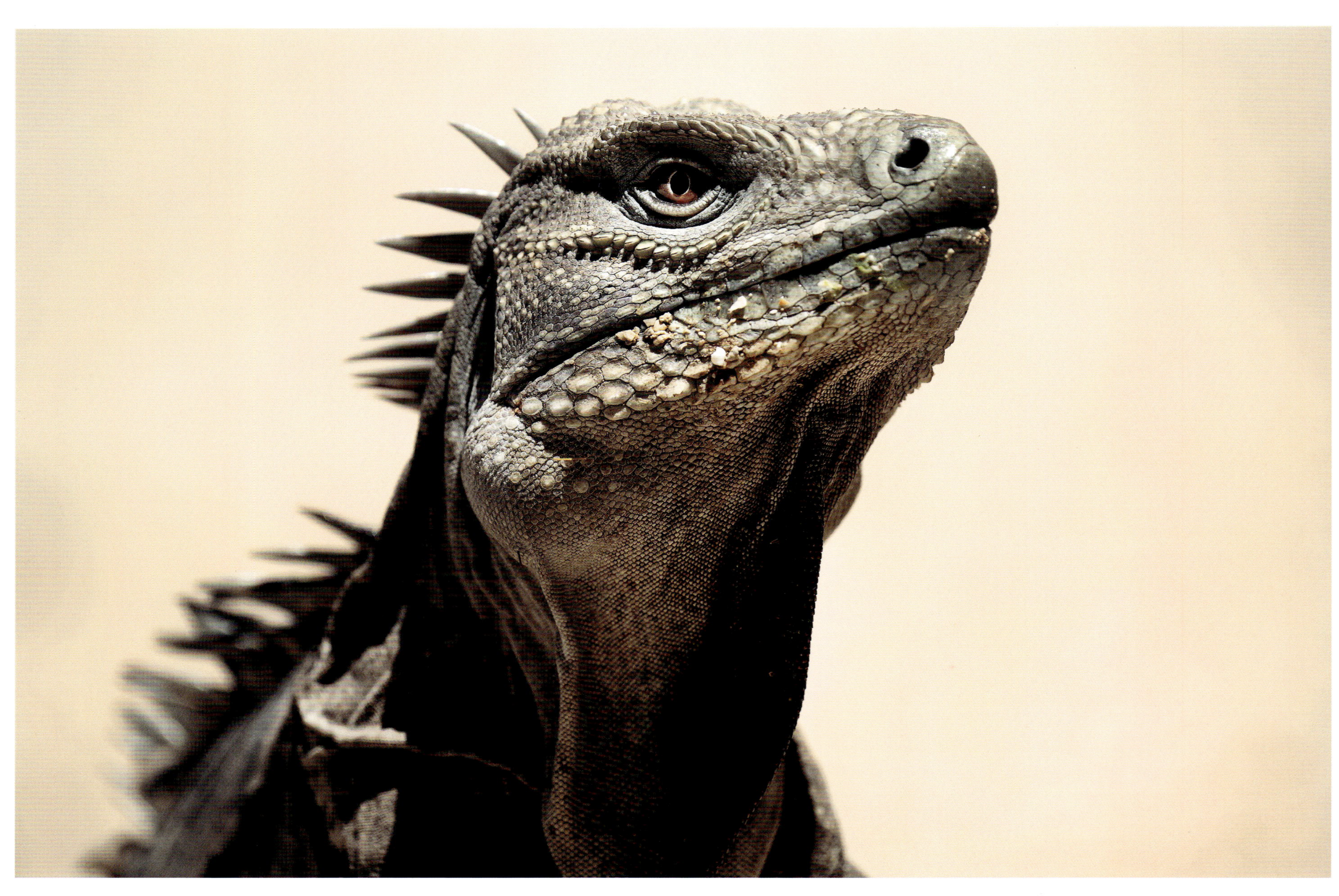

Tamara Blazquez Haik
Ricord's Rock Iguana
STATUS: ENDANGERED
Enriquillo Lake National Park,
Dominican Republic

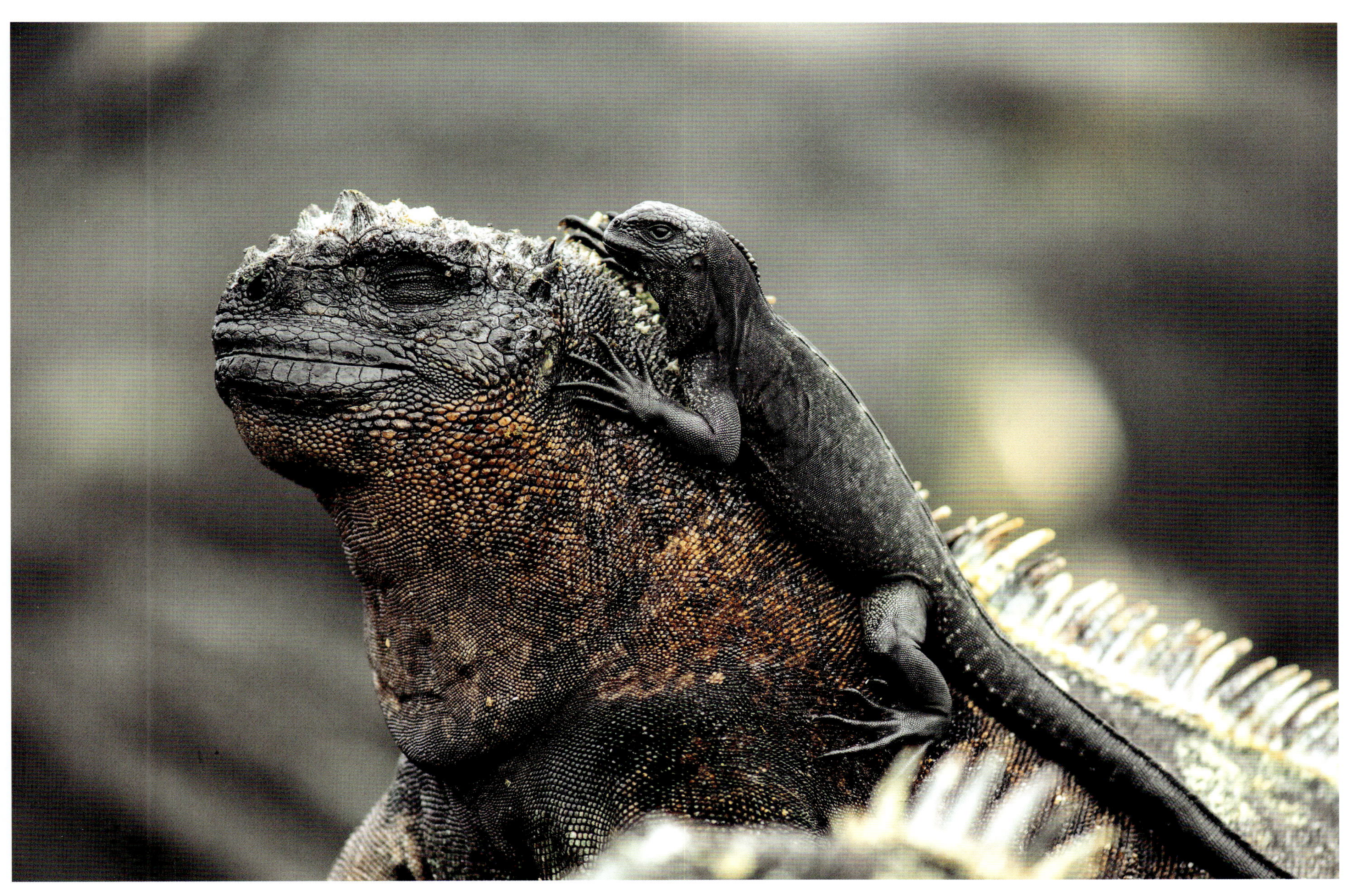

Sandesh Kadur
Marine Iguanas
STATUS: VULNERABLE
Galápagos National Park, Ecuador

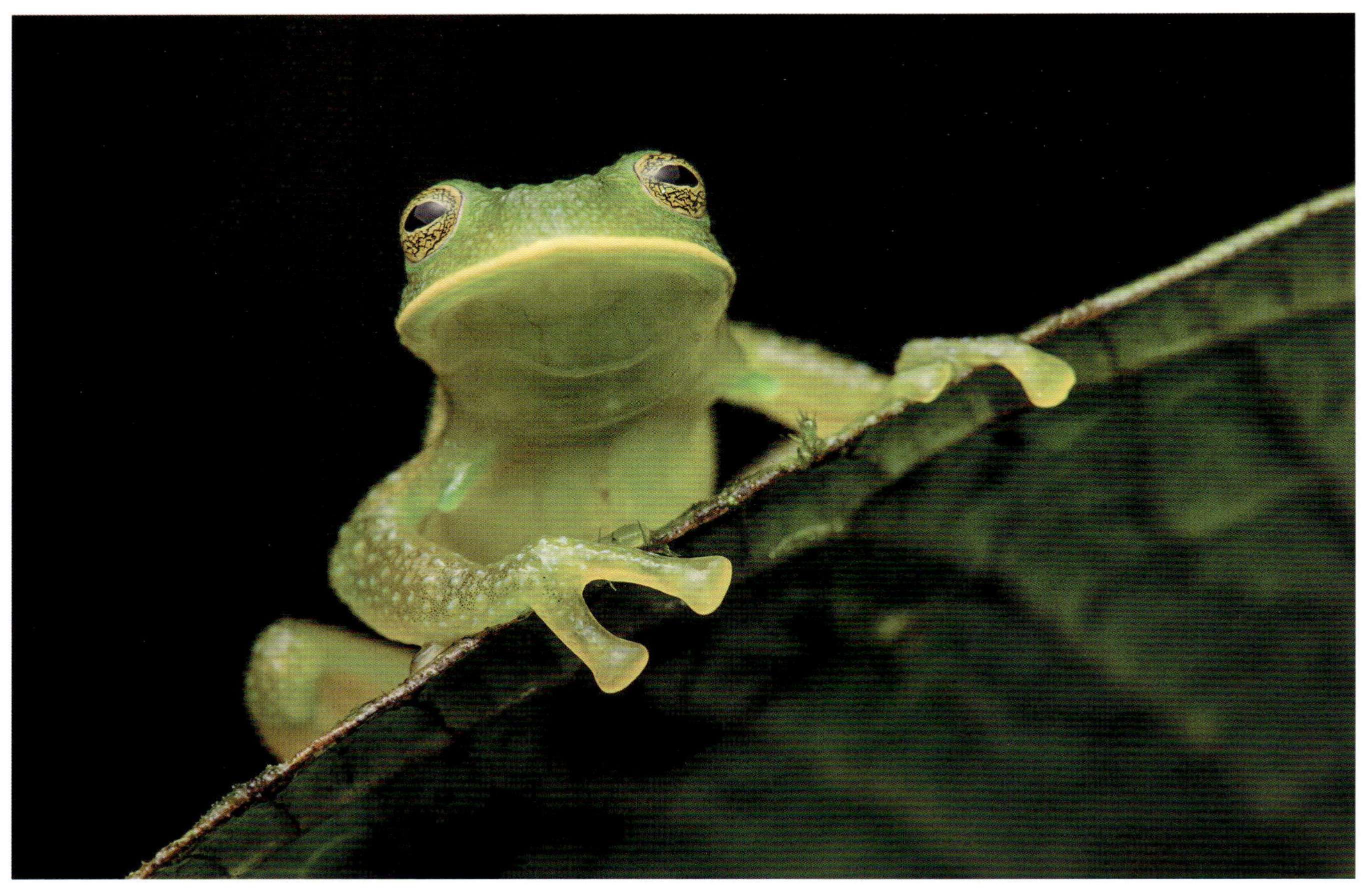

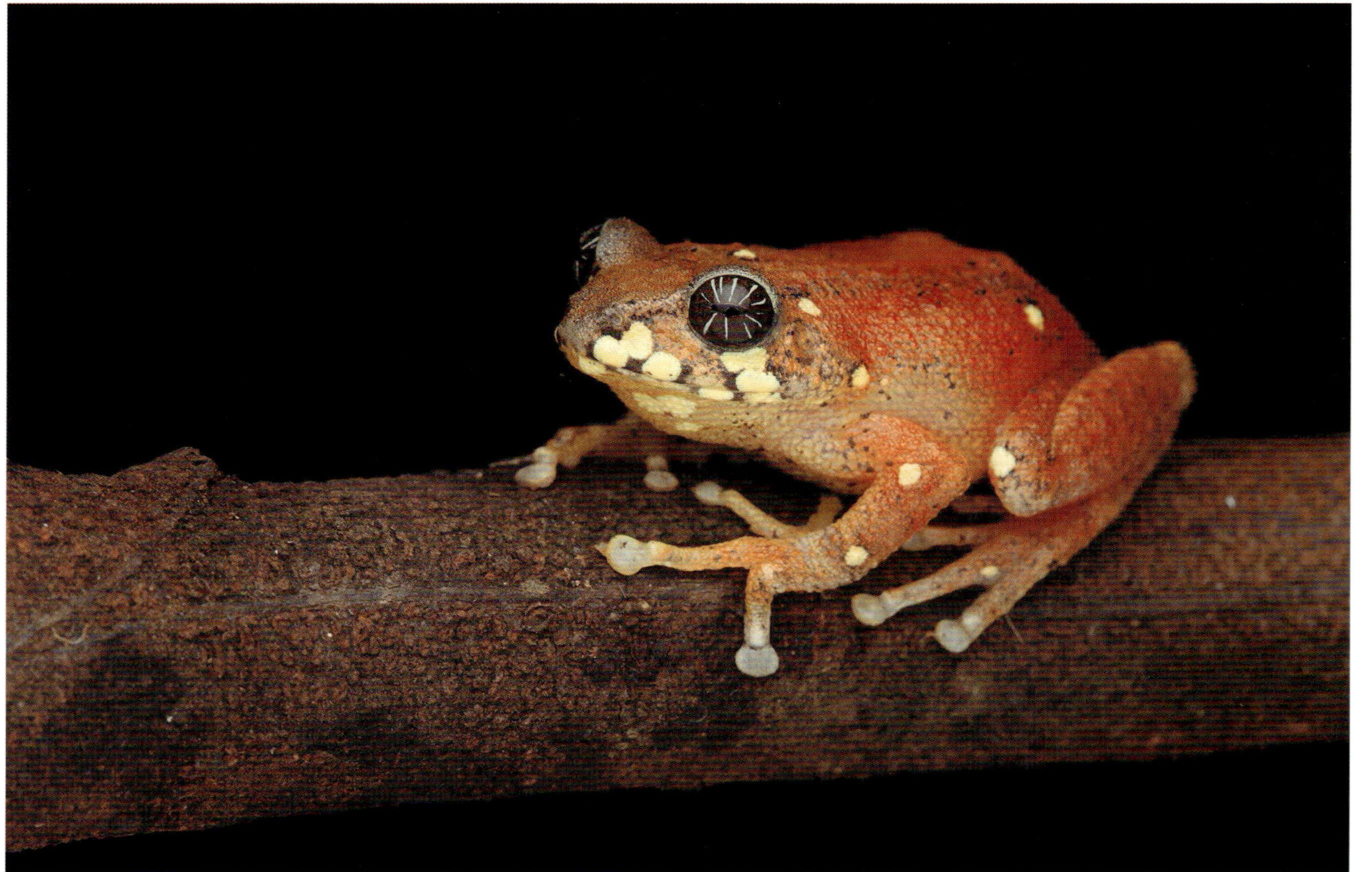

Anton Sorokin
Pichincha Giant Glass Frog
STATUS: VULNERABLE
Bellavista Cloud Forest
Reserve, Ecuador

Santhosh Krishnan
Star-eyed Bush Frog
STATUS: ENDANGERED
Nilgiri Biosphere Reserve,
India

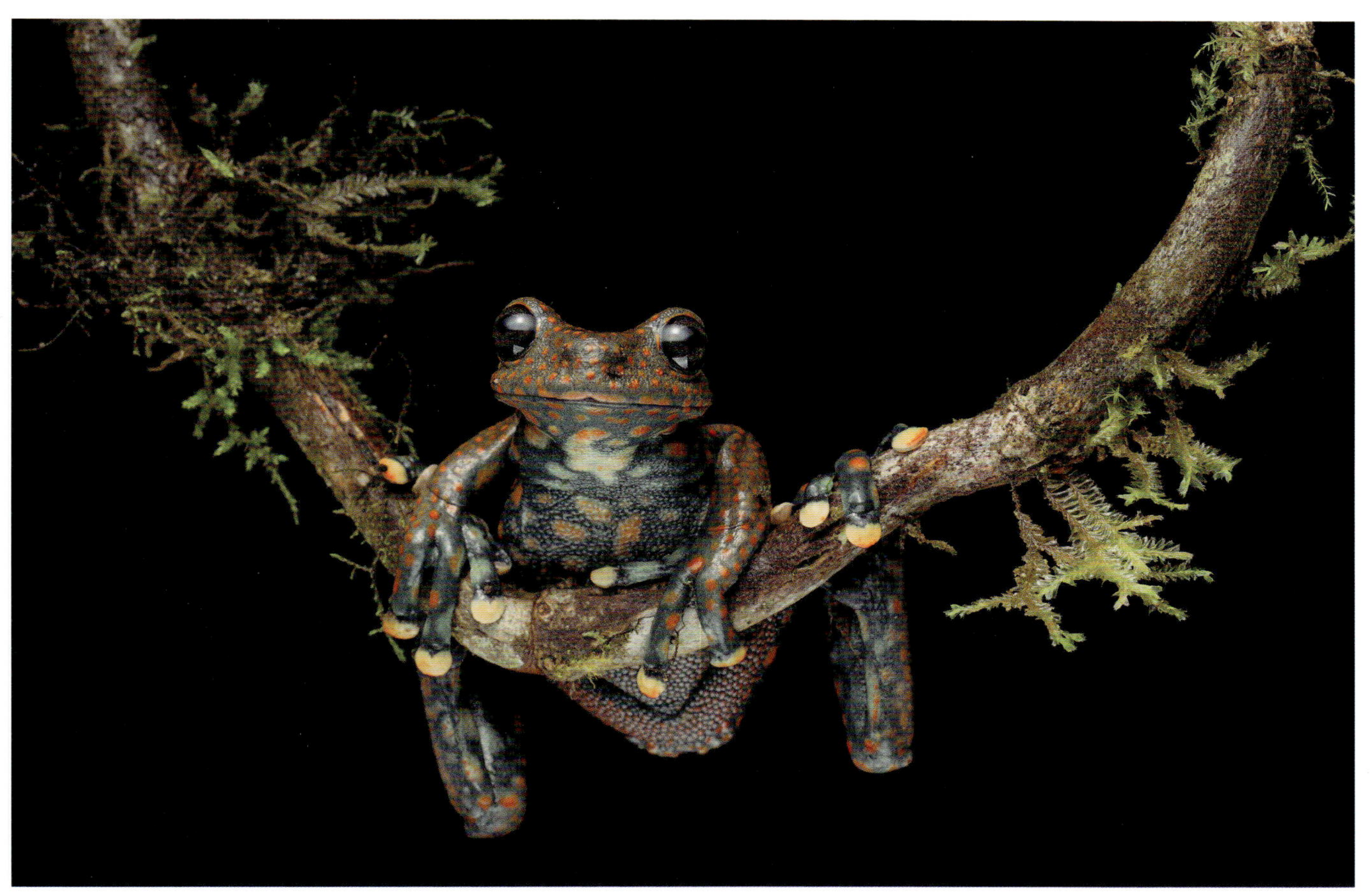

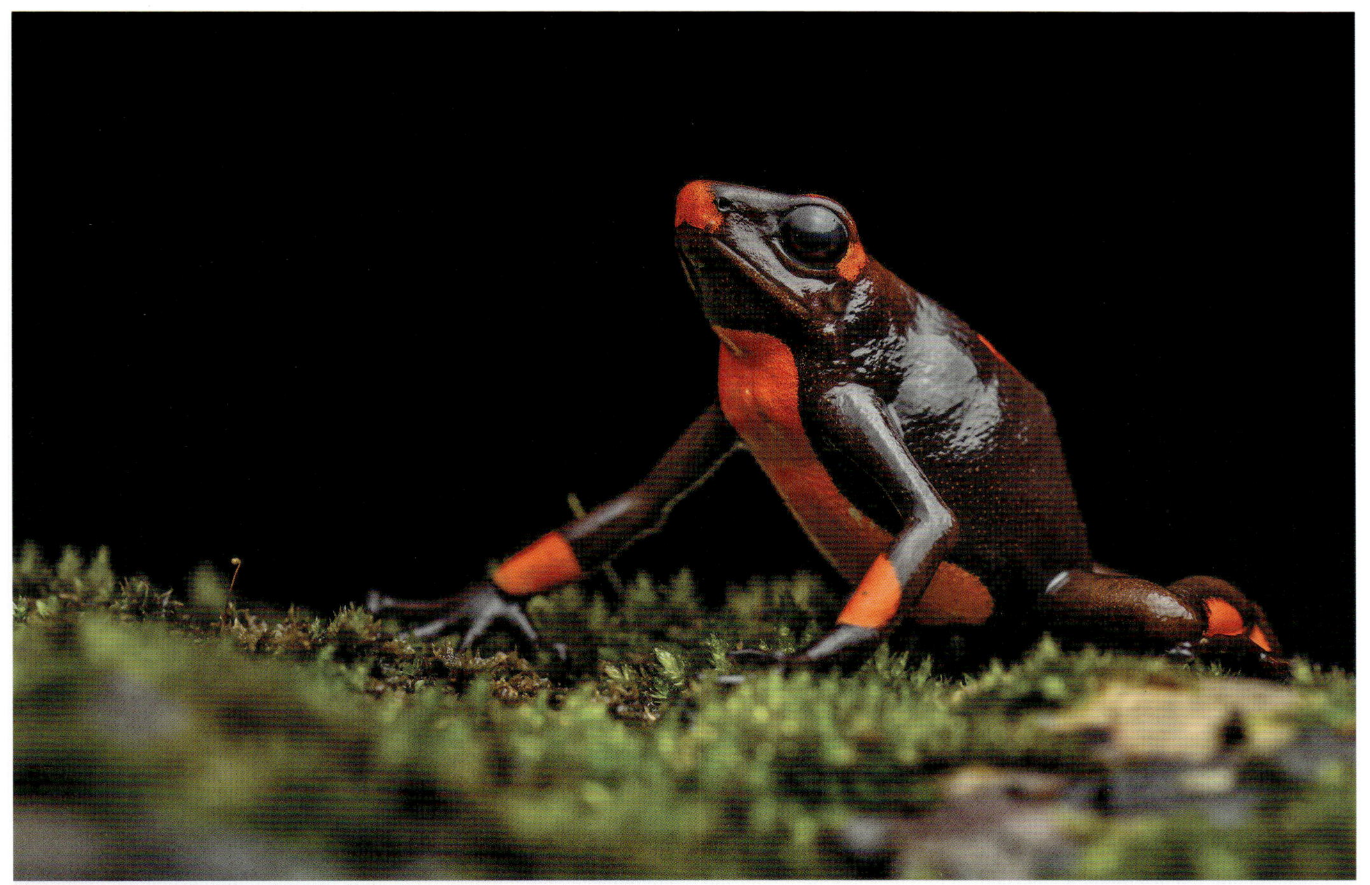

Lucas Bustamante
Spotted Torrent Frog
STATUS: CRITICALLY
ENDANGERED
Santa Barbara Park, Ecuador

Nick Kanakis
Harlequin Poison Frog
STATUS: CRITICALLY
ENDANGERED
Santa Cecilia, Colombia

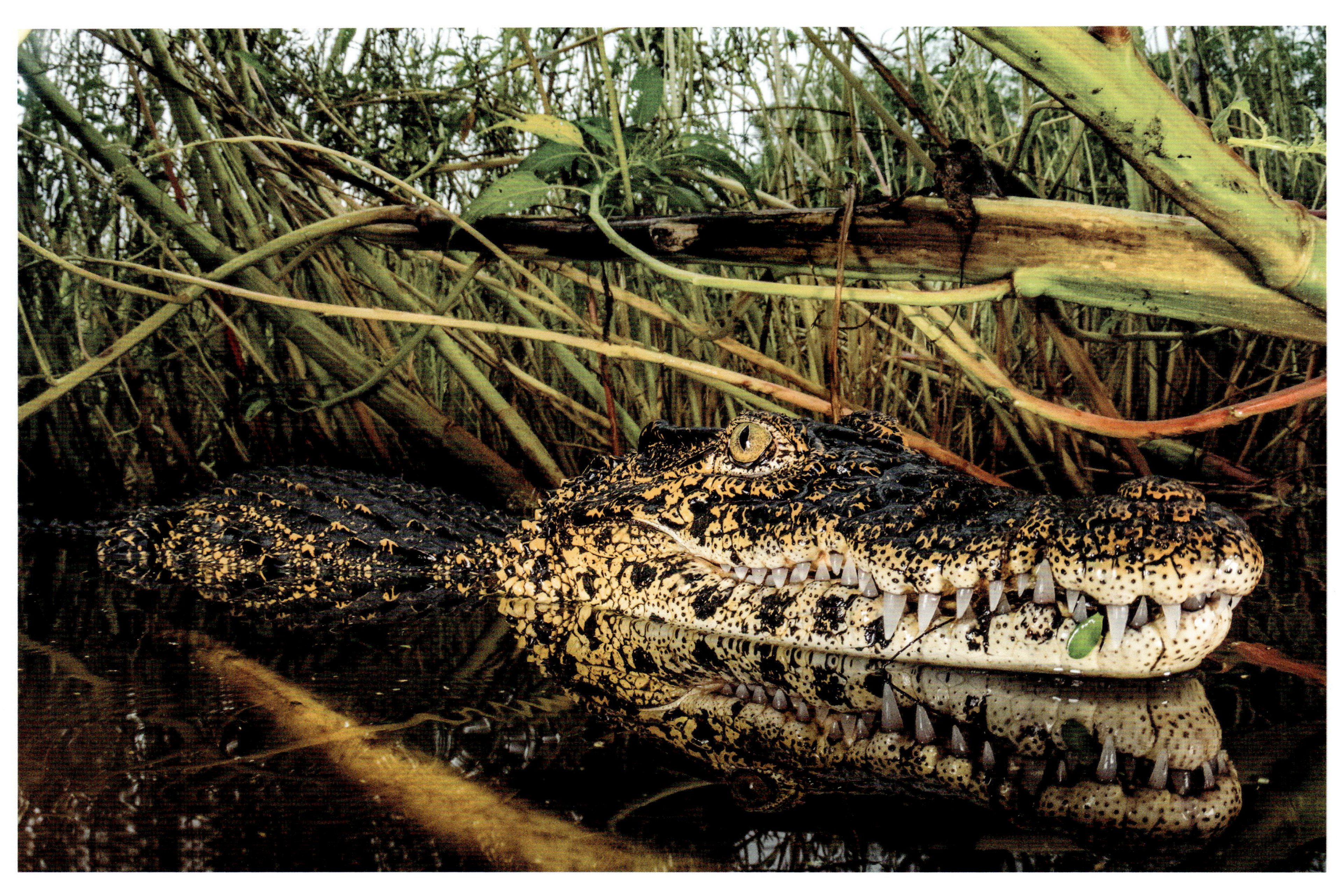

Shane Gross
Cuban Crocodile
STATUS: CRITICALLY ENDANGERED
Ciénaga de Zapata National Park, Cuba

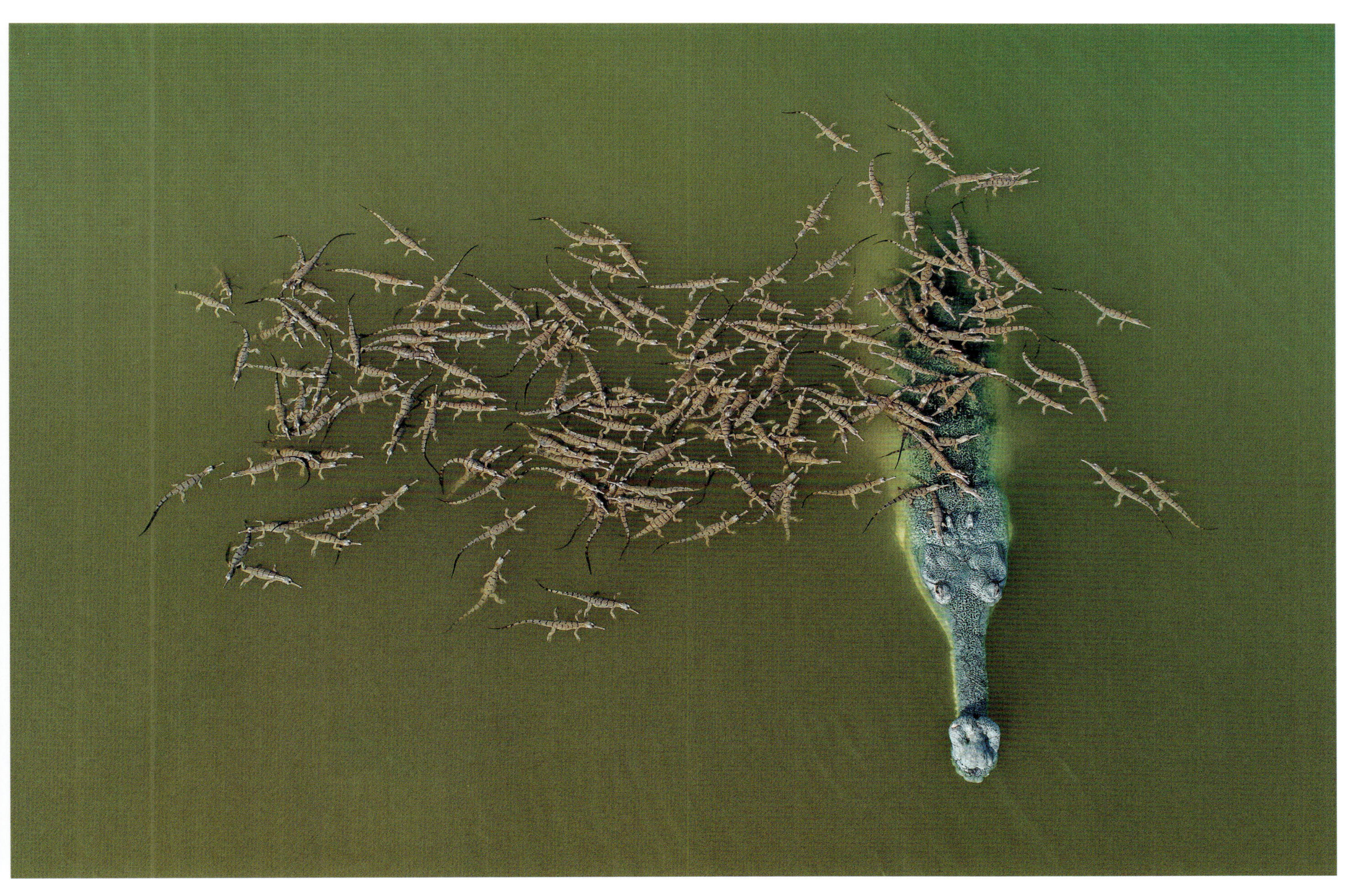

Dhritiman Mukherjee
Gharial
STATUS: CRITICALLY ENDANGERED
National Chambal Sanctuary, India

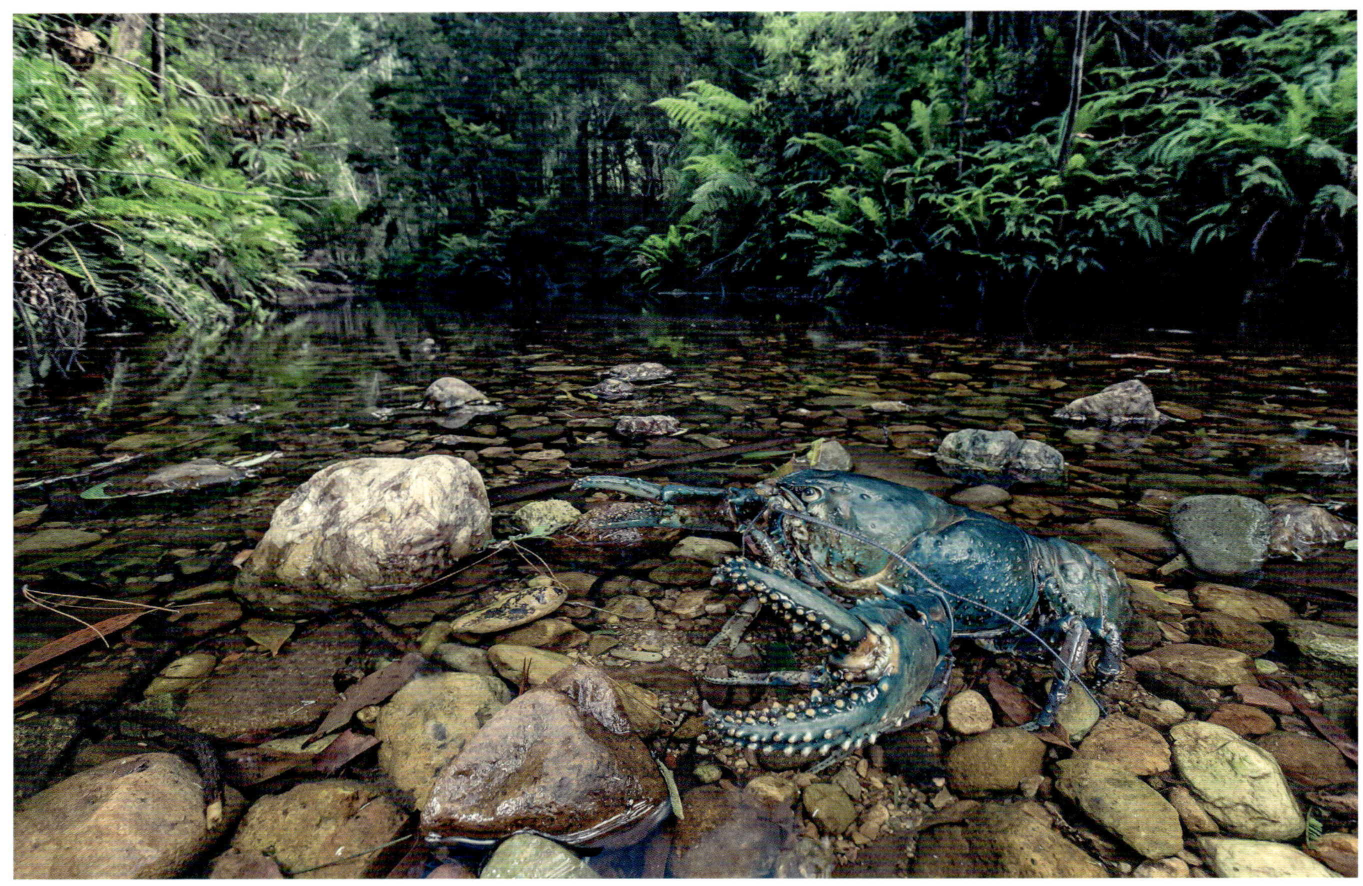

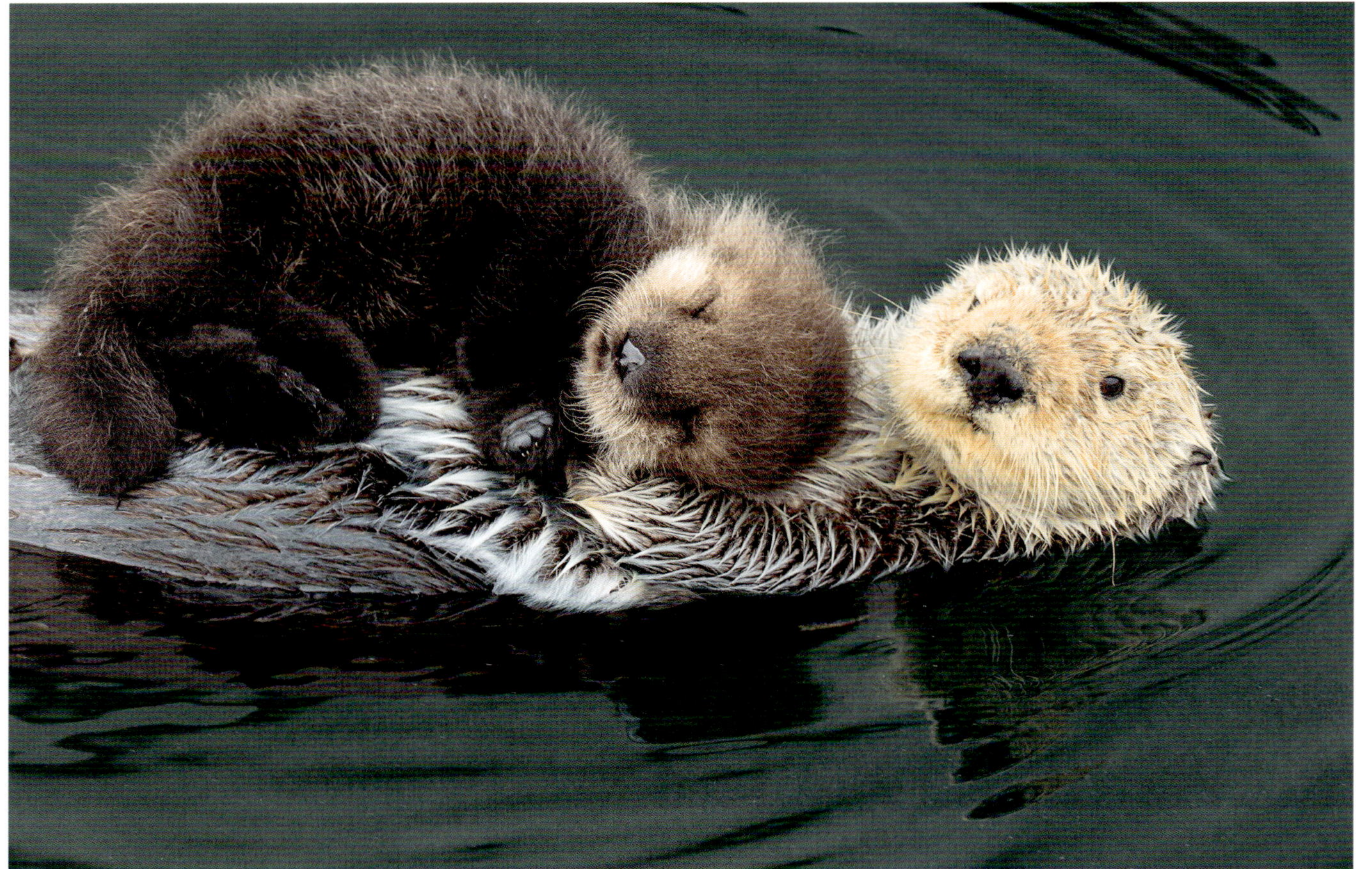

Ryan Francis
Tasmanian Giant
Freshwater Crayfish
STATUS: ENDANGERED
Tasmania, Australia

Suzi Eszterhas
Sea Otters
STATUS: ENDANGERED
Monterey Bay, California,
United States

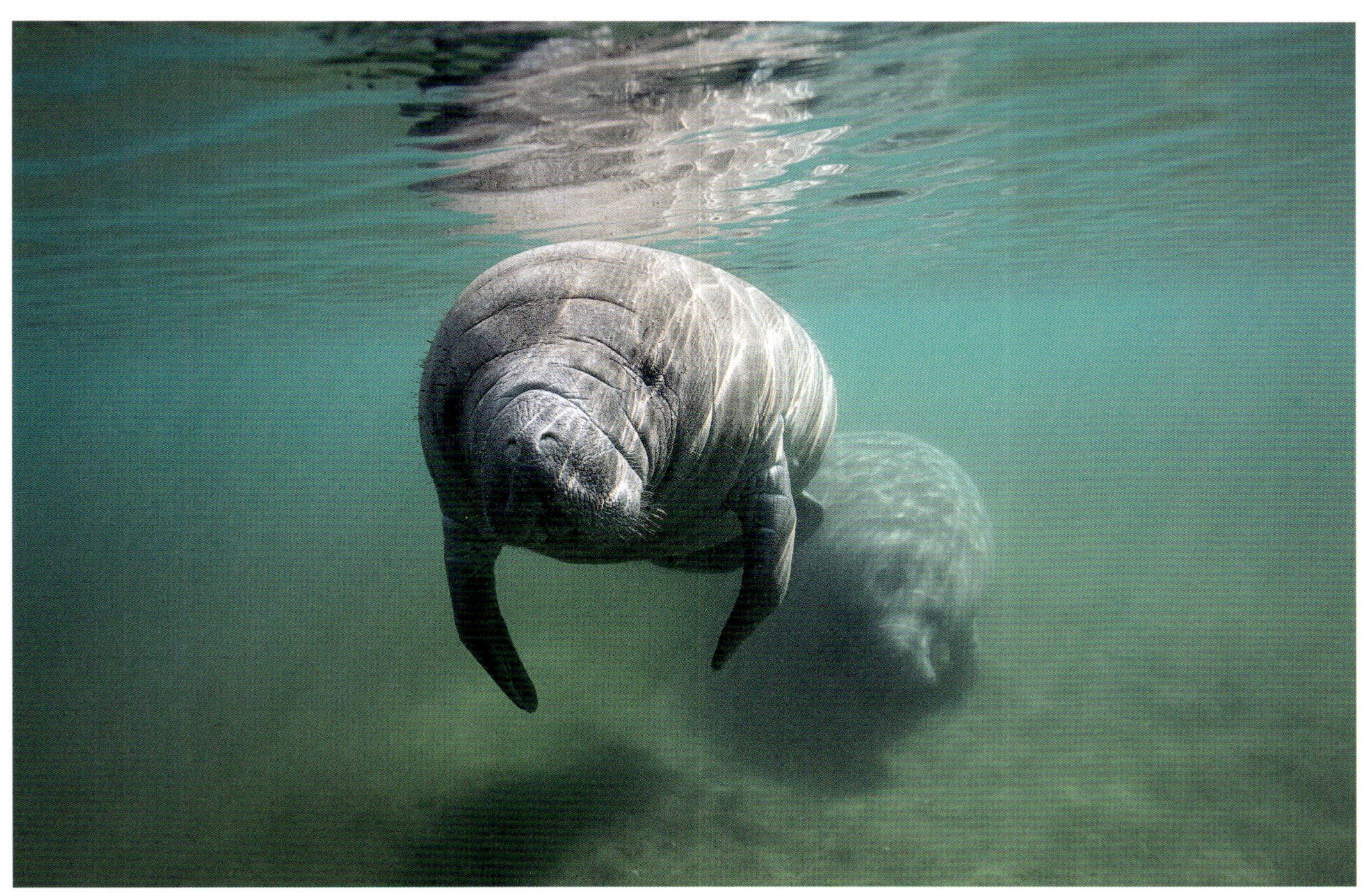

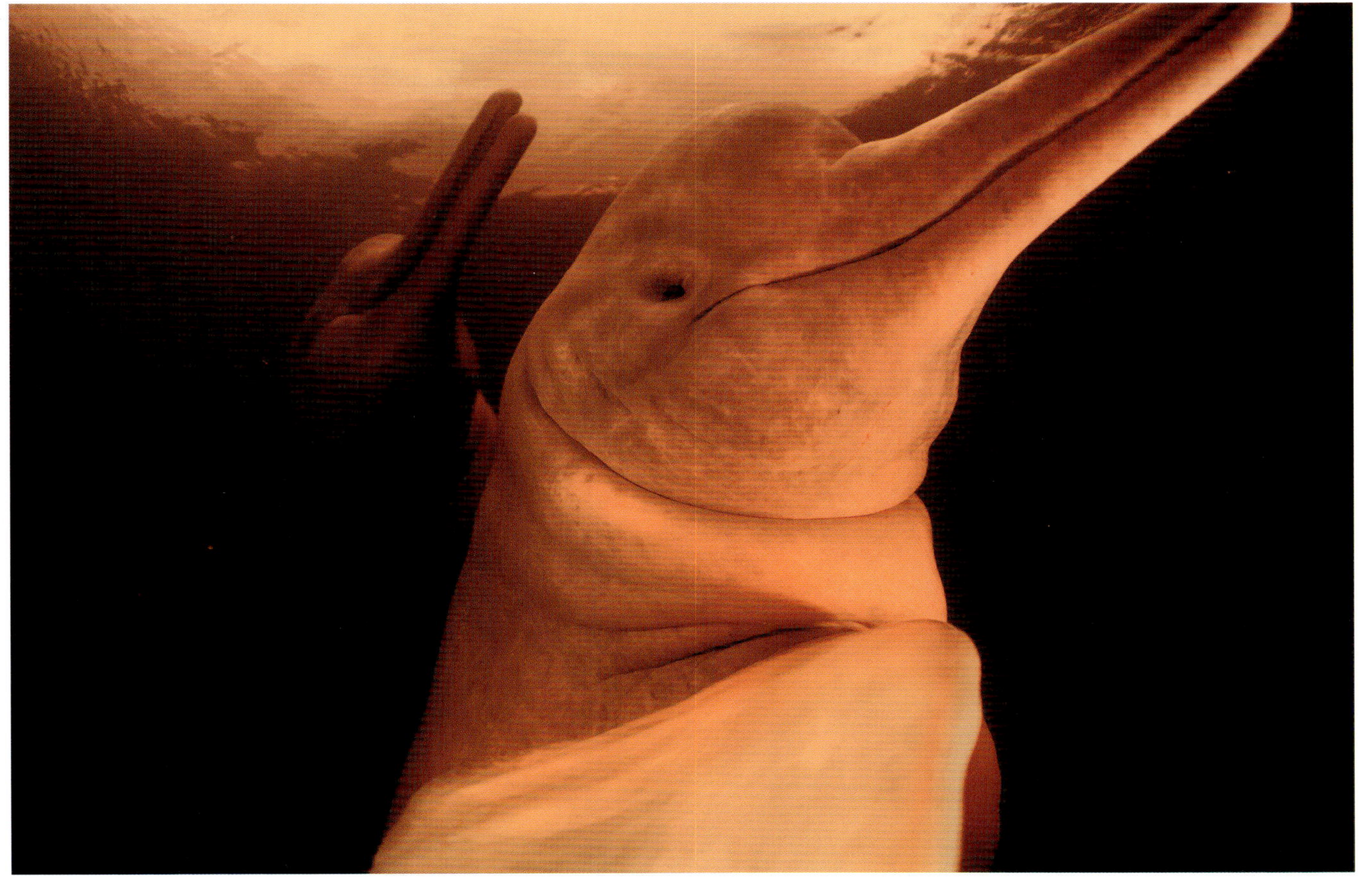

Gabby Salazar
Florida Manatee
STATUS: THREATENED
(UNDER U.S.
ENDANGERED SPECIES ACT;
VULNERABLE UNDER IUCN)
Florida, United States

Luciano Candisani
Pink River Dolphins
STATUS: ENDANGERED
Rio Negro, Brazil

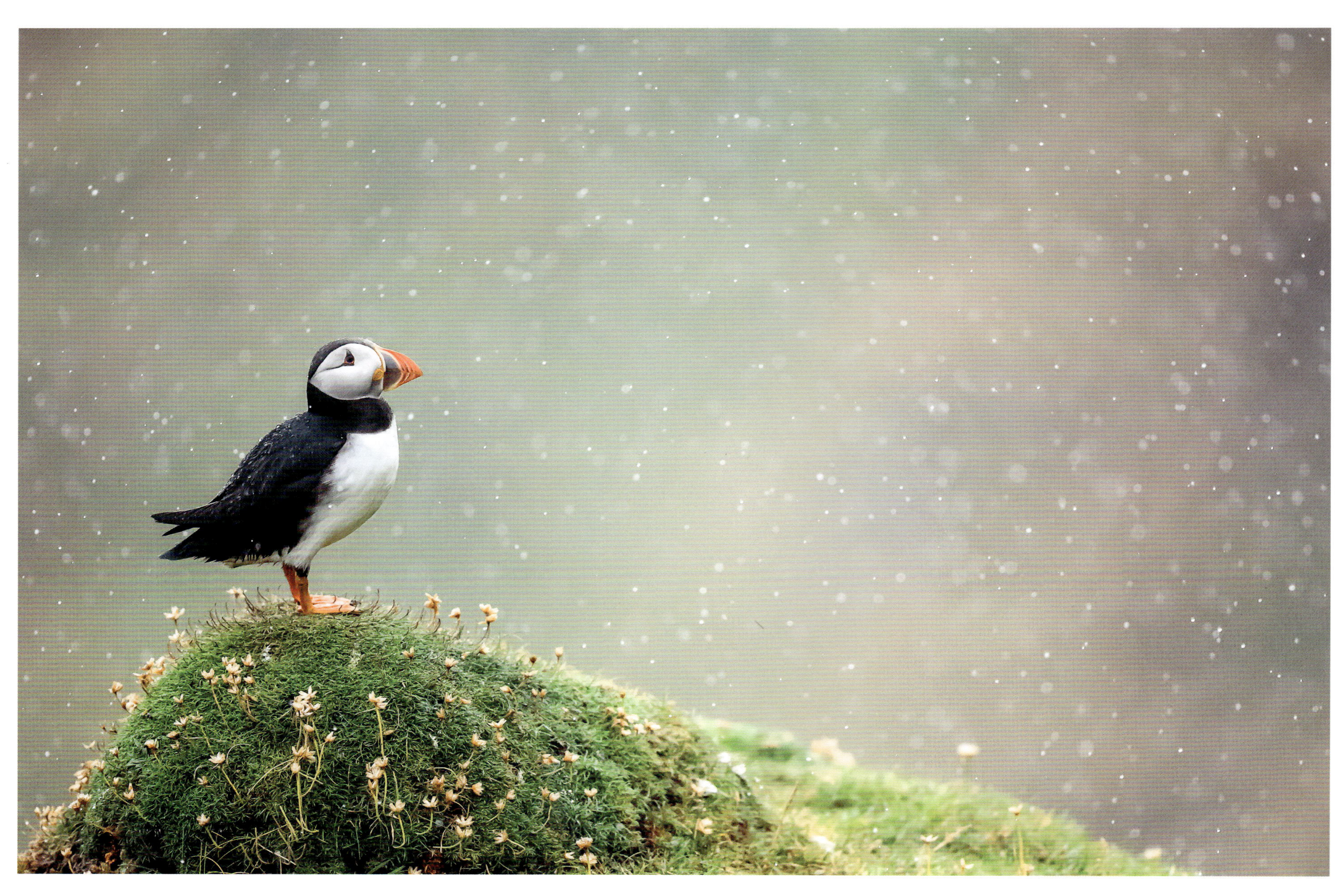

Kevin Morgans
Atlantic Puffin
STATUS: VULNERABLE
Hermaness National Nature Reserve,
Scotland

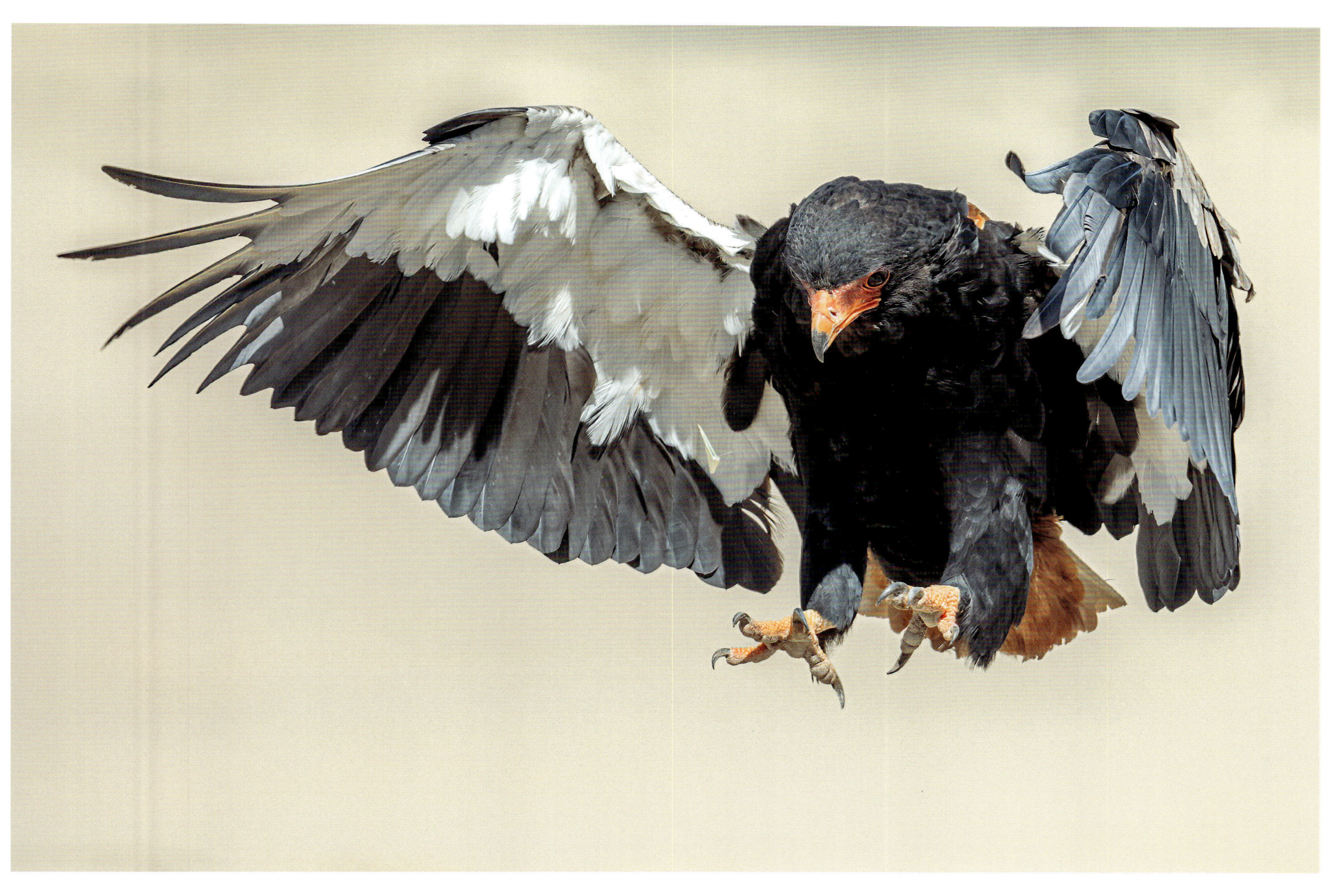

Willie van Schalkwyk
Bateleur
STATUS: ENDANGERED
Kgalagadi Transfrontier Park, South Africa

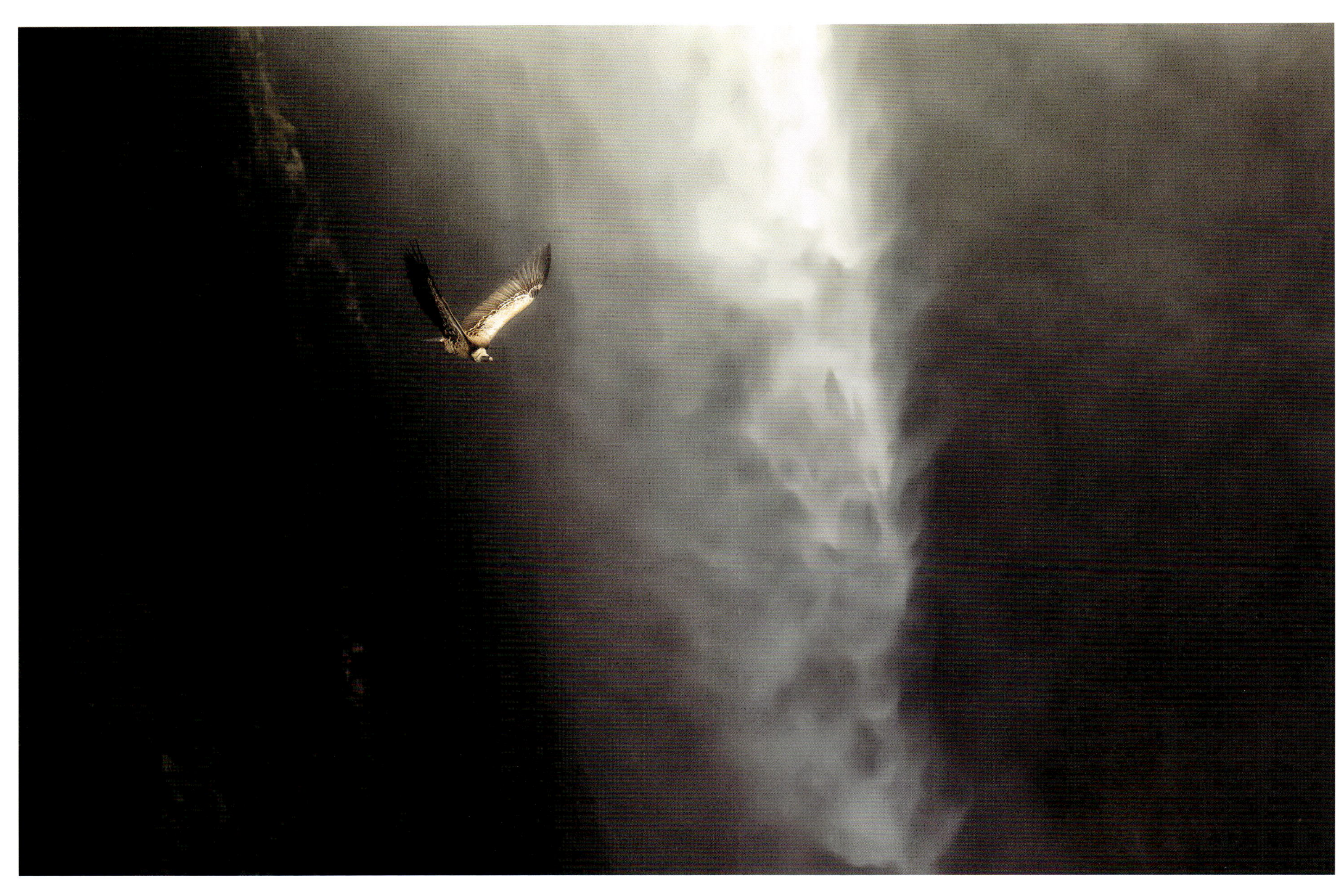

Marco Gaiotti
Rüppell's Vulture
STATUS: CRITICALLY ENDANGERED
Simien Mountains National Park, Ethiopia

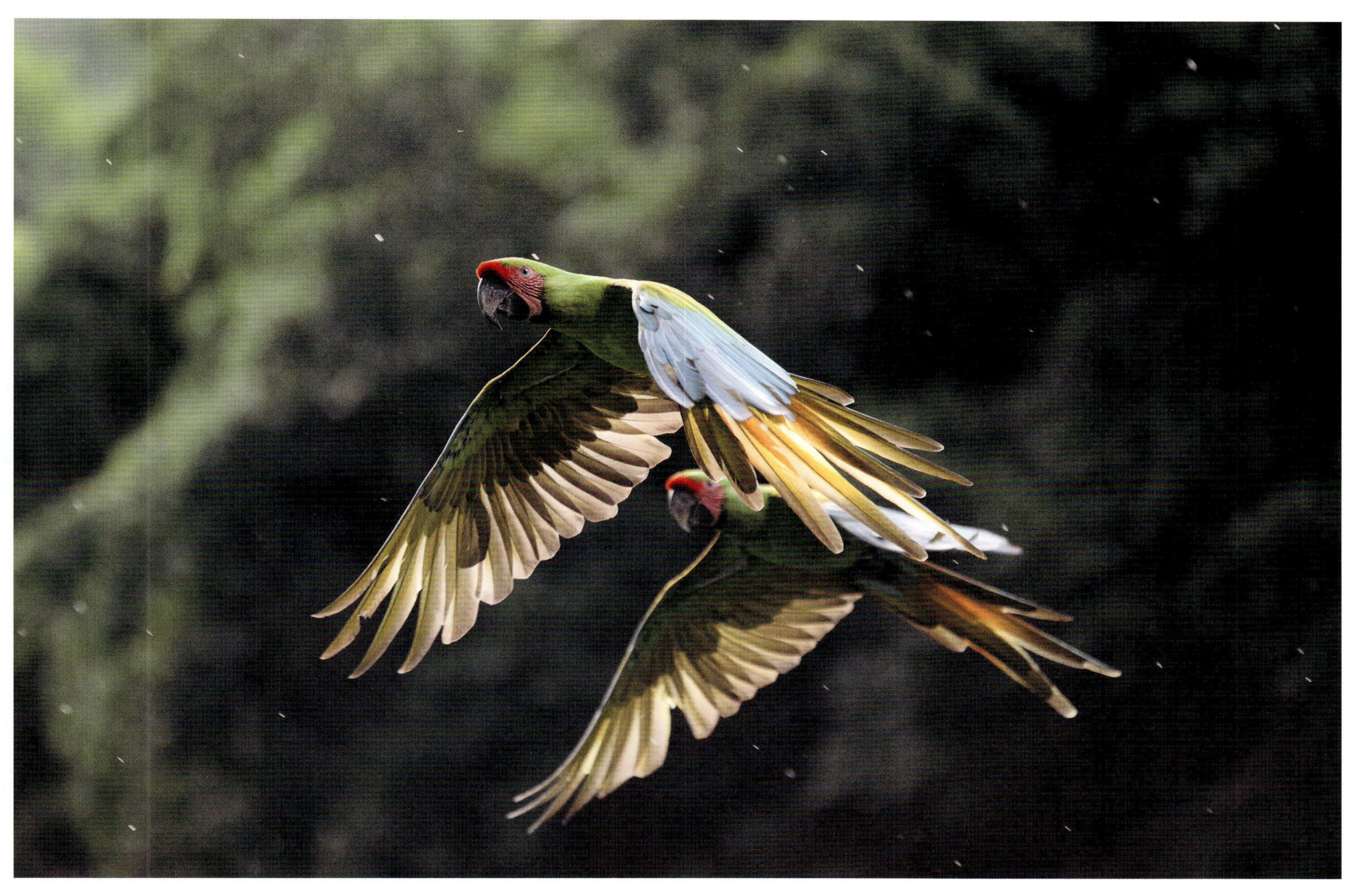

Molly Ferrill
Great Green Macaws
STATUS: CRITICALLY ENDANGERED
Limón, Costa Rica

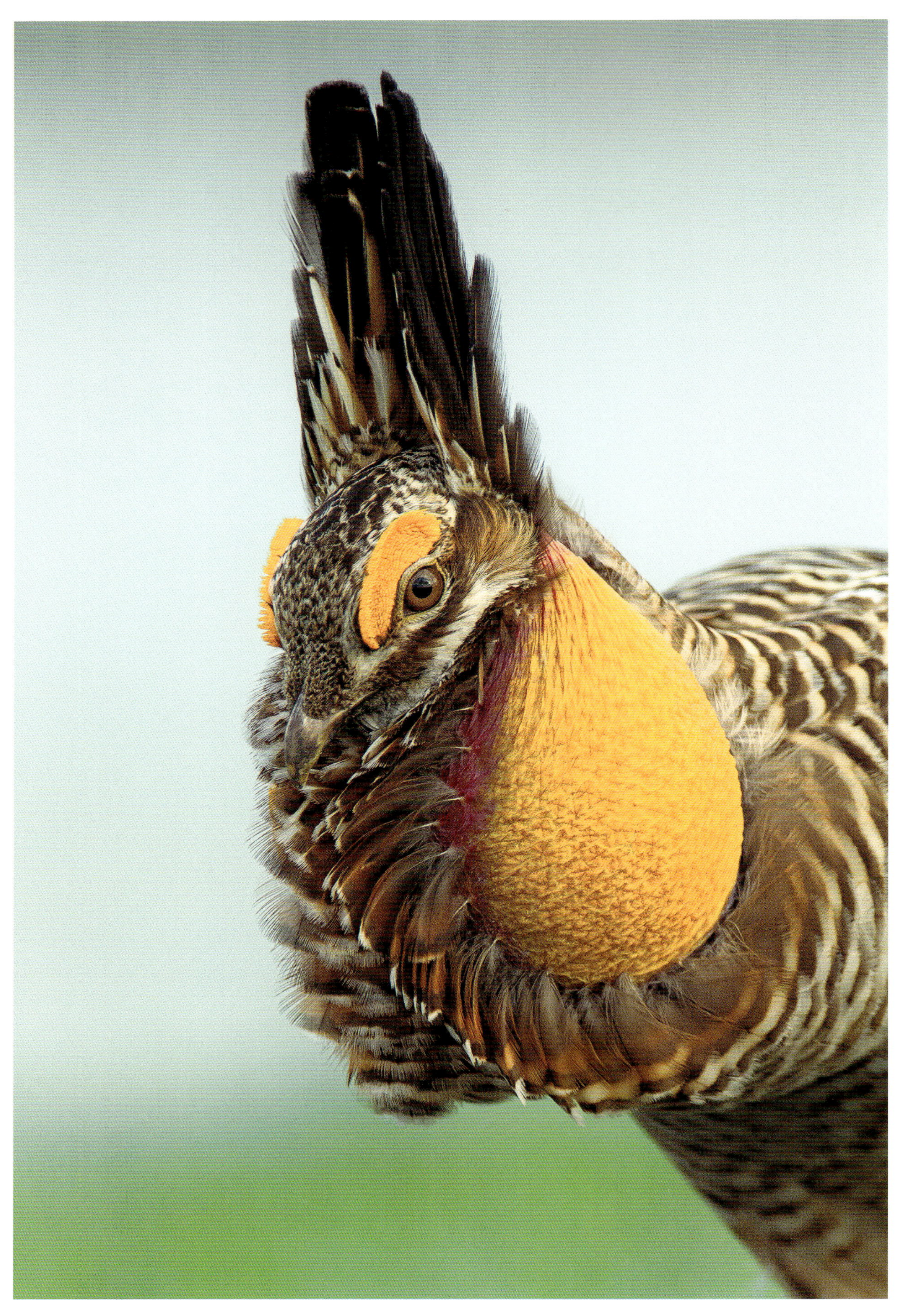

Noppadol Paothong
Attwater's Prairie Chicken
STATUS: ENDANGERED
(UNDER U.S. ENDANGERED SPECIES ACT)
Attwater Priaire National Wildlife Refuge,
Texas, United States

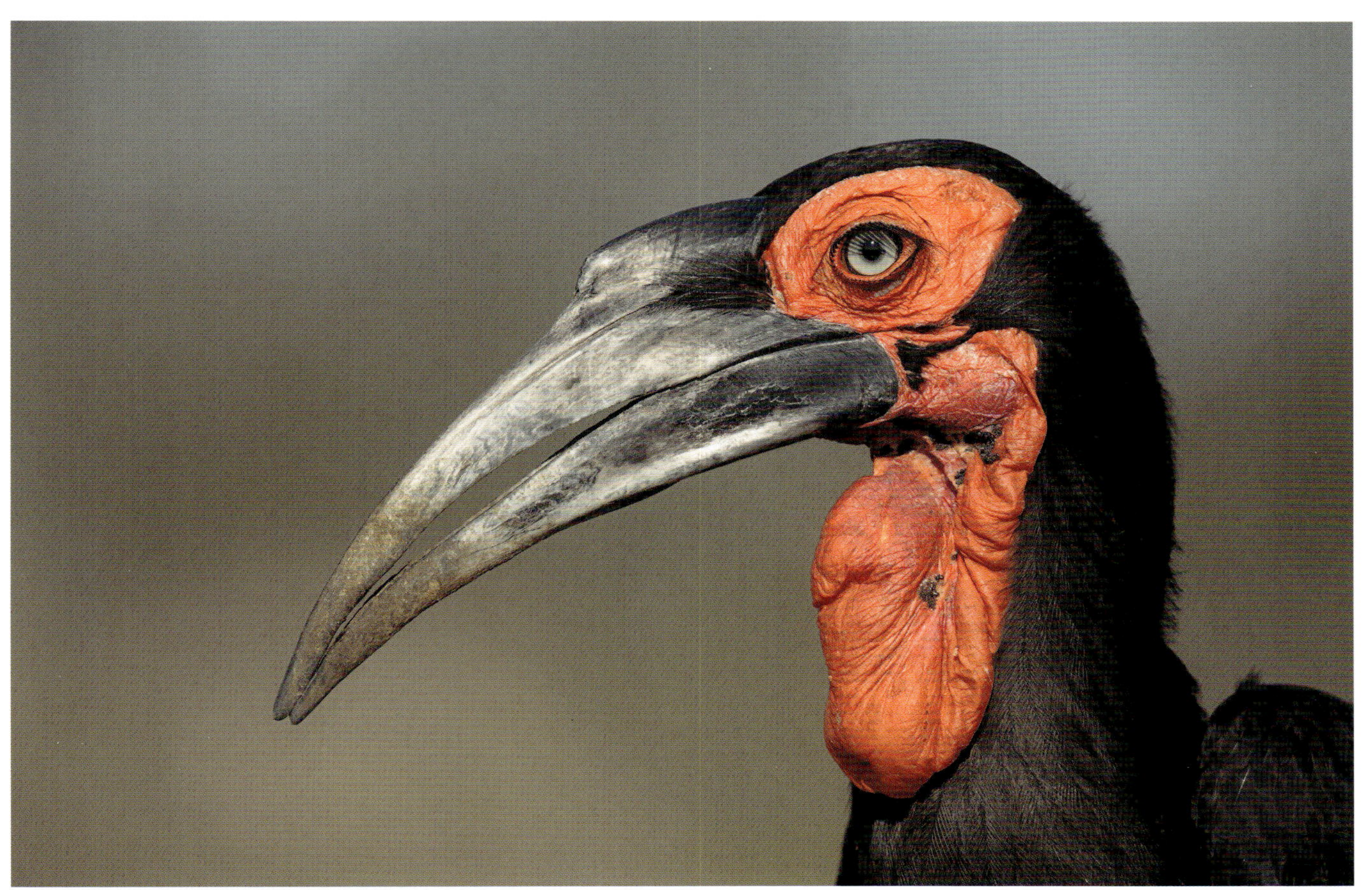

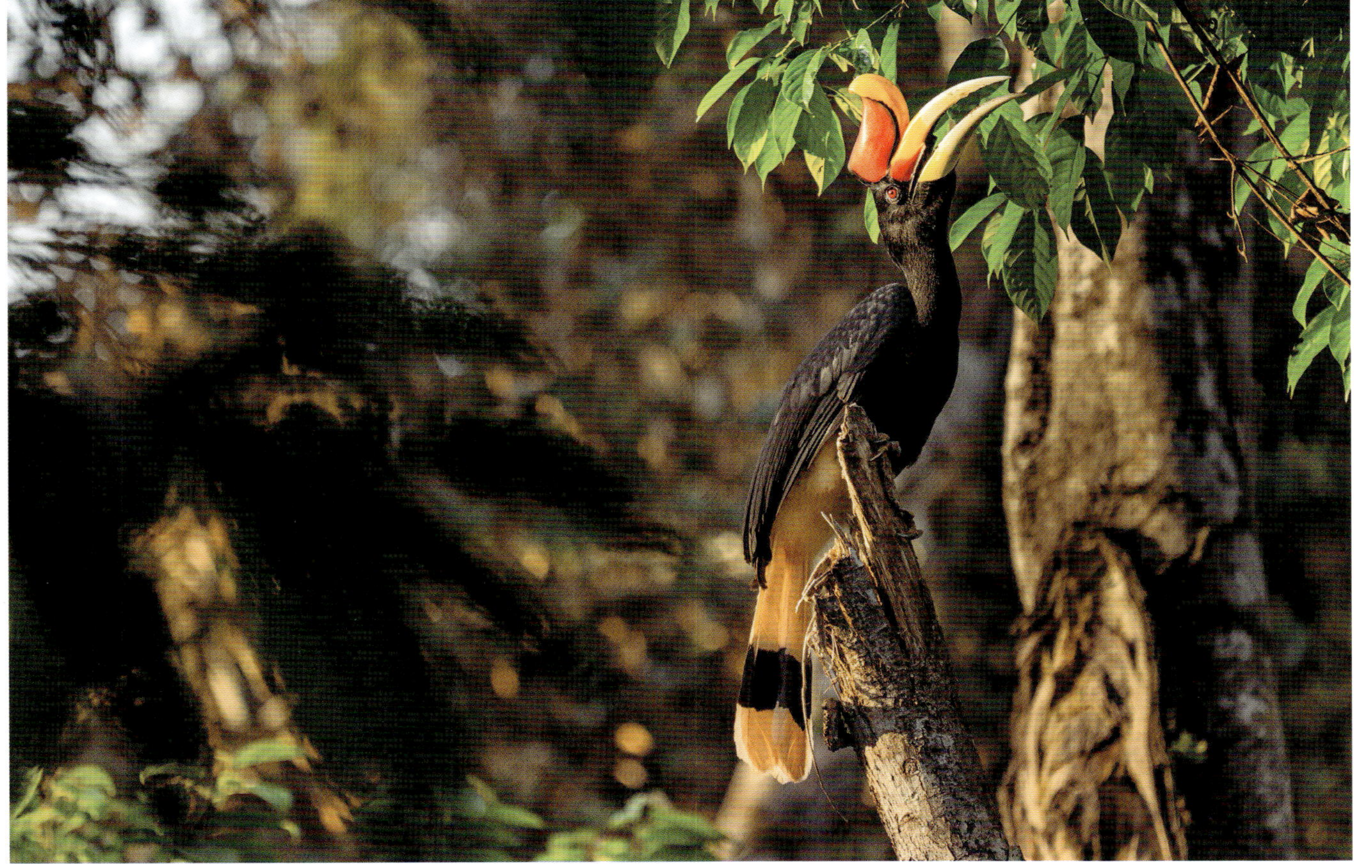

Gerda van Schalkwyk
Southern Ground-Hornbill
STATUS: ENDANGERED
(IN SOUTH AFRICA;
VULNERABLE GLOBALLY)
Kruger National Park,
South Africa

Celina Chien
Rhinoceros Hornbill
STATUS: VULNERABLE
Deramakot Forest Reserve,
Malaysia

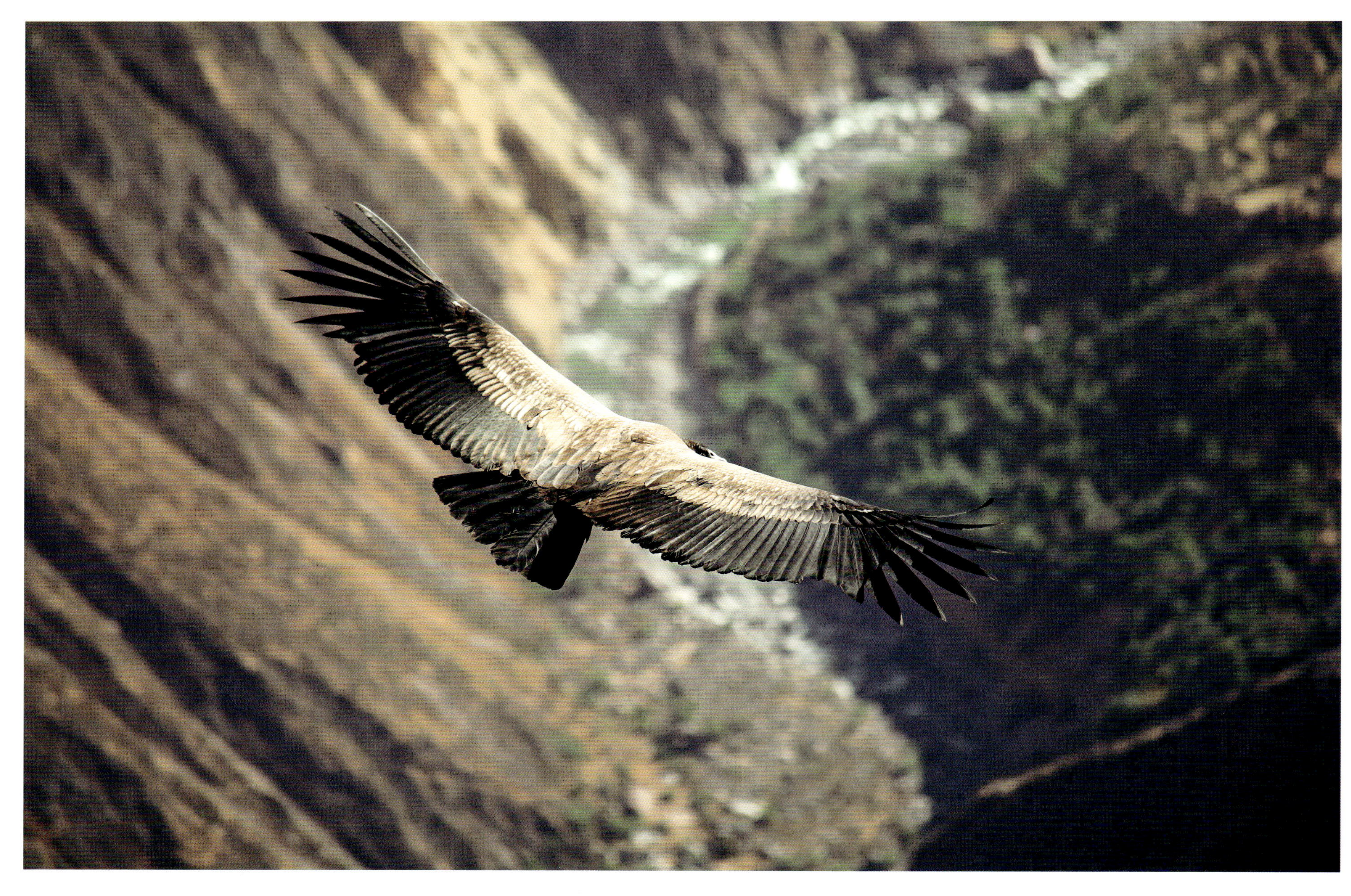

Graeme Green
Andean Condor
STATUS: VULNERABLE
Colca Canyon, Peru

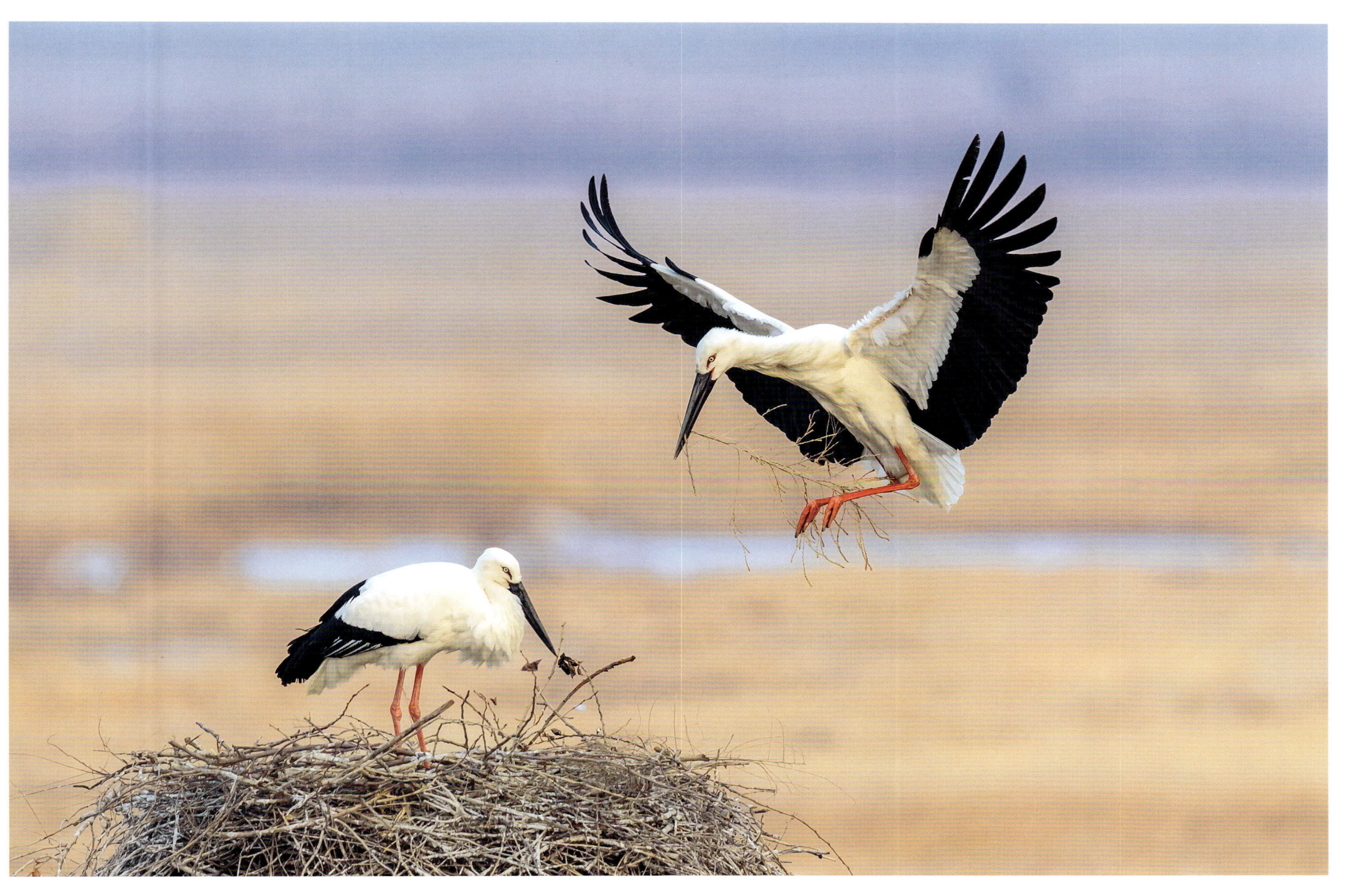

Xuedong Bai
Oriental Storks
STATUS: ENDANGERED
Heilongjiang, China

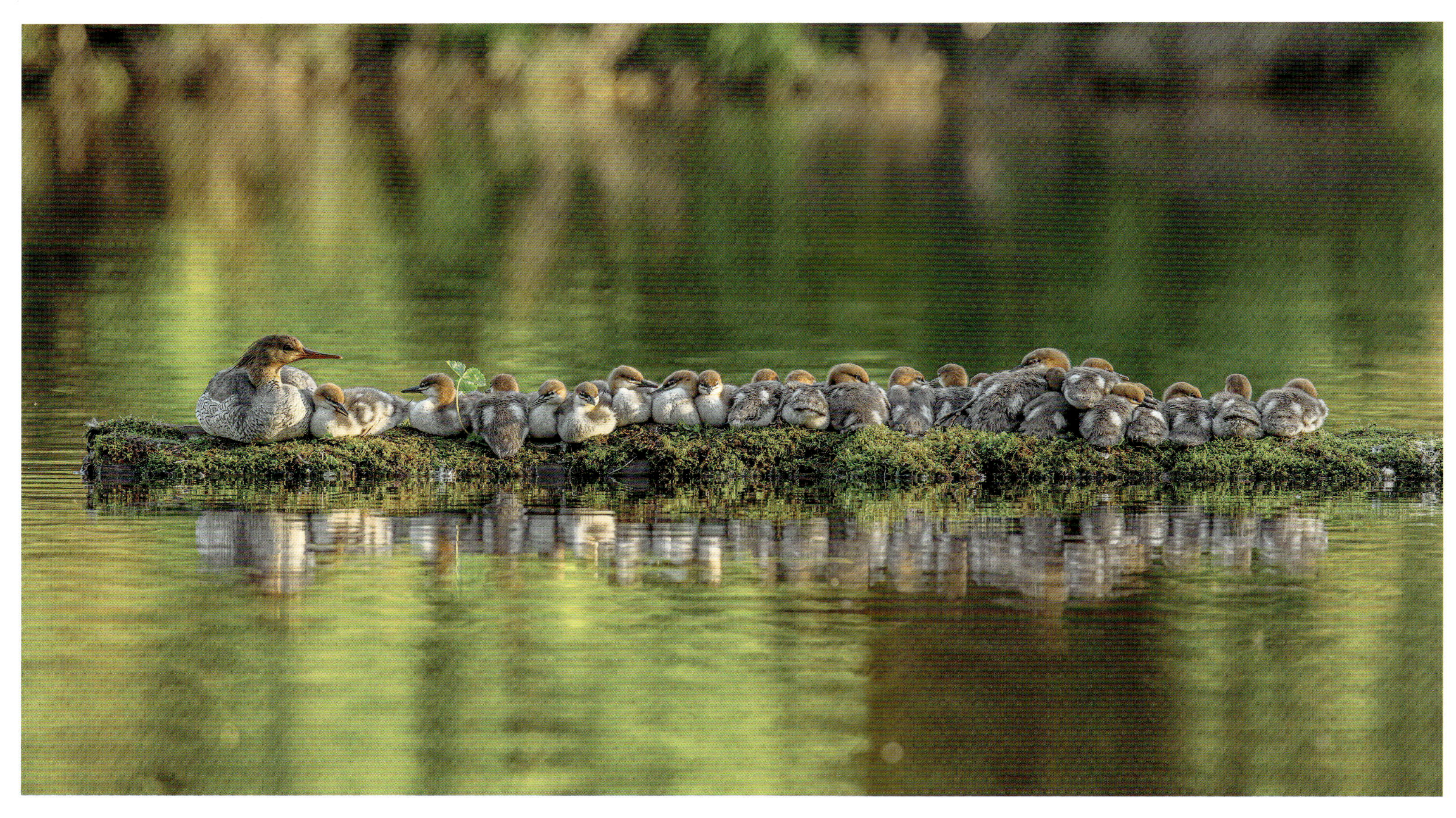

Qingshun Liu
Scaly-sided Mergansers
STATUS: ENDANGERED
Changbai Mountains, China

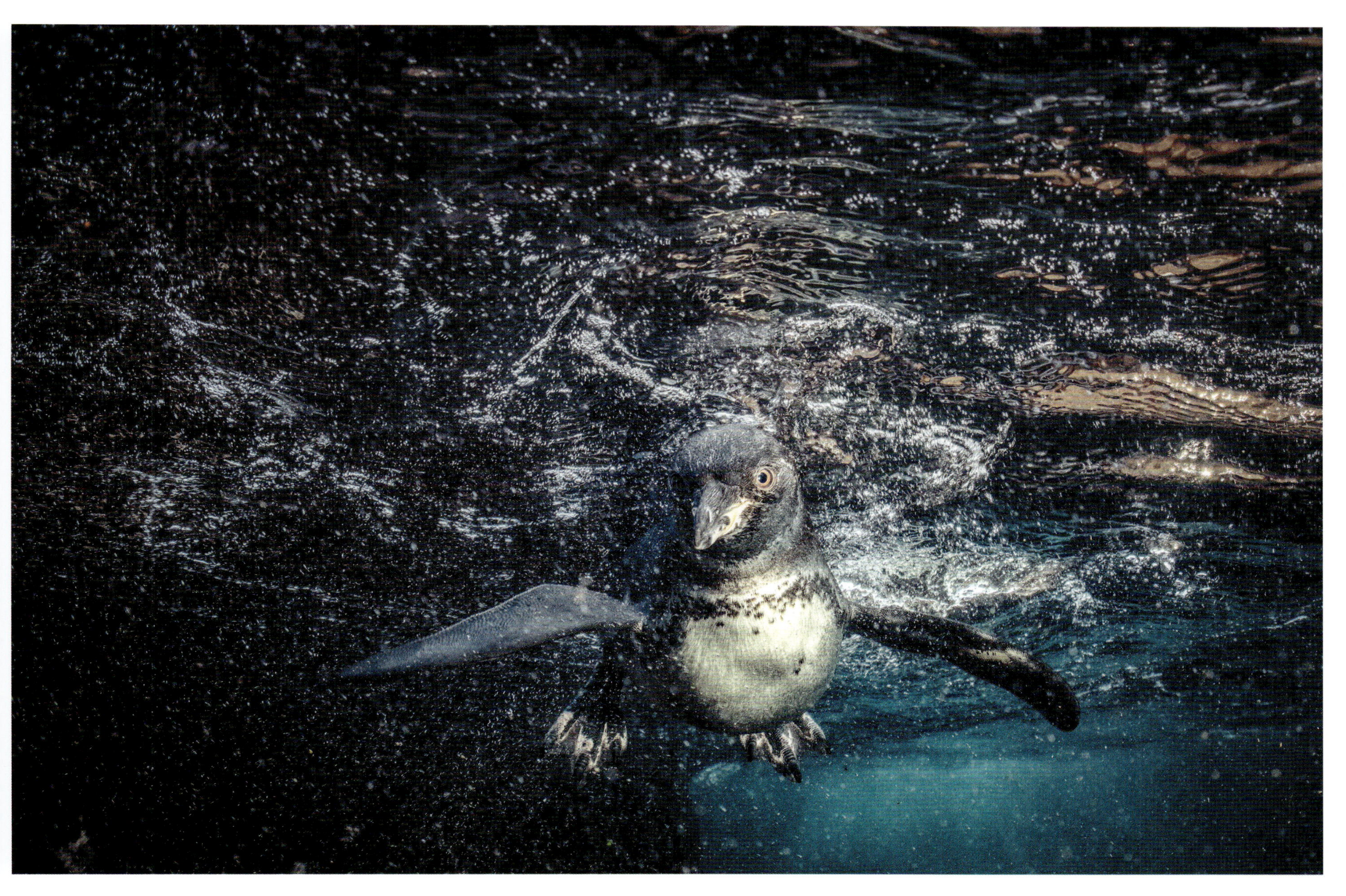

Cristina Mittermeier
Galápagos Penguin
STATUS: ENDANGERED
Galápagos National Park, Ecuador

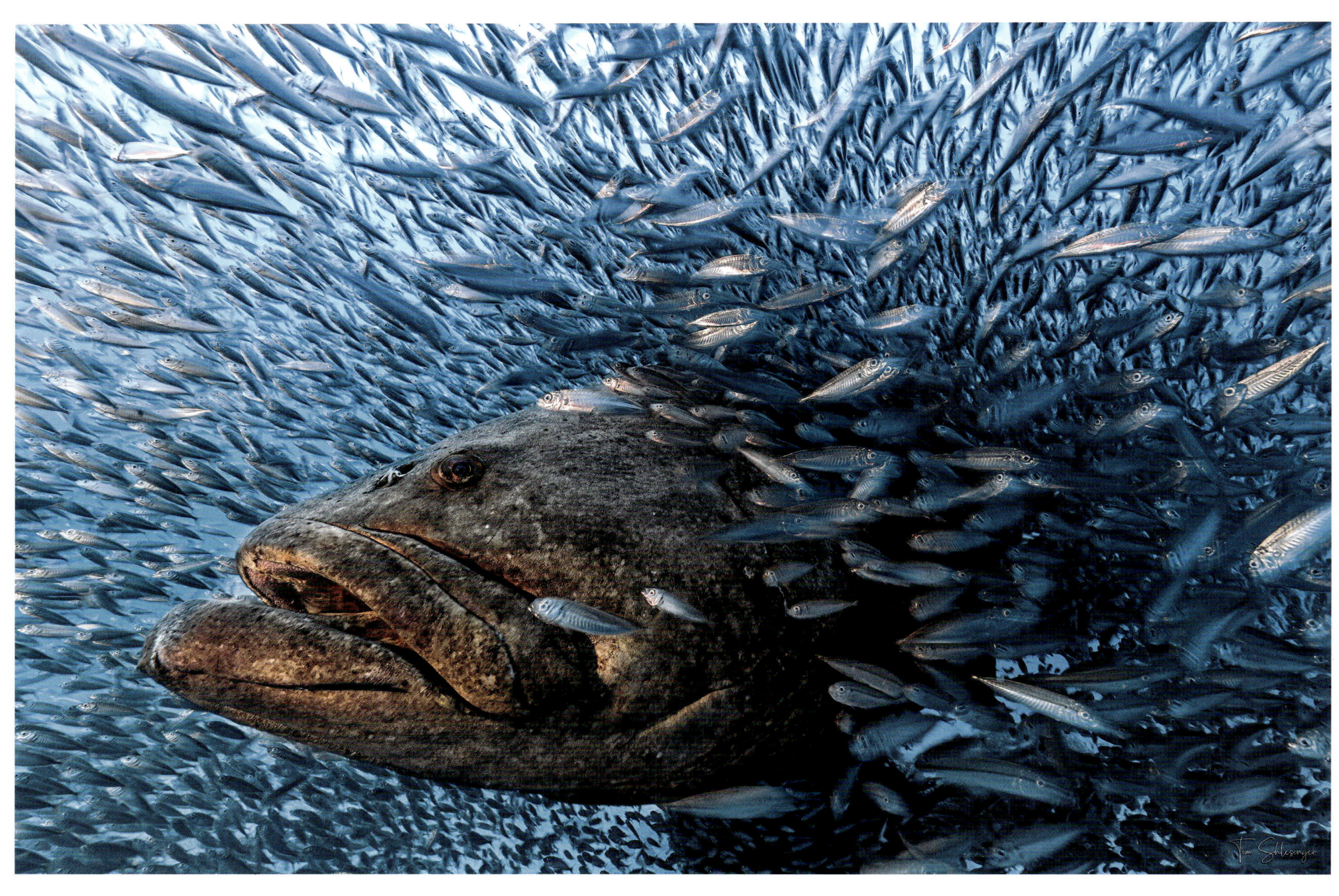

Tom Shlesinger
Atlantic Goliath Grouper
STATUS: VULNERABLE
Palm Beach, Florida, United States

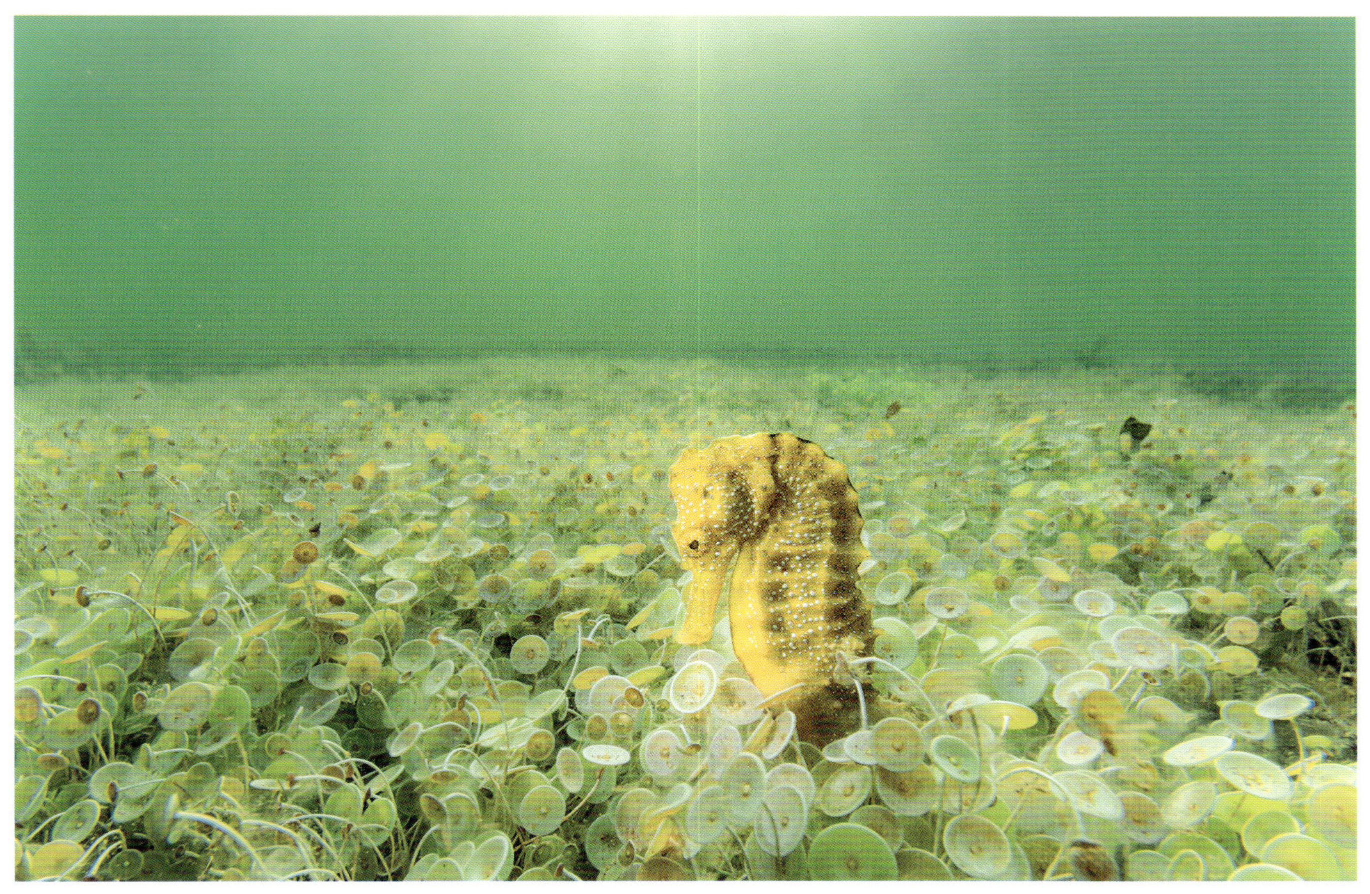

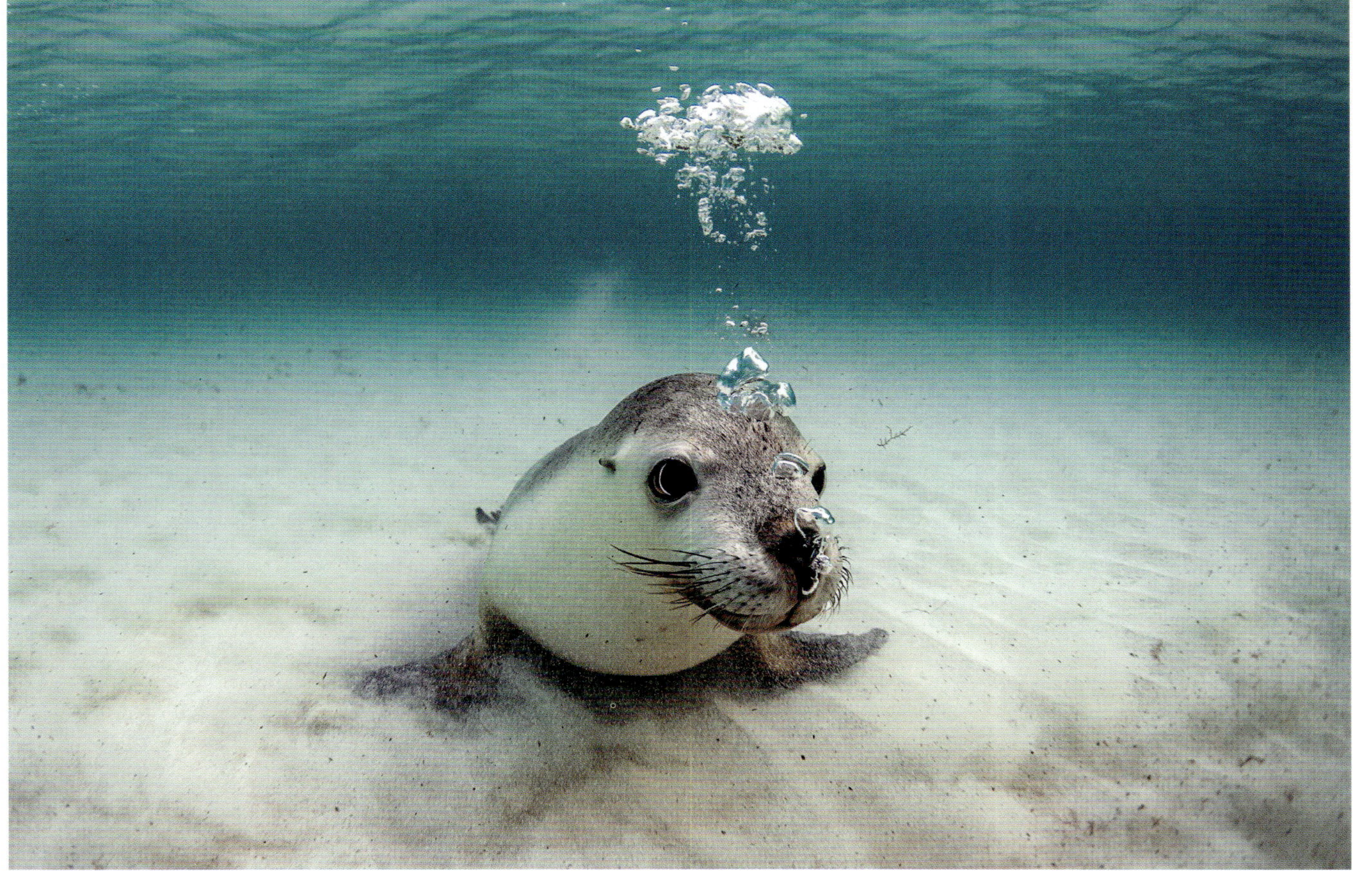

Angel Fitor
Long-snouted Seahorse
STATUS: NEAR THREATENED
(GLOBALLY; ENDANGERED
IN SPAIN)
Mar Menor, Spain

Scott Portelli
Australian Sea Lion
STATUS: ENDANGERED
Grindal Island, Australia

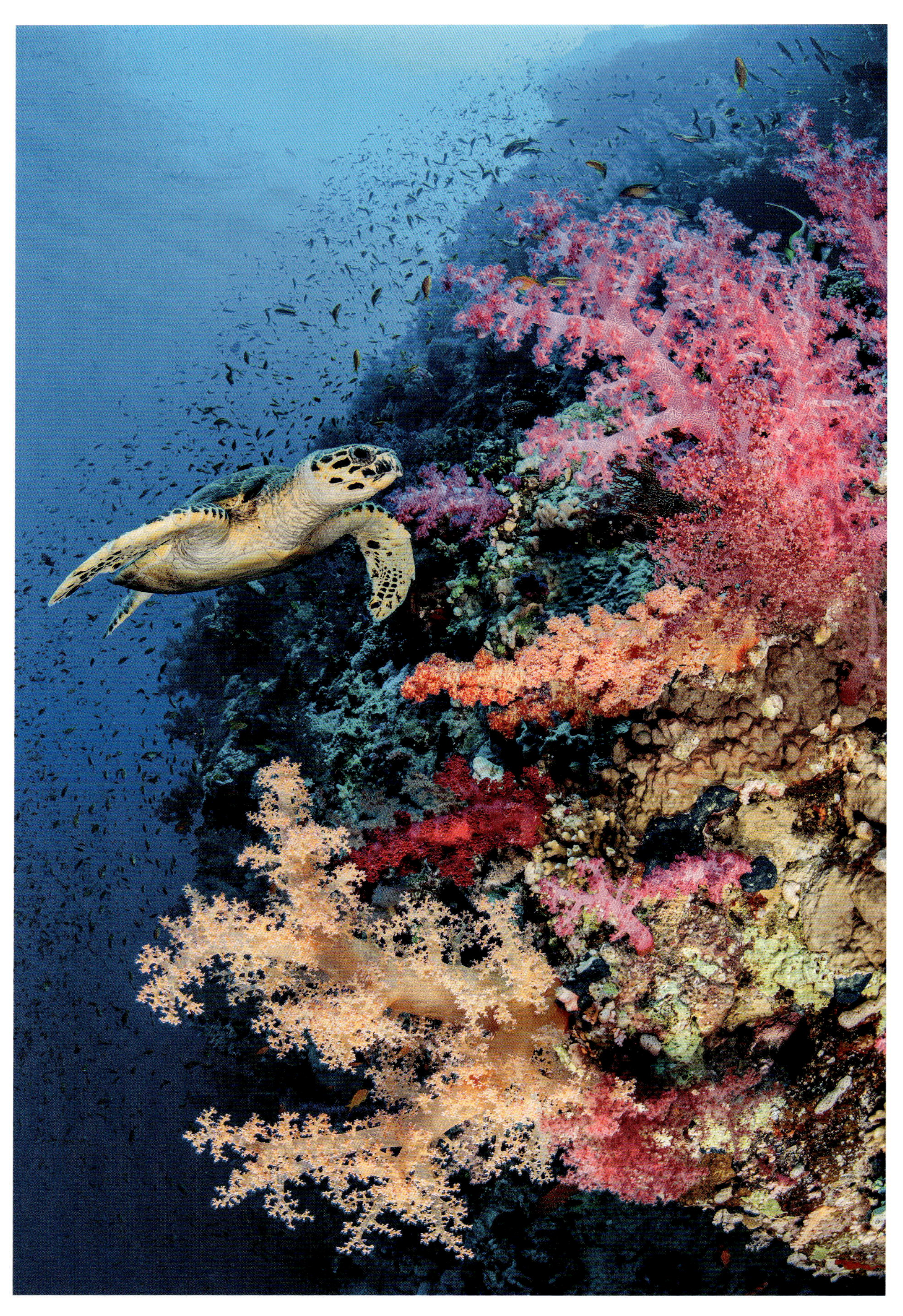

Alex Mustard
Hawksbill Turtle
STATUS: CRITICALLY ENDANGERED
Ras Muhammed National Park, Egypt

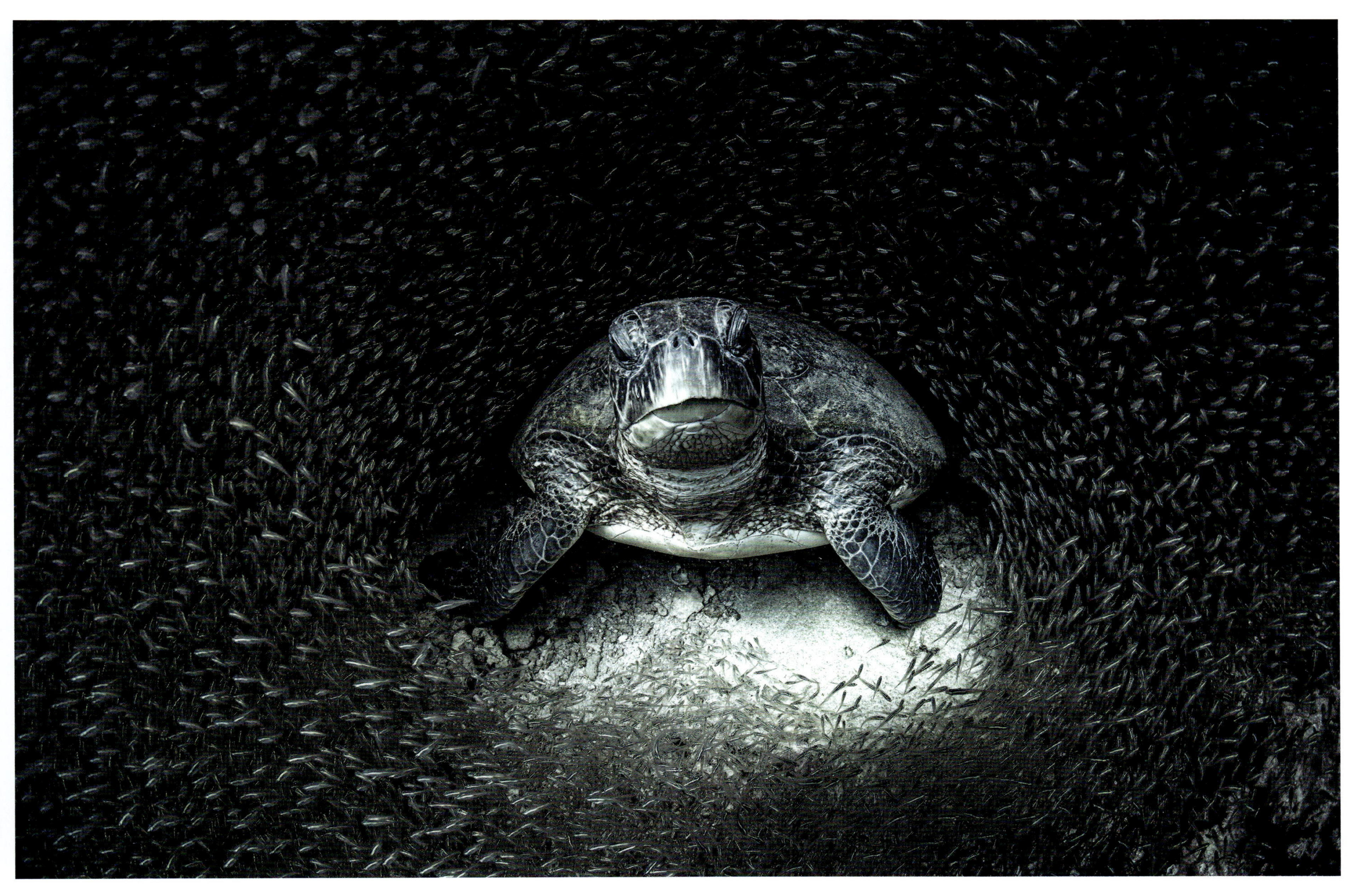

Aimee Jan
Green Sea Turtle
STATUS: ENDANGERED
Ningaloo Marine Park, Australia

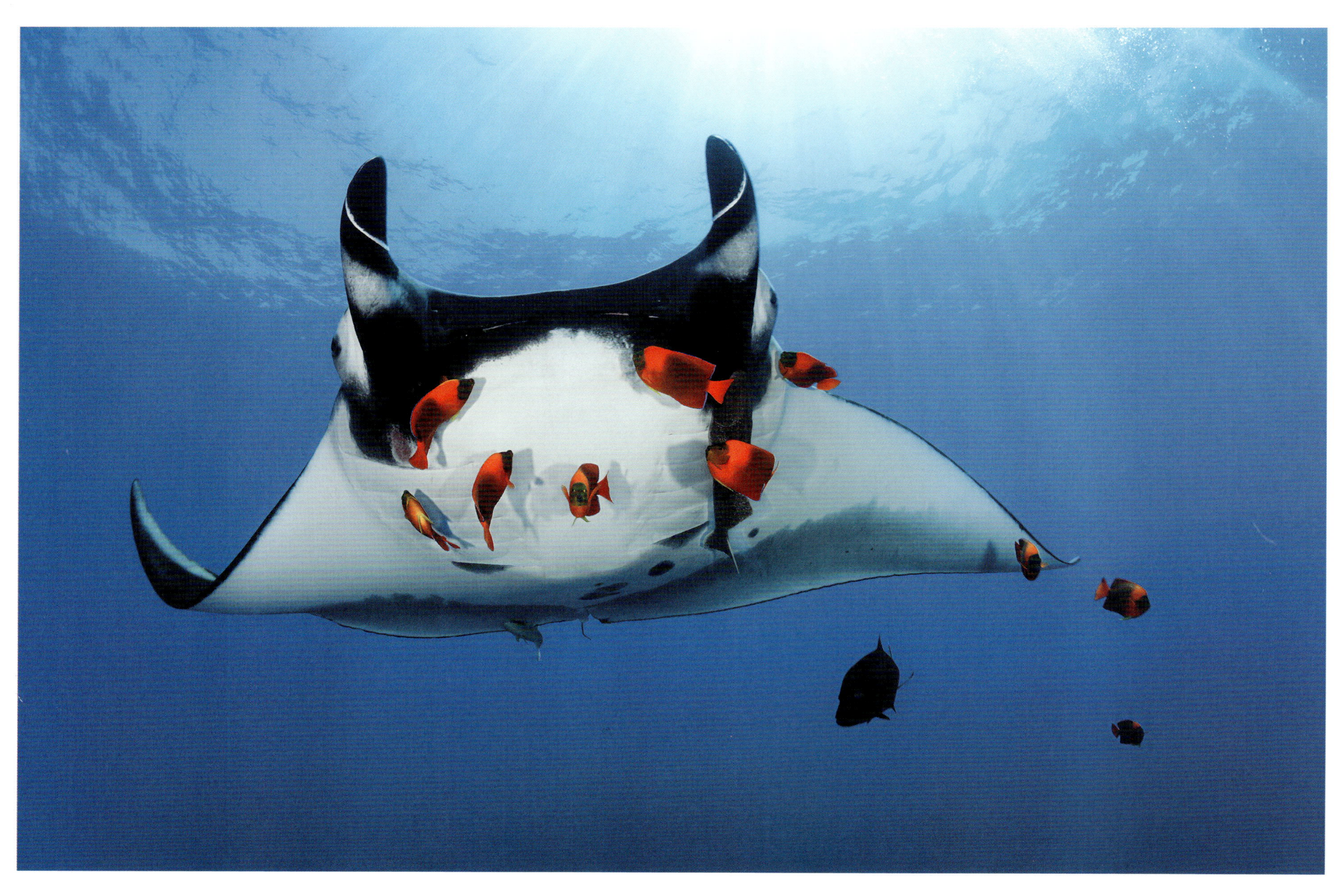

Claudio Contreras Koob
Giant Manta Ray
STATUS: ENDANGERED
Revillagigedo National Park, Mexico

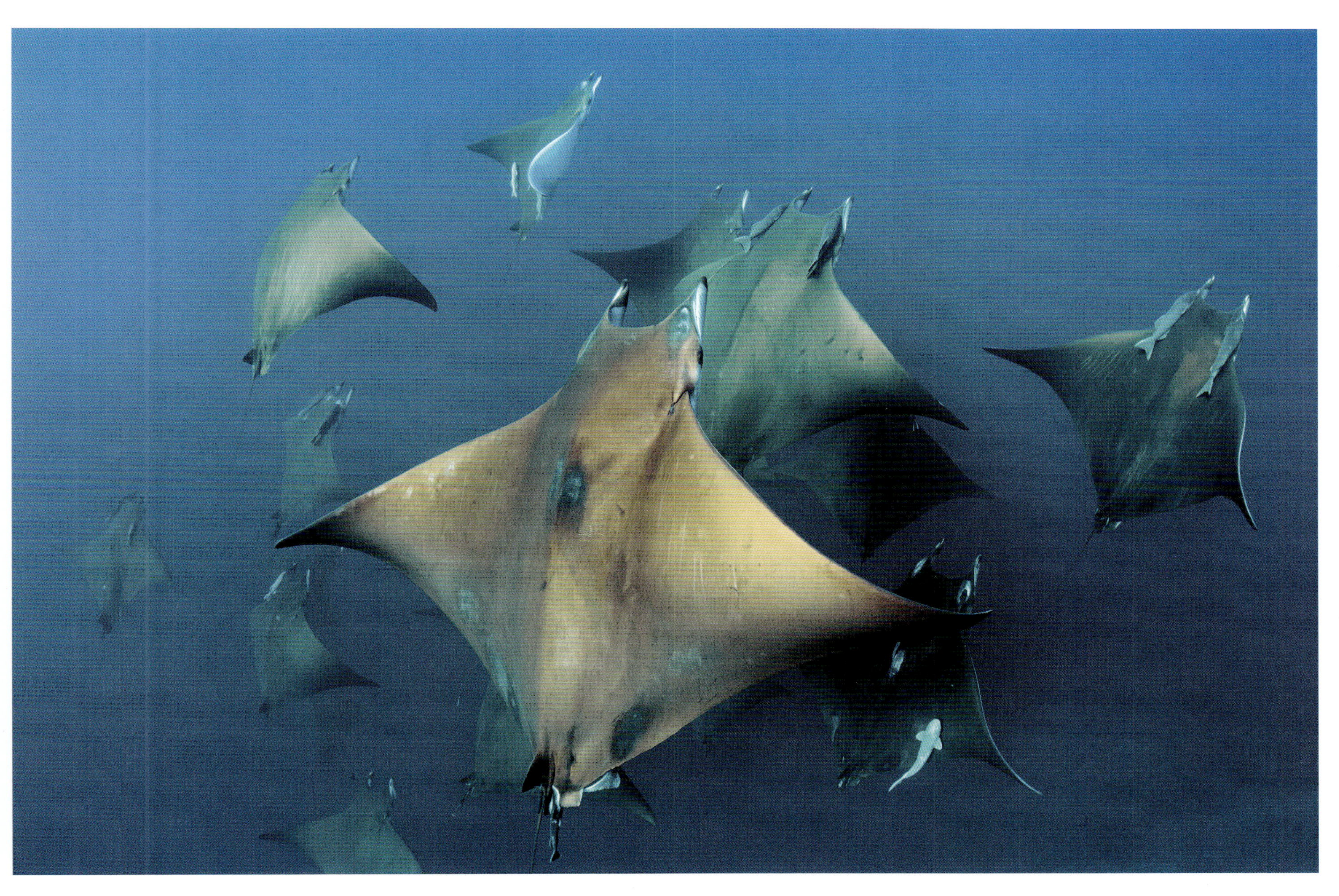

Magnus Lundgren
Chilean Devil Ray
STATUS: ENDANGERED
Azores, Portugal

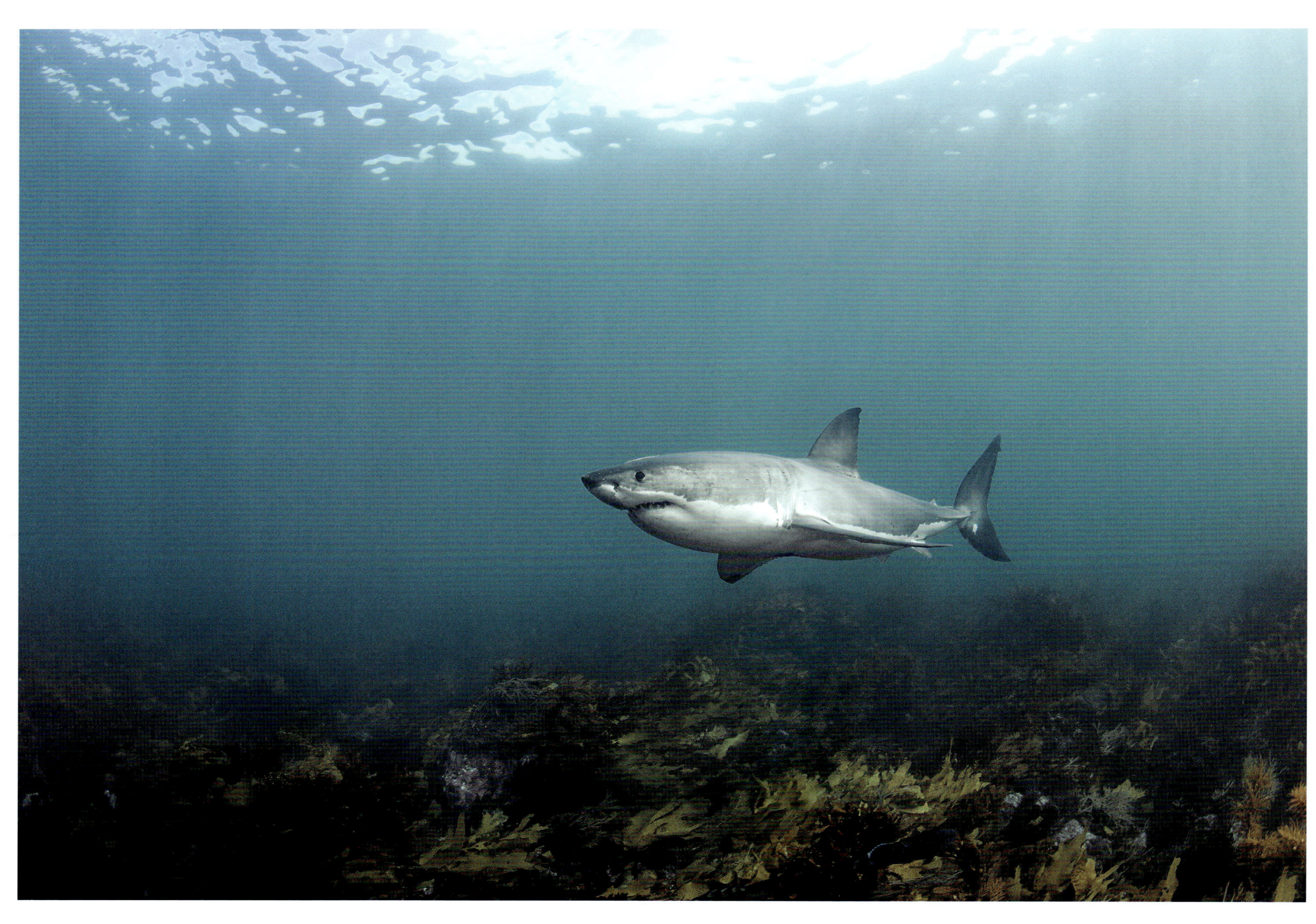

Chris Fallows
Great White Shark
STATUS: VULNERABLE
Stewart Island, New Zealand

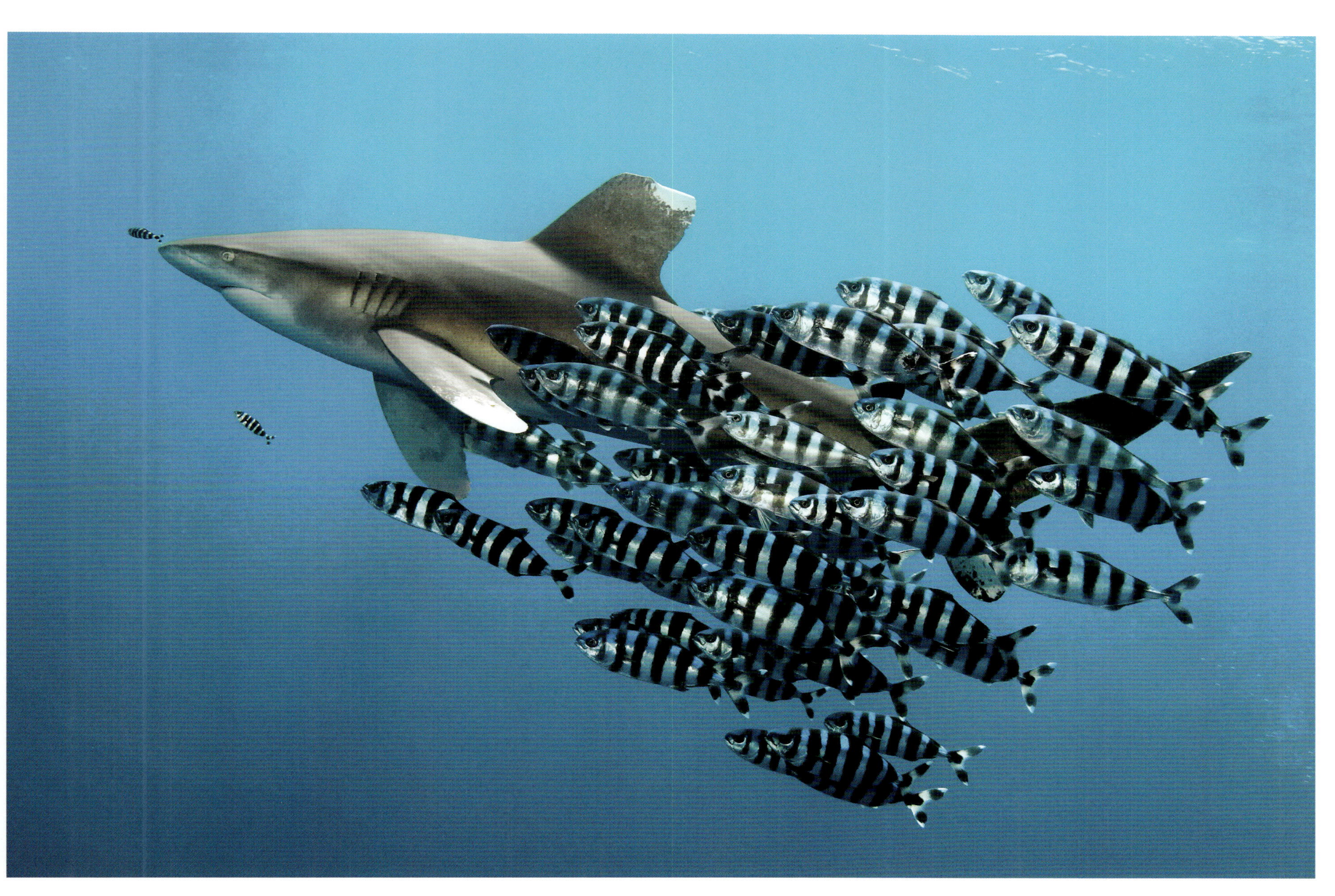

Magnus Lundgren
Oceanic Whitetip Shark
STATUS: CRITICALLY ENDANGERED
Elphinstone Reef, Egypt

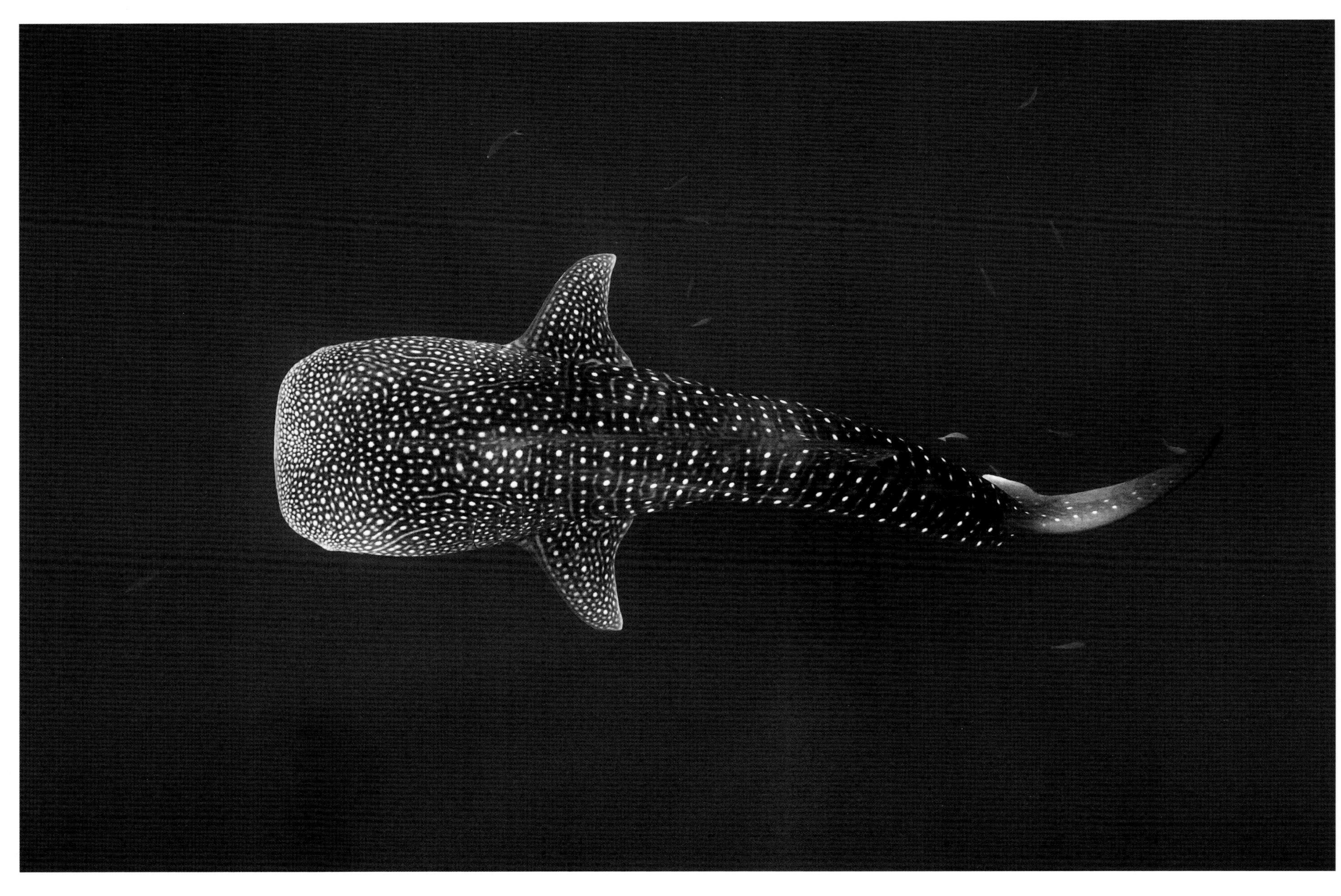

Jono Allen
Whale Shark
STATUS: ENDANGERED
Fuvahmulah, Maldives

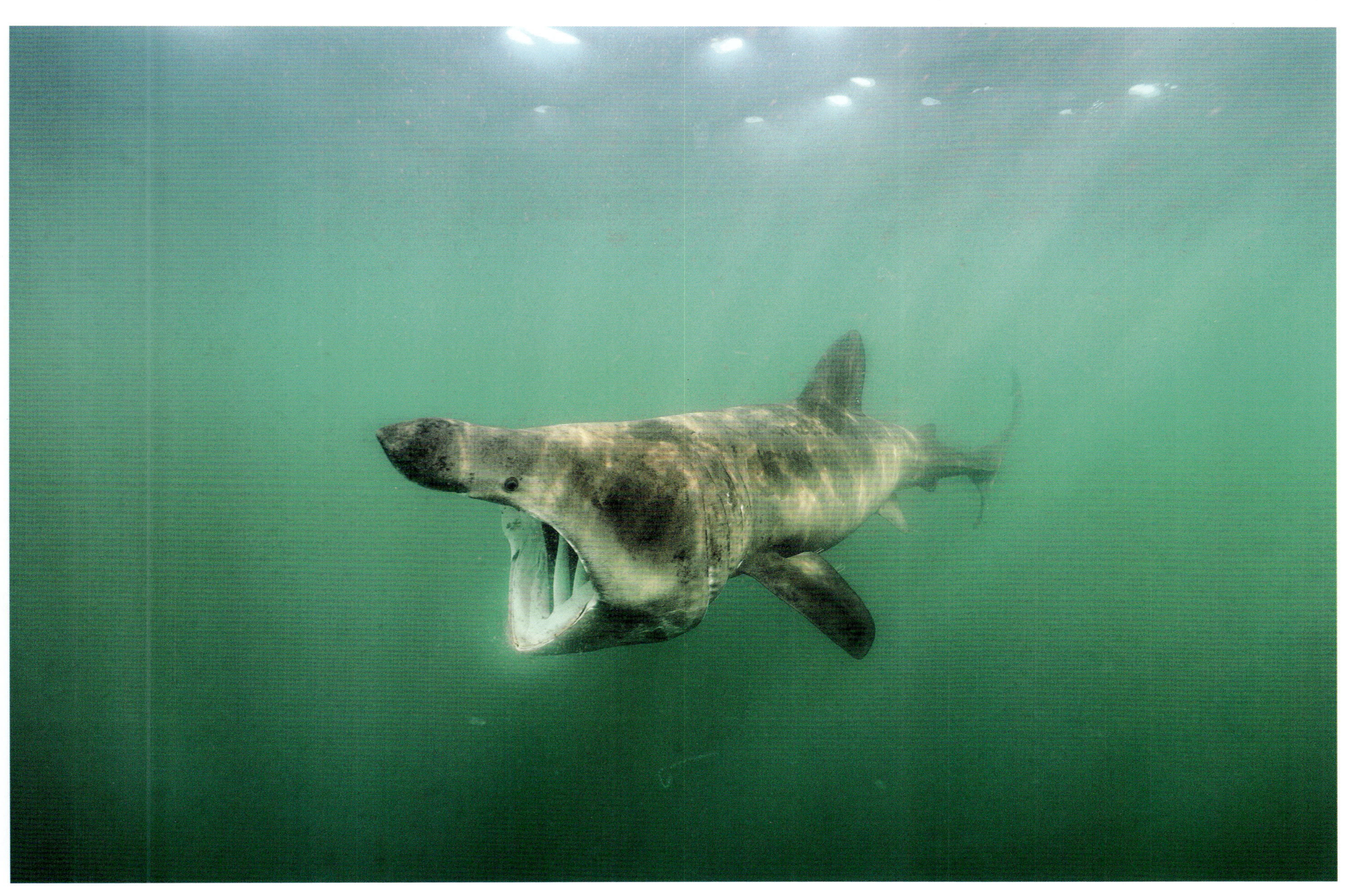

Brian Skerry
Basking Shark
STATUS: ENDANGERED
Chatham, Massachusetts, United States

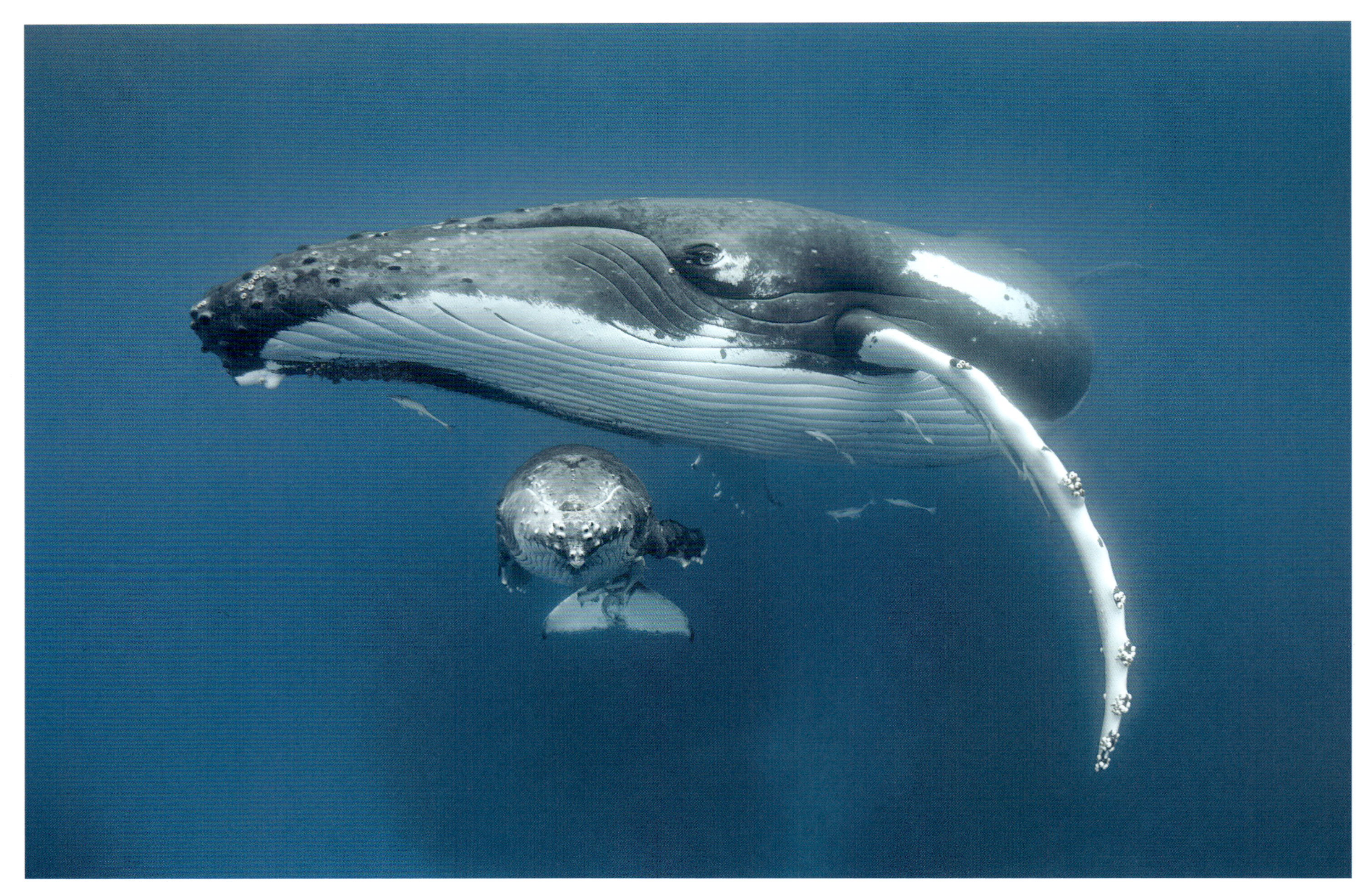

Tony Wu
Humpback Whale
STATUS: ENDANGERED (AMONG THE OCEANIA
POPULATIONS, OF WHICH TONGA FORMS A
SUB-POPULATION)
Vava'u, Tonga

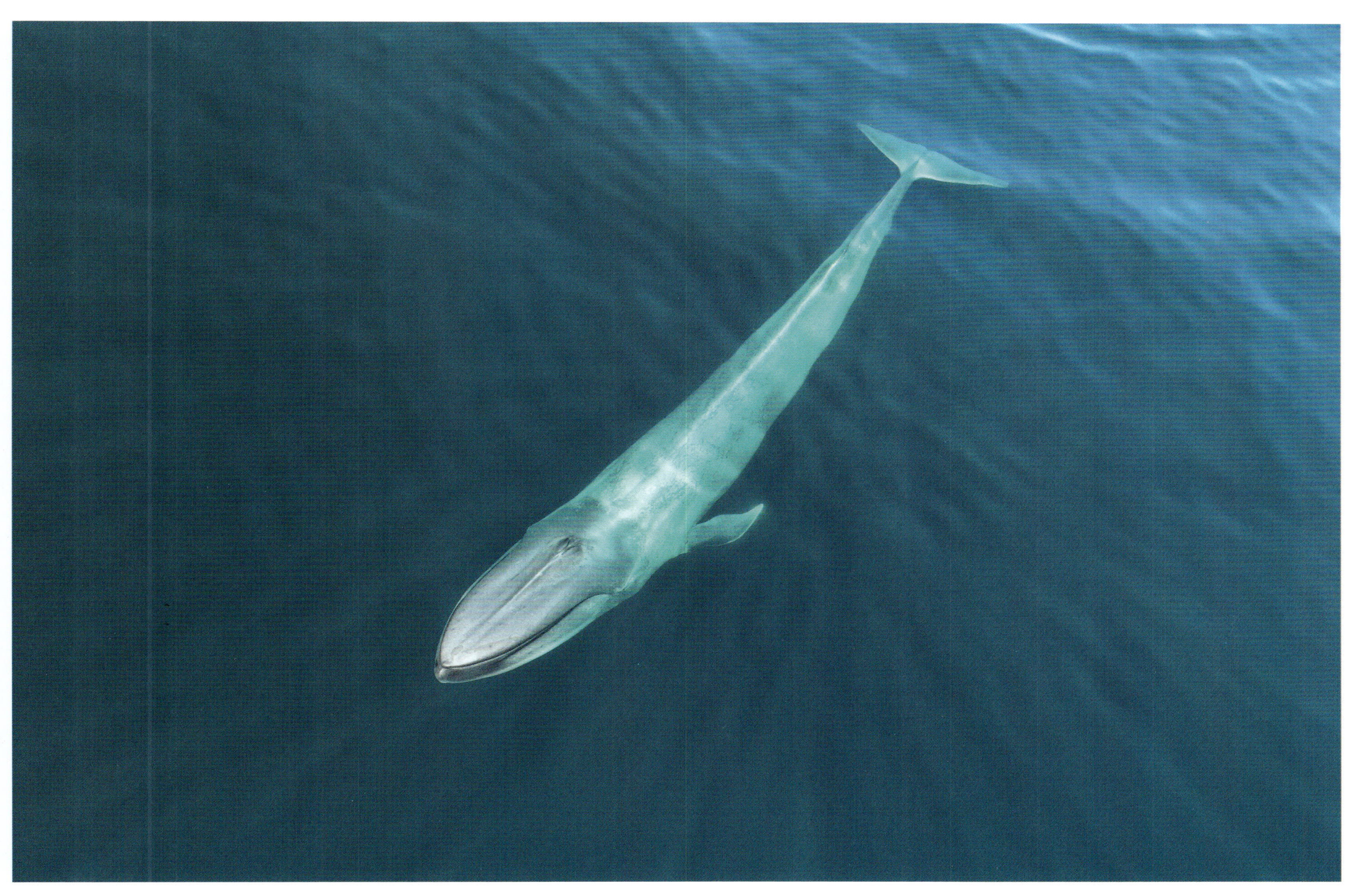

Mark Carwardine
Blue Whale
STATUS: ENDANGERED
Baja California, Mexico

Hope in Dark Times

Dr. Jane Goodall

Founder, The Jane Goodall Institute / UN Messenger of Peace

I WAS BORN LOVING AND BEING FASCINATED BY ALL ANIMALS. My heroes growing up were Dr. Doolittle and Tarzan. I dreamed of going to Africa, learning about wild animals, and writing books about them.

This passion led me to become the first person to study chimpanzees in the wild in Gombe National Park in Tanzania. One of the most fascinating discoveries was to find out how like us they are in so much of their behavior. They are, along with bonobos, our closest relatives in the animal kingdom, sharing 98.6 percent of our DNA.

This closeness allows us to stand back and ask what the main difference is between them and us. It is, I think, the explosive development of the human intellect. Animals are much more intelligent than was once thought, but none of them are capable of sending rockets into space or designing the Internet.

How bizarre, then, that the most intellectual creature that has ever walked the planet is destroying its only home: Planet Earth. In my lifetime, I have seen so many changes, as we destroyed forests; polluted land, air, and water; and poisoned the soil with agricultural chemicals and industrial, agricultural, and household waste. The natural resources of our planet are finite. In some places, we are using them up faster than Mother Nature can replenish them. At the same time, human populations are growing, along with our numbers of livestock. Too many people strive for short-term gain and unlimited economic growth at the expense of protecting the environment for future generations. Sometimes this is due to a desire to make more money and gain more power in an increasingly materialistic society. Sometimes it is due to poverty, as the poor will destroy the environment to make space to grow food or make money simply to survive.

Indigenous wisdom is being lost or ignored, the knowledge that we are part of the natural world and depend on it for clean air, water, food, and more. We depend on healthy ecosystems. An ecosystem is made up of diverse interrelated plants and animals, each one with a role to play. Every time a species goes extinct, it's like pulling a thread from a glorious living tapestry. If we pull too many threads, the tapestry will hang in tatters and the ecosystem will collapse.

It's our disregard and disrespect for the natural world that has led to climate change and the loss of biodiversity, both of which are existential threats to life on Earth as we know it. It is true that the challenges we face are formidable. We need to alleviate poverty, address the unsustainable lifestyles of so many people, think about human population growth, and stamp out corruption. Climate change is something that is affecting everyone, though the poor suffer the most. But it is so important that we do not lose hope. When people lose hope, they tend to give up, fall into apathy, and do nothing.

People often ask me if I really do have hope for the future. I believe we have a window of time during which we can start to heal some of the harm we have inflicted and slow down the heating of the planet. But only if we get together and take action now. We must protect our forests, plant trees, and address the terrible pollution of the ocean, air, and land. There also needs to be increased education and empowerment, particularly of girls and women.

There are reasons to have hope and keep going, including the commitment, energy, and passion of young people when they understand the problems and are empowered to think of solutions and take action. Young people everywhere are changing the world.

There is also the remarkable human brain. An increasing number of scientists are designing innovative technologies that are already helping us live in greater harmony with the natural world, such as solar, wind, and tide power; ways of controlling pest insects without the use of poisonous pesticides; and plant-based alternatives to meat, eggs, and milk that will hopefully bring industrialized or "factory" farming, which is having such a negative impact on the environment, to an end. People are also beginning to realize that they make an impact on the planet every day and that millions of small ethical choices in what they buy, wear, and eat can cumulatively lead to big change.

Then there is the fact that nature is amazingly resilient. Places that humans have destroyed can and have been restored. When I arrived in Gombe to study chimpanzees in 1960, the park was part of the equatorial forest belt that stretched to the west coast. By the late 1980s, it was a tiny island of forest surrounded by bare hills, the farmland overused and infertile, with people struggling to survive. It hit me that unless we could help people find ways of making a living without destroying the environment, we couldn't save chimpanzees, forests, or anything else. As we worked with people, they came to realize that protecting the environment was not just for wildlife, but also for their own future. There are no more bare hills around Gombe. Nature has been restored.

All around the world, many animals and plants on the brink of extinction have been given another chance because of rewilding programs, captive breeding, and education. The black robin in New Zealand was reduced to only one fertile male and one fertile female, but Don Merton wouldn't give up his efforts to save them, and there are some 250 black robins today.

Everywhere, there are examples of this indomitable spirit, people who tackle what seems impossible, refuse to give up, and often succeed. Rachel Carson, for example, fought against huge commercial and political interests until she got the pesticide DDT banned, despite the fact that toward the end she was battling cancer.

It is these positive stories, of which there are many around the world, that give people hope. Especially when these stories can be brought to life by photography and documentaries, more and more people start to feel hopeful.

There are so many incredible animals in the world. Of the animals in *The New Big 5*, I've spent hours watching elephants: young ones playing in a water hole; a group walking in a long line, each holding the tail of the individual in front; an adolescent male, so full of energy, mock-charging anything that moved. I've also spent time with lowland gorillas in Congo. The adults were sitting in the water but a juvenile male was trying not to get his feet wet, jumping from one tussock of grass to another, like a little clown. Lions used to be everywhere—I'm thinking in particular of two magnificent black-maned lions I saw on the Serengeti.

I've never seen a polar bear or a tiger in the wild, but I've seen so many images, such as a mother relaxing as her cubs play around her, or two young play-wrestling males standing upright, or a tiger moving silently through the forest.

This is why photographs are so important. For many people, it's only through such images that they can develop a deep respect and love for animals in the wild, as they haven't had the opportunity to spend time with them.

Photographers are also able to show the reality of why some animals are endangered, such as dead elephants, their trunks cut off to make it easier for poachers to hack out the tusks, or thousands of ivory carvings for sale in a tourist market in Asia. I'm also thinking of the haunting photos of a polar bear standing on a small piece of sea ice where once the ice sheet provided a way to reach the seals on which he depends—a real-life symbol of the effects of climate change.

It's not easy getting great wildlife photos or films. It takes infinite patience and determination. It may require spending days in hot tropical climates, plagued by insects, or in Arctic conditions, waiting for just the right shot—a photo that will move viewers and touch their hearts.

I hope that the photos in this *The New Big 5* book will lead people into the wonderful worlds of these iconic species and encourage them to explore the lives of so many other fascinating creatures, many of which are also endangered. Then, perhaps, other people will become involved in helping to create a world where wildlife can flourish for future generations to enjoy. We can all make a difference, but it's up to us the kind of difference we choose to make.

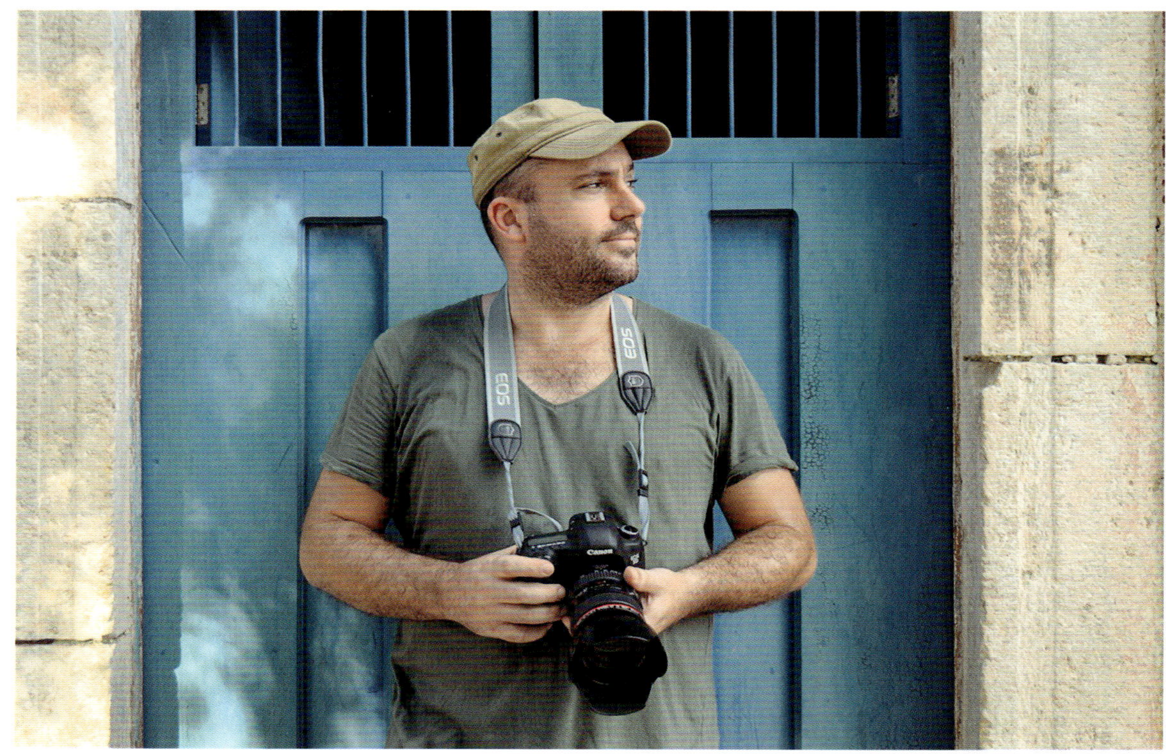

About the Author

Graeme Green is a British photographer and journalist. His work has appeared in international publications and other media outlets, including the Guardian, BBC, CNN, the *Sunday Times*, the *Sunday Telegraph*, *British Journal of Photography*, *National Geographic Traveler*, *Royal Photographic Society Journal*, *Forbes*, *Outdoor Photography*, *USA Today*, *Outside*, *Wanderlust*, the *New Daily*, *Digital Camera*, and the *South China Morning Post*. He has covered wildlife, conservation, and environmental issues in countries including Rwanda, India, Peru, and Japan, as well as stories about human rights, poverty, and other subjects.

Graeme is the founder of the New Big 5 project, an international conservation initiative supported by more than 300 of the world's photographers, conservationists, and wildlife charities. He lives in Derbyshire, England.

www.graeme-green.com.

Acknowledgments

I'm extremely grateful to all the photographers from around the world who supported the New Big 5 project and whose incredible pictures appear in this book. More than 16,000 photos were submitted, which made my job of selecting around 200 very difficult. These photographers' time, creativity, and dedication to wildlife is what gives this book its power.

I'm also thankful to Dr. Paula Kahumbu for writing such an insightful foreword, to Dr. Jane Goodall for her hopeful closing comments, and to all the contributors who shared their expertise, experiences, and ideas in the book's essays, including Dominique Gonçalves, Krista Wright, Dr. Tara Stoinski, Dr. Moreangels Mbizah, Dr. Anish Andheria, and Dr. Wes Sechrest. I'm also grateful to all the people who gave their time to be interviewed, and to the many experts, friends, colleagues, and conservation organizations who helped by providing information and resources during the course of researching this book.

Thanks to all the conservationists, wildlife experts, community members, and other people I've spent time with and worked with during assignments over the years for conversations and experiences that all fed into this book.

Thanks also go to the people at Earth Aware for their faith in the New Big 5 project and for making working on this book such an enjoyable collaborative process, including senior editor Karyn Gerhard, Katie Killebrew, Raoul Goff, Amanda Nelson, designer Allister Fein, and production manager Joshua Smith.

Sincere thanks to Samantha Roberts for her support, and for giving her time and skills to build the New Big 5 website.

Thank you to my wife, Andrea, who has helped decide many of the featured images, and who has given her patience, strength, and support during the long, difficult period it took to work on this book.

A final thank-you to everyone working today to protect wildlife and the world we live in for future generations.

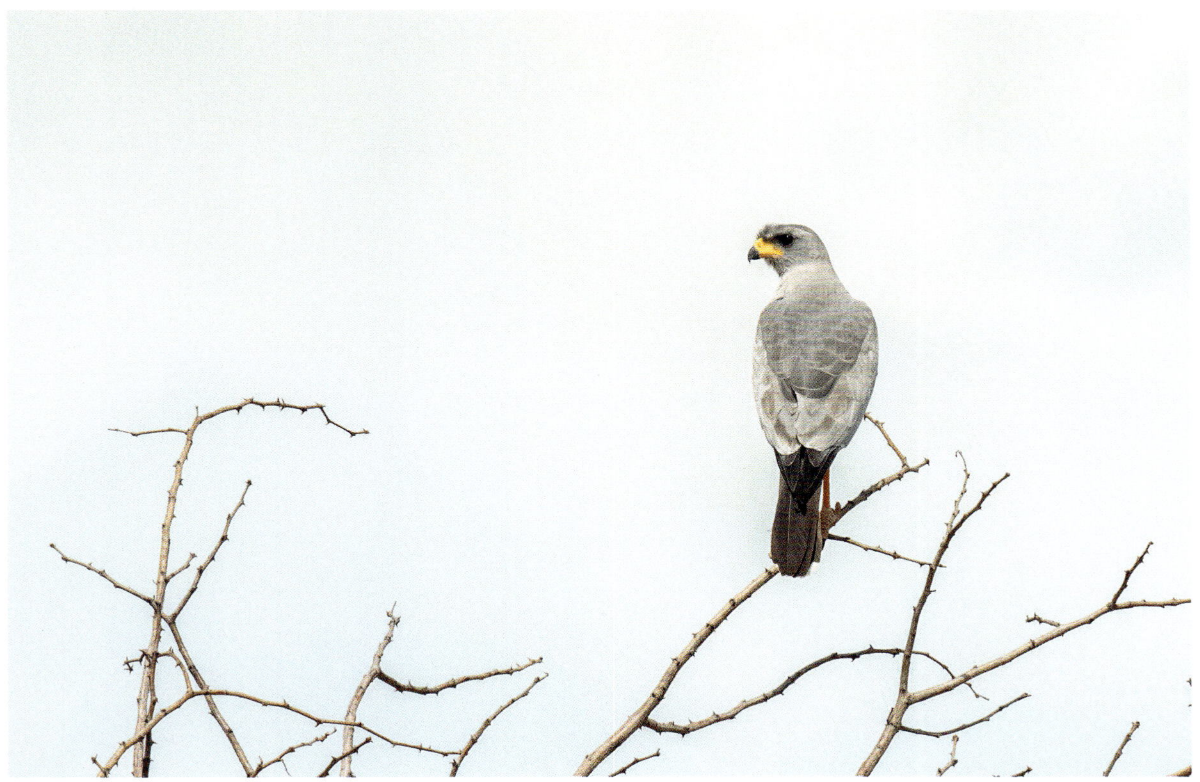

Graeme Green
Eastern Chanting Goshawk
Ruaha National Park, Tanzania

The Photographers

Karine Aigner (United States)
Instagram: @kaigner
www.karineaigner.com

Ramakrishnan Aiyaswamy (India)
Instagram: @ramakrishnan_aiyaswamy
www.ramakrishnanaiyaswamy.com

Jono Allen (Australia)
Instagram: @jonoallenphotography
www.jonoallen.com

Majed Alzaabi (Kuwait)
Instagram: @majedphotos
www.majedphotos.com

Irene Amiet (Switzerland)
Instagram: @ireneamiet
www.ireneamiet.com

Shogo Asao (Japan)
Instagram: @shogoasao
www.rakuensanka.com

Priyanshi Bachhawat Nahata (India)
Instagram: @priyanshi.wildographs
www.wildographs.com

Xuedong Bai (China)
www.tqstar.cn

Daryl and Sharna Balfour (South Africa)
Instagram: @darylbalfourwildphotos
www.wildphotossafaris.com

Alessandro Beconi (Italy)
Instagram: @beconialessandro
www.alessandrobeconi.com

Emanuele Biggi (Italy)
Instagram: @emanuele_biggi
www.anura.it

Tamara Blazquez Haik (Mexico)
Instagram: @tamarablazquezhaik
www.tamarablazquez.com

Clay Bolt (United States)
Instagram: @claybolt
www.claybolt.com

Will Burrard-Lucas (United Kingdom)
Instagram: @willbl
www.willbl.com

Lucas Bustamante (Ecuador)
Instagram: @luksth
www.saviafund.org

Luciano Candisani (Brazil)
Instagram: @lucianocandisani
www.lucianocandisani.com.br

Marina Cano (Spain)
Instagram: @marinacano
www.marinacano.com

Mark Carwardine (United Kingdom)
Instagram: @markcarwardinel
www.markcarwardine.com

Vladimir Cech, Jr. (Czech Republic)
Instagram: @vladimir_cech_jr
www.vladimircechjr.com

Celina Chien (China)
Instagram: @celinaxchien
www.celinaxchien.com

Mia Collis (Kenya)
(courtesy of the Sheldrick Wildlife Trust)
Instagram: @mia_collis
www.miacollis.live

Claudio Contreras Koob (Mexico)
Instagram: @claudio_contreras_koob
www.sulazul.com

Jaime Culebras (Spain)
Instagram: @jaime_culebras
www.photowildlifetours.com

Rupayan Datta (India)
Instagram: @rupayan_datta

Joan de la Malla (Spain)
Instagram: @joandelamalla
www.joandelamalla.com

Mangesh R. Desai (India)
Instagram: @gowildforlife
www.gowild.in

Carole Deschuymere (Belgium)
Instagram: @carolewildlife
www.caroledeschuymere.com

Jasper Doest (Netherlands)
Instagram: @jasperdoest
www.jasperdoest.com

Ronan Donovan (United States)
Instagram: @ronan_donovan
www.ronandonovan.com

Suzi Eszterhas (United States)
Instagram: @suzieszterhas
www.suzieszterhas.com

Chris Fallows (South Africa)
Instagram: @chrisfallowsphotography
www.chrisfallows.com

Molly Ferrill (United States)
Instagram: @mollyferrill
www.mollyferrill.com

Angel Fitor (Spain)
Instagram: @angelfitor
www.seaframes.com

Tim Flach (England)
Instagram: @timflachphotography
www.timflach.com

Sascha Fonseca (Germany)
Instagram: @sascha.fonseca
www.saschafonseca.com

William Fortescue (United Kingdom)
Instagram: @willfortescue
www.williamfortescue.com

Ryan Francis (Australia)
Instagram: @ryanfrancisphotography
www.flickr.com/photos/ryanfrancis

Marco Gaiotti (Italy)
Instagram: @marcogaiotti_naturephotography

Sujuaan Gasim (Maldives)
Instagram: @sujugasim

Françoise Gervais (Canada)
Instagram: @francoisegervaisphotography
www.fgervaisgallery.com

Daisy Gilardini (Switzerland)
Instagram: @daisygilardini
www.daisygilardini.com

Paul Goldstein (United Kingdom)
Instagram: @paulgoldstein
www.paulgoldstein.co.uk

Sergey Gorshkov (Russia)
Instagram: @sergey_gorshkov_photographer

Graeme Green (United Kingdom)
Instagram: @graeme.green
www.graeme-green.com

Martin Gregus (Slovakia)
Instagram: @mywildlive
www.matkopictures.com
www.martingregusjr.com

Shane Gross (Canada)
Instagram: @shanegrossphoto
www.shanegross.com

Amy Gulick (United States)
Instagram: @amy_gulick
www.amygulick.com

Jen Guyton (Germany)
Instagram: @jenguyton
www.jenguyton.com

Drew Hamilton (Canada)
Instagram: @drewhh
www.drewhh.com

Usha Harish (India, Kenya)
Instagram: @usha.harish.photography
www.ushaharish.com

Mark Edward Harris (United States)
Instagram: @markedwardharrisphoto
www.markedwardharris.com

Paul Hilton (United Kingdom)
Instagram: @paulhiltonphoto
www.paulhiltonphotography.com

Heath Holden (Australia)
Instagram: @heathholdenphoto
www.heathholden.com

Joshua Holko (Australia)
Instagram: @joshuaholko
www.jholko.com

Richard I'Anson (Australia)
Instagram: @richianson
www.richardianson.com

Lara Jackson (United Kingdom)
Instagram: @lara_wildlife
www.larawildlife.co.uk

Aimee Jan (New Zealand)
Instagram: @oceanaimee
www.oceanaimee.com

Vicki Jauron (United States)
Instagram: @vicjauron
www.babylonandbeyond.com

Sara Jenner (United Kingdom)
Instagram: @sara.jennerl

Hao Jiang (China)
Instagram: @haojiang00629
www.1x.com/member/HaoJiang

Beverly Joubert (South Africa)
Instagram: @beverlyjoubert
www.beverlyjoubert.com

Sandesh Kadur (India)
Instagram: @sandesh_kadur
www.sandeshkadur.com

Nick Kanakis (United States)
Instagram: @nick_kanakis
www.nickkanakis.com

Ketan Khambhatta (India)
Instagram: @ketankhambhatta

Aarzoo Khurana (India)
Instagram: @aarzoo_khurana
www.aarzookhurana.com

Clement Kiragu (Kenya)
Instagram: @clement.wild
www.clementwild.com

Stephanie-Emmy Klarmann (South Africa)
Instagram: @our_african_voyage
www.stephanie-emmy.myportfolio.com

Dmitry Kokh (Russia)
Instagram: @master.blaster
www.dmitrykokh.com

Santhosh Krishnan (India)
Instagram: @santhosh_krishnan01

Tim Laman (Japan)
Instagram: @timlaman
www.timlaman.com

Frans Lanting (Netherlands)
Instagram: @franslanting
www.lanting.com

Florian Ledoux (France)
Instagram: @florian_ledoux_photographer
www.florian-ledoux.com

Antonio Liebana (Spain)
Instagram: @liebanafot
www.antonioliebana.es

Ole J. Liodden (Norway)
Instagram: @ojlwildphoto
www.oleliodden.com

Qingshun Liu (China)
www.tqstar.cn

David Lloyd (New Zealand)
Instagram: @davidlloyd
www.davidlloyd.net

Hannes Lochner (South Africa)
Instagram: @hannes_lochner
www.hanneslochner.com

Magnus Lundgren (Sweden)
Instagram: @magnuslundgrenphotography
www.magnuslundgren.com

Xiaoyun Luo (China)
www.99encounters.com

Piper Mackay (United States)
Instagram: @piper_mackay
www.pipermackayphotography.com
www.facebook.com/piper.mackay

Nili Mahendra Gudhka (Kenya)
Instagram: @thejunglechic
www.thejunglechic.com

Thomas D. Mangelsen (United States)
Instagram: @thomasdmangelsen
www.mangelsen.com

Andy Mann (United States)
Instagram: @andy_mann
www.andymann.com

Brian W. Matthews (United Kingdom)
Instagram: @bwmphoto
www.bwmphoto.com

Steve McCurry (United States)
Instagram: @stevemccurryofficial
www.stevemccurry.com

Shivang Mehta (India)
Instagram: @shivang.mehta
www.naturewanderers.com

Cristina Mittermeier (Mexico)
Instagram: @mitty
www.cristinamittermeier.com

Karabo LeBronpeter Moilwa (Botswana)
Instagram: @karabo_lebronpeter

Robin Moore (United Kingdom)
Instagram: @robindmoore
www.robindmoore.com

Kevin Morgans (United Kingdom)
Instagram: @kevmorgans
www.kevinmorgans.com

Anette Mossbacher (Germany)
Instagram: @anette_mossbacher
www.anettemossbacher.com

Dhritiman Mukherjee (India)
Instagram: @dhritiman_mukherjee
www.dhritiman.com

Alex Mustard (United Kingdom)
Instagram: @alexmustard1
www.amustard.com

Latika Nath (India)
Instagram: @latikanath
www.latikanath.com

Paul Nicklen (Canada)
Instagram: @paulnicklen
www.paulnicklen.com

Noppadol Paothong (Thailand)
www.npnaturephotography.com

Andy Parkinson (United Kingdom)
Instagram: @andyparkinsonphoto
www.andrewparkinson.com

Teeku Patel (Kenya)
Instagram: @teekupatelfotofilm
www.teekupatel.com

Richard Peters (United Kingdom)
Instagram: @richardpetersphoto
www.richardpeters.co.uk

Sergio Pitamitz (Italy)
Instagram: @segiopitamitz
www.pitamitz.com

Scott Portelli (Australia)
Instagram: @scott.portelli
www.scottportelli.com

Shibu Preman (India)
Instagram: @shibu.preman
www.shibunair.com

Scott Ramsay (South Africa)
Instagram: @scottramsay.africa
www.scottramsay.africa

Jim Richardson (United States)
Instagram: @jimrichardsonng
www.jimrichardsonphotography.com

Marco Ronconi (Italy)
Instagram: @marcoronconi_
www.marcoronconi.com

Jay Roode (South Africa)
Instagram: @jayroode
www.jayroode.com

Gurcharan Roopra (Kenya)
Instagram: @gurcharan
www.gurcharanroopra.com

Jenny E. Ross (United States)
www.lifeonthinice.org
www.jennyross.com

Rahul Sachdev (India)
Instagram: @rahulsphotography
www.rahulsachdev.net

Gabby Salazar (United States)
Instagram: @gabbyrsalazar
www.gabbysalazar.com

Dave Sandford (Canada)
Instagram: @davesandford
www.davesandfordphotos.com

Chris Schmid (Switzerland)
Instagram: @schmid_chris
www.schmidchris.com

Yaron Schmid (Israel)
Instagram: @yswildlifephotography
www.yswildlifephotography.com

Jonathan Scott (Kenya, United Kingdom)
and **Angela Scott** (Egypt)
Instagram: @thebigcatpeople
www.jonathanangelascott.com

Sudhir Shivaram (India)
Instagram: @sudhirshivaram
www.sudhirshivaramphotography.com

Tom Shlesinger (Israel)
Instagram: @tom_shlesinger

Brian Skerry (United States)
Instagram: @brianskerry
www.brianskerry.com

Anton Sorokin (Russia)
Instagram: @antonsrkn
www.antonsorokin.com

Aishwarya Sridhar (India)
Instagram: @chikoo_wild
www.aishwaryasridhar.com

Tom Svensson (Sweden)
Instagram: @tomsvensson1
www.tomsvensson.se

Pinkesh C. Tanna (India)
Instagram: @pinkesh_tanna

Scott Trageser (United States)
Instagram: @scott.trageser.photo
www.naturestills.com

Victor Tyakht (Russia)
Instagram: @v.tyakht

Michelle Valberg (Canada)
Instagram: @michellevalbergphotography
www.michellevalberg.com

Lance van de Vyver (New Zealand)
Instagram: @panthera_photo_safaris
www.pantheraphotosafaris.com

Gaël R. Vande weghe (Belgium)
Instagram: @gael.world
www.gael.world

Marsel van Oosten (Netherlands)
Instagram: @marselvanoosten
www.squiver.com

Gerda van Schalkwyk (South Africa)
www.flickr.com/photos/gerdavs

Willie van Schalkwyk (South Africa)
www.flickr.com/photos/willievs

Federico Veronesi (Italy)
Instagram: @federico_veronesi
www.federicoveronesi.com

Thomas Vijayan (Canada)
Instagram: @thomasvijayan
www.thomasvijayan.com

Ami Vitale (United States)
Instagram: @amivitale
www.amivitale.com

Berndt Weissenbacher (South Africa)
Instagram: @berndtweissenbacher
www.bekahawe.co.za

Marcus Westberg (Sweden)
Instagram: @marcuswestbergphotography
www.marcuswestberg.photo

Staffan Widstrand (Sweden)
Instagram: @staffanwidstrand
www.staffanwidstrand.se

Shannon Wild (Australia)
Instagram: @shannon_wild
www.shannonwild.com

Steve Winter (United States)
Instagram: @stevewinterphoto
www.stevewinterphoto.com

Art Wolfe (United States)
Instagram: @artwolfe
www.artwolfe.com

Nelis Wolmarans (South Africa)
Instagram: @neliswolmarans_photo_safaris
www.neliswolmarans.com

Jenny Wong (Canada)
Instagram: @jdubcaptures
www.jennwong.ca

Tony Wu (Japan)
Instagram: @tonywu98
www.tony-wu.com

Qiang Zhang (China)

Xingchao Zhu (China)
www.tqstar.cn

Christian Ziegler (Germany)
Instagram: @christianziegler
www.christianziegler.photography

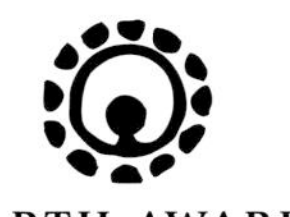

EARTH AWARE

An Imprint of MandalaEarth
PO Box 3088
San Rafael, CA 94912
www.MandalaEarth.com

Find us on Facebook: www.facebook.com/MandalaEarth
Follow us on Twitter: @MandalaEarth

CEO Raoul Goff
Associate Publisher Phillip Jones
Editorial Director Katie Killebrew
Senior Editor Karyn Gerhard
VP Creative Chrissy Kwasnik
Art Director Allister Fein
VP Manufacturing Alix Nicholaeff
Production Manager Joshua Smith
Sr Production Manager, Subsidiary Rights Lina s Palma-Temena

Text © 2023 Graeme Green

Earth Aware wishes to thank copyeditor Bob Cooper, proofreader Margaret
Parrish, and editorial assistants Amanda Nelson and Jon Ellis, for their
tireless work in helping to bring this beautiful and important book to life.

ISBN: 978-1-64722-870-5

Manufactured in India by Insight Editions
10 9 8 7 6 5 4 3 2 1

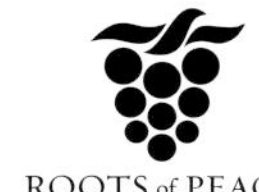 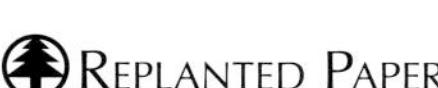

ROOTS of PEACE   REPLANTED PAPER

Insight Editions, in association with Roots of Peace, will plant two trees
for each tree used in the manufacturing of this book. Roots of Peace is an
internationally renowned humanitarian organization dedicated to
eradicating land mines worldwide and converting war-torn lands into
productive farms and wildlife habitats. Roots of Peace will plant two
million fruit and nut trees in Afghanistan and provide farmers there with
the skills and support necessary for sustainable land use.